Nail Structure and Product Chemi~

Nail Structure and Product Chemistry
Second Edition

Douglas D. Schoon

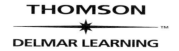

THOMSON
™
DELMAR LEARNING

Australia   Canada   Mexico   Singapore   Spain   United Kingdom   United States

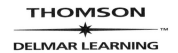

Nail Structure and Product Chemistry
Douglas D. Schoon

MILADY STAFF
President:
Dawn Gerrain

Director of Editorial:
Sherry Gomoll

Developmental Editor:
Judy Aubrey Roberts

Editorial Assistant:
Jessica Burns

Director of Production:
Wendy A. Troeger

Production Editor:
J.P. Henkel

Production Assistant:
Angela Iula

Composition:
ATLIS Graphics

Director of Marketing:
Wendy E. Mapstone

Channel Manager:
Sandra Bruce

Marketing Coordinator:
Kasmira Koniszewski

Cover Design:
Joseph Villanova

Library of Congress Cataloging-in-Publication Data
Schoon, Douglas D.
  Nail structure and product chemistry / Douglas D. Schoon.—2nd ed.
      p. cm.
  Rev. ed. of: Milady's nail structure & product chemistry. Albany, N.Y : Milady Pub., c1996.
  Includes index.
  ISBN 1-4018-6709-X (pbk.)
  1. Manicuring. 2. Nails (Anatomy)—Care and hygiene. 3. Fingernails. I. Schoon, Douglas D. Milady's nail structure & product chemistry. II. Milady Publishing Company. III. Title.
  TT958.3.S36 2005
  646.7'27—dc22
                        2004023016

ISBN-13: 978-1-4018-6709-6
ISBN-10: 1-4018-6709-X

NOTICE TO THE READER

Publisher does not warrant or guarantee any of the products described herein or perform any independent analysis in connection with any of the product information contained herein. Publisher does not assume, and expressly disclaims, any obligation to obtain and include information other than that provided to it by the manufacturer.

The reader is expressly warned to consider and adopt all safety precautions that might be indicated by the activities described herein and to avoid all potential hazards. By following the instructions contained herein, the reader willingly assumes all risks in connection with such instructions.

The publisher makes no representations or warranties of any kind, including but not limited to, the warranties of fitness for particular purpose or merchantability, nor are any such representations implied with respect to the material set forth herein, and the publisher takes no responsibility with respect to such material. The publisher shall not be liable for any special, consequential, or exemplary damages resulting, in whole or part, from the reader's use of, or reliance upon, this material.

To Mom and Dad—you bought me a chemistry set and a telescope and then taught me to open my mind and dream. Those were the greatest gifts I've ever received. Thank you for everything.

And to Judy and Tinker, the coolest person and cutest dog in the world!

Contents

Preface

As a nail technician, what is the most important thing you can possess? It's something so important that you cannot succeed without it! It can make you financially successful while making your job more fun and enjoyable. It can solve your problems and give your clients more satisfaction from their nails. It can identify problems and quickly find solutions. What one thing can do so much for a professional nail technician? It's called *information*, and it is easily your most important tool.

Information is knowledge. Without it you couldn't keep a set of nail enhancements on your clients and you wouldn't know a safe practice from a damaging one. You certainly wouldn't know what to tell your clients when their nail plates started forming ridges, becoming brittle, splitting, or starting to turn strange colors. Information is the key to your success and earning potential. The more you know, the better your services will be and the more successful you will become in your career. Knowledge can give clients beautiful, long-lasting, and durable nail enhancements while protecting and nurturing the fingernail. With the proper knowledge your manicures and pedicures will be more beneficial and your clients will have a better understanding of their nails. Most important, they'll have a greater appreciation for your skills and training.

This book is designed to give you that information. But only you can turn it into your own personal knowledge. Only when the knowledge becomes yours can you use it to become a better nail professional. That is your challenge. Learn all you can! Take the time to really understand this information and it will serve you well. If you do, I promise that you'll grow and prosper in more ways than you imagine.

A STUDY TIP

This book is not set up like most textbooks, and you should read it a little differently. The information in this book is presented in story form. This is the story of the natural nail and nail enhancement products. Why is this book written like a story? To make it easier to understand. How is it like a story? You will see that information learned in the first few chapters will pop up throughout the book. Also, what you learn in later chapters will help better explain ideas discussed in earlier chapters. Each chapter is connected and dependent on the others parts of the book. So my best advice is don't read this like a book—read it like a story and you'll find it will be easier to learn and understand the information.

There are several features included that will help you gain a better understanding of the many subjects you will learn about. In each chapter you will find terms that are highlighted in bold. These terms may be unfamiliar in some cases, but they are in bold because this is the first time they have been used and they are important. You should take time to learn their meaning and understand the concepts behind them. That should be your most important goal when you study. Finally, at the end of each chapter you will find a Fast Track section, a list of the most important concepts in the chapter. But don't just memorize the bulleted points—make sure you understand the concepts behind them. That's why the concept for each Fast Track item has been marked with (FT). Use both the Fast Track concepts and the boldface terms as study guides. They are at the heart of each chapter.

ABOUT THE AUTHOR

Doug Schoon has over 30 years of scientific experience and a master's degree in organic chemistry and is considered to be the leading research scientist in his field. His unique expertise focuses on the science of both natural and artificial

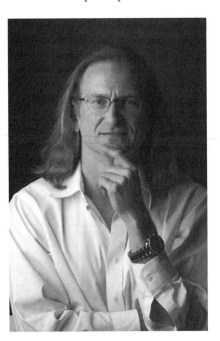

nails. He is a well-known and respected author, as well as an internationally renowned lecturer and educator. Schoon is a strong advocate for salon safety. As co-chair of the Nail Manufacturer Council, he frequently represents the entire nail industry on scientific and technical issues in Europe, Canada, and the United States, and is often called upon to serve as an expert witness in legal cases involving cosmetic safety and health.

Additionally, dermatologists frequently call Mr. Schoon to assist them in writing books and scientific papers concerning fingernails. For the last 16 years he has led the scientific research team for Creative Nail Design, Inc., and presently serves as the company's vice president of science and technology. He currently resides in Dana Point, California.

Acknowledgments

REVIEWERS

Below is a list of the highly knowledgeable reviewers that I was fortunate to have as readers of the original manuscript of this book. I am very grateful to them for their keen insights and observations, their wonderful suggestions, and the significant improvements they have made to this edition.

Mary Duran, Phoenix, Arizona

Agneta Moden, Stockholm, Sweden

Tiffany Greco, Vista, California

Amanda Reevell, Oxford, United Kingdom

Kristina Saindon, Denver, Colorado

Nikki Birch, Scottsburg, Indiana

Debbie Waite, Carlsbad, California

Nancy King, Phoenix, Arizona

Sam Sweet, Leeds, United Kingdom

Lynn Denis, Québec, Canada

The publishers would like to thank the following reviewers and contributors for their assistance with this edition:

Angela Sharp, Sharp's Academy of Hairstyling, Inc., Grand Blank, Michigan

Martha Phillips, Ford Beauty Academy, Boardman, Ohio

Beth Wallace, Allen Thornton Career Technical Center, Killen, Alabama

Patricia Martin, International School of Beauty, New Port Richey, Florida

Linda Craig, Looking Good Hair & Nail Salon, Redding, California

Linda Fishel, La'James International College & Day Spa, Iowa

Kerry Stroman, College of Hair Design, Lincoln, Nebraska

Robin Ratliff, Gainesville Hairstyling, Gainesville, Florida

Edward Tezak, Westminster, Colorado

Leesa Myers, Academy of Career Training, Kissimmee, Florida

Betty Walker, Kings Mountain, North Carolina

Robert Morey, Flint, Michigan

CONTRIBUTORS

Each of the following people contributed written material that appears in this book. I'm sure you will agree when you read their contributions that each of them made highly useful and very interesting additions to the book.

Nancy King, Scottsdale, Arizona

Debbie Doerrlamm, Ronkonkoma, New York

Jana Wright, Newport Beach, California

Miho Nagasato, Osaka, Japan

Takara-Belmont Education Team, Tokyo, Japan

Hanne Gruer, Oslo, Norway

Olga Miroshnichenko, Almaty, Kazakhstan

Samantha Sweet, Leeds, United Kingdom

Galina Zelenova, Moscow, Russia

Adri Roelofse, Namibia, Africa

Justine Hartel, Los Angeles, California

Sonette van Rensburg, Dubai, United Arab Emirates

Evelyn Wang, Taipei, Taiwan

PHOTOGRAPHY AND ARTWORK

Much of the photography and artwork appearing in this book is a work of an extremely talented and innovative photographer and graphic artist, Paul Rollins, who resides in Laguna Niguel, California. Mr. Rollins was also the principal photographer and graphic artist for the original 1995 edition of this same book.

Also, a very special thank-you to those who contributed photographic images from their dermatological practices and medical research:

Dr. Robert Baran

Dr. Nancy Satur

Dr. Josette André

Dr. Ted Reid

TRANSLATIONS

Thanks to Yelena Klinova for translating the Russian contribution in Chapter 16 into English and to Miho Nagasato for her Japanese translation.

SPECIAL THANKS

If I have seen further than most men, it is because I stood on the shoulders of giants.

—Sir Isaac Newton, 1676

No one can "know it all." There is just too much to know. The information in this book comes from hundreds of different sources, including my own research and that of the extremely talented team of scientists and staff at Creative Nail Design with whom I am fortunate to work. However, I also owe a very deep debt of gratitude to several doctors and researchers who have dedicated their lives to the study of the natural nail. Their prolific writings and informative discussions have influenced me greatly and taught me much of what I know about the natural nail, and I gratefully thank each of them.

Dr. Robert Baran

Dr. Nardo Zaias

Dr. Richard K. Scher

Dr. Howard Maibach

Dr. Phoebe Rich

Dr. C. Ralph Daniel

Dr. Peter Samman

Dr. David A. Fenton

Dr. Oscar Mix

Dr. Nancy Satur

Finally, a most special thank-you to the Nordstrom family: Mary, Jan, Tom, and especially Jim, who patiently mentored me during the first decade of my career in the professional nail industry. Without this family's dedication, vision, and passion, I would never have been introduced to this wonderful industry, and I would not have written this book.

ART CONTRIBUTORS

CRC Press, Boca Raton, Florida

Dr. Josette André, Brussels, Belgium

Dr. Robert Baran, Cannes, France

Dr. Nancy Satur, Encinitas, California

Ted Reid, Selenium Technology, Lubbock, Texas

Creative Nail Design, Vista, California

Paul Rollins, Photographer, Laguna Niguel, California

Chapter 1

Fingernail Anatomy

Objective

In this chapter you will learn about the many parts of the fingernail and toenail. You'll see how all of the parts work together to support the growth of the nail plate. You will then have the basic information you need to understand the anatomy and structure of the natural nail.

THE FINGERNAIL AND TOENAIL

Ask someone to show you a fingernail or toenail. Usually the person will point to the hard keratin structure growing over the tip of the finger or toe. If you look at Figure 1–1, you'll see that this is actually called the **nail plate.** You will also see that the nail plate is only a single part of the overall nail structure. Each part of the structure is vital to nail growth and development. Clearly, the health of each part is essential to maintaining a healthy nail.

What you will learn in this book about the parts of the fingernail will also apply to the toenail in many cases. Seeing things from this point of view, you'll discover that the toenail and fingernail are very much alike. In fact, they are more similar than different. Each of your fingernails or toenails can be divided

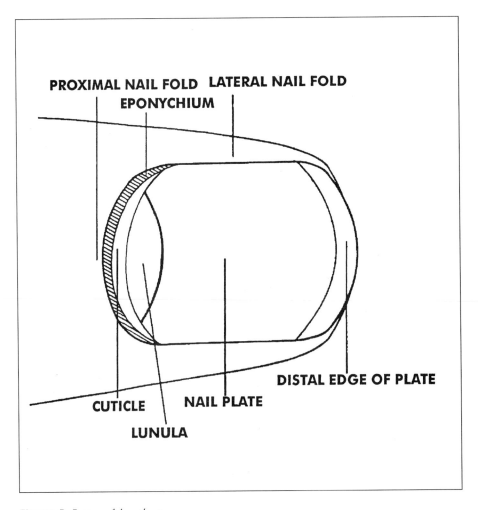

Figure 1-1 *Parts of the nail unit*

into several major sections. Each of these separate parts cooperates with the others to form what dermatologists call the **nail unit.** The rest of this chapter will focus on these various parts. You will learn how each part interacts with the others to keep the nail healthy.

Nail Folds: The Guardians of Your Nails

Examine the area on your finger where the skin touches the nail plate (Figure 1–2). The skin does not end where it meets the plate. Instead, the skin makes a U-turn and folds back underneath itself. This fold of skin pushes up against the nail plate, creating a tight seal that prevents **bacteria** and **chemicals** from getting underneath. There are four of these seals surrounding the nail plate from all sides. Their function is to protect the underlying nail bed from infection and injury. They are the "guardians" of the natural nail. When a **guardian seal** *(FT)* is broken, infection can result. These important seals protect the nail bed and matrix area from the outside world. In this chapter we will learn how important it is for nail professionals to protect these seals and keep them healthy. Bacteria, **fungi,** or **viruses** can attack and create an infection if even one of these folds is damaged or broken.

Examine the base of your nail at the point where the skin meets the emerging nail plate. This skin folds underneath itself, and the underside rests on top of the unexposed nail plate. The eponychium (defined below) covers the newly forming natural nail with a roof of living skin. The area where the skin folds is called the **proximal nail fold** *(FT)* (PROHK-sih-mul nail fold). *Proximal* is a medical term meaning "nearest"—in this case referring to the fold nearest the point where the nail attaches *(FT)*, so you can see where the skin fold gets its name. On

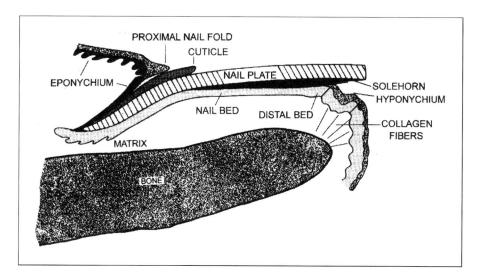

Figure 1-2 *Cross section of the major parts of the nail plate*

each side of the plate, two more folds form tight seals along the sidewalls. These sidewall seals are called the **lateral nail folds** *(FT)* (LAH-ter-uhl nail folds). *Lateral* means "to the side" *(FT)*. The two lateral nail folds are important guardian seals. We will learn about the other seals in a moment. But first, let's focus our attention on the base of the nail plate.

Eponychium and Cuticle

Living skin covers approximately 20 percent of the nail plate. The skin that lies directly on top of the newly developing nail plate is called the **eponychium** *(FT)* (epp-uh-NICK-ee-um). Normally the uppermost, visible part of the eponychium has the appearance of smooth, healthy skin. Cuts, nicks, bruises, irritating substances, or other injuries to the eponychium can cause permanently lost or damaged nail plates. Clearly, this is an important part of the nail unit. Not surprisingly, the tissue that sits upon the nail plate is very different from the visible eponychium. The underside of the eponychium nail fold has a strange, sticky texture.

The word *cuticle* is loosely and often incorrectly used. Ask clients to point to their cuticle and they'll most likely point vaguely to the skin at the base of the nail plate—the visible part of the living eponychium—instead of the nonliving tissue that adheres to the nail plate. How did this misconception get started? Surprisingly, it probably started because of some medical text. These few references often simply state that the cuticle is the eponychium, without explaining to the reader that the cuticle sheds from the underside of the eponychium.[1] But the cuticle is only a part of the eponychium. In fact, it is found on the underside of the eponychium, where the tissue sits against the newly forming nail plate. This tissue sticks very tightly to the freshly made nail plate. The tissue binds so tightly that the growing nail plate pulls off a thin layer and drags it along. In other words, the detached tissue "rides" on the nail plate, seeming to grow from under the edge of the nail fold. This thin layer of colorless tissue is the **cuticle** *(FT)*, the dead

1. Experts disagree on the exact location of the eponychium. Some use this term to describe only the underside of the proximal nail fold area. In this book I use this term to indicate the visible portion of the nail fold area as well.

WHAT'S IN A NAME?

Over the years, much confusion has been caused by a misunderstanding of nail anatomy. Some state regulations tell students they can't cut the cuticles, when really they mean the living tissue of the eponychium. Cutting the fold can break the seal and lead to infection. These regulations aren't meant to prevent you from cleaning the nonliving tissue (cuticle) from the nail plate.

Clearly, the confusion can be avoided if we teach clients about the anatomy of the natural nail. While they are marveling at your knowledge, you will be helping eliminate the confusion. And you'll be making a positive contribution to our industry.

tissue on the nail plate, not the living tissue that surrounds the nail plate (Figure 1–3 and Color Plate 1). In the cross section shown in Figure 1–3, the cuticle can be seen separating from the underside of the eponychium. The underside of the eponychium is constantly shedding thin layers of this colorless tissue. As this shed skin emerges with the nail plate it creates one of the most important of the four nail plate guardian seals.

During a properly performed manicure, the eponychium is gently pushed back to expose the cuticle. The cuticle must be carefully removed. Improperly performed, this part of the manicure can cause problems for clients. For example, applying artificial nail products over this thin layer of skin will prevent proper adhesion, causing the artificial nail to separate and lift from the surface of the natural nail plate. Many hours of valuable time are lost to repairs made necessary by careless removal of the cuticle. Not only can improperly removing the cuticle contribute to artificial nail service breakdown, it can also lead to infection or nail deformities. This is why it is very important to avoid removing cuticle from underneath the nail fold. It is fine to push back the eponychium first, but do not place any instrument underneath the nail fold itself. This can lead to injury and infection.

Sharp instruments can inflict serious injury, so avoid them during manicures. Finally, follow manufacturer's directions, using cuticle removers exactly as directed. It will make your job easier if you use the product correctly. These products are potentially irritating and may cause skin and nail damage if not used

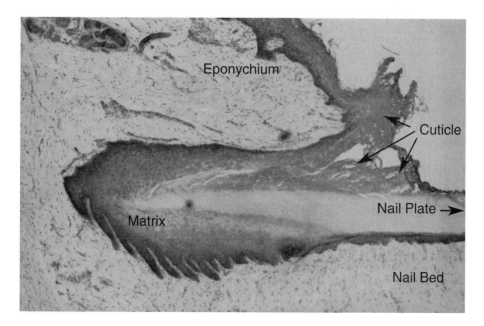

Figure 1-3 *Cuticle*

properly. It is important for nail professionals to respect the cuticle. It is an important part of the seal that guards and protects the nail matrix.

The Matrix

Directly below the eponychium is a small area of living tissue called the **matrix** (MAY-tricks). This small, glistening white patch of tissue is the most important part of the entire nail unit. Why? The matrix produces a super-tough protein called **keratin** (KAIR-uh-tin). These **keratin cells** are the building blocks of the nail plate. You will soon see that keratin cells create the layers of the nail plate. This makes the matrix the official birthplace of the nail plate. The matrix is an opaque, bluish white, almost rectangular area of highly specialized cells. These special cells are designed to take the nutrients that we eat and turn them into an amazingly tough and durable substance called keratin. If the matrix becomes damaged, the effects are usually seen in the nail plate. In Chapter 4 you will see how damage to the matrix area can cause splits, ridges, white spots, and other deformities of the natural nail plate. If damage to the matrix is severe, it could lead to permanent deformity.

The size and shape of the matrix determine the thickness, width, and curvature of the nail plate (FT). A wider matrix creates a wider nail plate. The thumbs therefore have a wider matrix than the other fingers. Also, longer matrixes make thicker nail plates, as you will learn in the next chapter, and so you'll discover that people with naturally thin nail plates must have short matrix areas.

The Nail Plate

The nail plate is mostly made of keratin, the same chemical substance that hair is made from. Keratin is a special protein that creates the bulk of the nail plate. In nature, there are over 30 different types of keratin, ranging from very soft Hungarian goose down to extremely hard desert turtle shells and even rigid porcupine quills. Keratin is a very tough and flexible material well suited to withstand the rigors of the environment. Ancient peoples relied on their natural nails as tools as well as for protection, so their nails had to be tough and durable. Collagen and keratin serve similar functions, but for differing parts of the body. Collagen is the building or **structural protein** for skin, and keratin is the structural protein for nails. Like all proteins, keratin is made of long chains or strands of **amino acids** (uh-MEE-noh acids), joined together like pearls on a microscopic necklace. A typical **keratin strand** contains between 300 and 500 amino acids linked into a long chain. These single chains prefer to exist as loosely coiled strands. Almost two-thirds of the keratin found inside nail cells exist as extremely tiny, coiled strands. Dozens of these coiled strands stack neatly into tight bundles to create tiny fibers or **fibrils** of keratin. These fibrils can be seen only under the most powerful electron microscopes. At these extremely high magnifications they look like tiny whiskers embedded in a semisolid gel. All of this is encased in a clear sac to create a nail cell. These fibrous filaments are so narrow that a bundle of 2,000 would only be as thick as a single human hair. Even so, each fibril contains approximately half a million amino acid molecules, and each nail plate contains hundreds of millions of fibrils. That's a lot of amino acids in each nail!

The remaining one-third of the keratin is much softer and more gel-like in consistency. This type of keratin does not form fibers, but instead creates a firm supporting bed that encases and supports the fibrils. The keratin fibers are arranged inside the cells in neatly stacked rows of "logs" (i.e., like logs in a log cabin) that lie parallel to the free edge of the nail. The logs would seem to be rolling along toward the tip of the plate as the cells slowly flow toward the free edge.

You will learn in Chapter 2 that the creation of the nail plate is similar to skin and hair growth. The fingernail plate is made of about 100 layers of dead, flattened keratin cells. The toenail is thicker and can have up to 150 layers. The layers form a plate that resembles a brick-and-mortar wall. The nail plate is also often referred to as the **natural nail.**

ABRADING PERSONALITIES

Respect the nail plate—it protects the nail bed and fingertip. Thicker, stronger nail plates give the best protection. Nail plates that are overly thin cannot properly protect the delicate tissue lying underneath. This weakening is seen if the nail plate is overfiled. This is one of the easiest and most common ways to damage nails in the salon. Incorrect filing is the top cause of nail plate thinning and destruction.

A nail technician's main job is to keep the client's plates as thick and healthy as possible. Don't file away your client's nails—nurture them and keep them thick and healthy. Avoid using a coarse abrasive (less than 180 grit), and always use a very light touch when filing on the natural nail. Electric files can seriously damage the natural nail if used incorrectly. It is best to avoid using them on the natural nail unless you have advanced, specialized training on their proper and safe use.

Sticky substances between the cells, as well as tight rivetlike connections, hold the nail plate cells together. Many natural oils and proteins are found in the nail plate. Research shows that the main oils found in the nail plate are cholesterol and squalene. Both are found in skin oil (sebum). However, in the nails they are found in greater abundance.

After keratin cells are formed in the matrix, they are pushed upward and outward by the rhythmic, predictable flow of new cells. A fresh crop of keratin-containing nail cells is constantly being manufactured, pushing the older cells along a predetermined path. The new growth emerges from under the proximal nail fold of the eponychium. As new cells leave the matrix, they push the older cells toward the fingertips. Eventually, each keratin cell will reach the end of the finger. The part of the nail plate that grows beyond the fingertip is called the **free edge** or the **distal nail plate** Ⓕⓣ (DISS-tuhl nail plate). *Distal* means "farthest" Ⓕⓣ. It is important to remember the difference between *distal* and *proximal*. *Proximal* means "nearest." Therefore, *distal* is the opposite of *proximal*. These words may seem strange at first, but they are important to understand.

When the new keratin cells leave the matrix they are plump and whitish in appearance. Before emerging from under the eponychium the cells flatten, become transparent, and lose their whitish color. This explains why nail plates are normally colorless, except for the white half-moon peeking out from under the proximal nail fold.

The Lunula

The opaque, bluish white half-moon at the base of the nail plate is called the **lunula** (luh-NOO-luh) Ⓕⓣ. The lunula is the front part of the matrix we can see, or in other words, the visible matrix. Not all fingers have a visible lunula. The lunula outlines the front part of the matrix and on some fingers it is located underneath the eponychium. Usually, it is easiest to find a lunula on a thumb or index finger. You can tell if a person is right- or left-handed by examining the person's lunulas. The thumb with the largest lunula is on the dominant, writing hand. Try this on your friends and you'll find it almost always holds true.

The lunula also determines the shape of the nail plate Ⓕⓣ. Look at the shape of your lunula and compare it to the natural shape of your nail's free edge. You can see how closely they match. Both the lunula and free edge will have the same crescent shape. This is because the lunula shows how the front edge of the matrix is shaped. The shape of the matrix's front edge determines the free edge shape. Animals with differently shaped lunulas have nails or claws that match. Figure 1–4 shows the claw and lunula shapes of six different primates. In every case you'll see how closely they match.

In fetuses, the first nail plates begin to form on the fingers at 12 or 13 weeks. Strangely, the first new growth of nail plate starts at the lunula. It isn't until the fetus is 20 weeks old that the entire matrix is functioning and producing mature, fully formed nail plate. In a sense, the nail plate starts its life by growing in the opposite direction, at least until normal growth patterns are established. But even

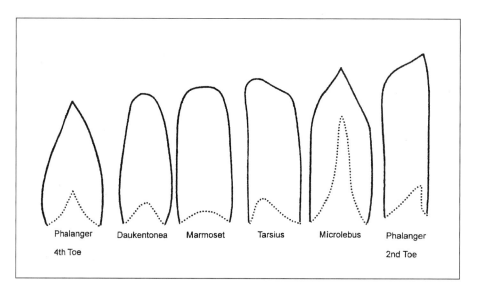

Figure 1–4 *Shape of lunula determines the free edge shape of the nail plate*

Drawing from W. E. Le Gros Clark, "The Problem of the Claw in Primates," *Proc. Zool. Soc. Lond.* 1936, 1–24.

after nail growth reaches full maturity, the area over the lunula is the thinnest part of the plate and is the easiest part to damage or puncture, especially with sharp implements. Care must be taken to prevent damage in this sensitive area. Injury to the underlying matrix can cause permanent nail deformities.

Nail Plate Cross Section

Each of the three parts (front, middle, and back) of the matrix produces a slightly different type of keratin. As a result, three distinct layers can be seen when the nail plate is highly magnified (Figure 1–5). This image was taken with a highly advanced, scientific tool called a **scanning electron microscope (SEM).** This type of microscope provides the very best high-magnification images of the nail plate. You will see several such images in this book. Use them to build a mental image of the nail plate. It will help in understanding this microscopic world if you use your mind's eye. Try to envision yourself small enough to see a molecule or a cell. Imagine what they really look like and you will gain a better picture of how it all works and how everything fits together.

The upper, dense layer of the nail plate comes from the back of the matrix. The center of the plate is fibrous and is made in the middle of the matrix. Finally, the thin layer on the bottom of the plate is derived from the lunula area. In the next chapter, you will see how these layers work together to give the nails their unique properties.

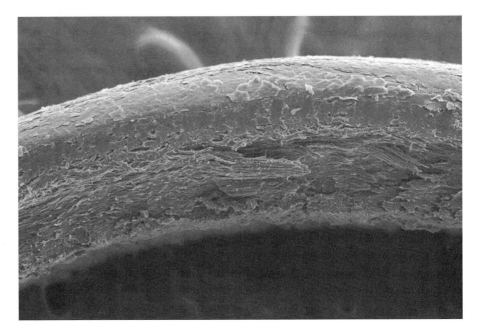

Figure 1-5 *Cross section of the nail plate reveals three distinct layers*

The Nail Bed

Until the 1980s many scientists believed a large portion of the nail plate's keratin cells came from the nail bed. Now we know that these cells come from the matrix. Even so, the importance of the nail bed has not diminished. The **nail bed** is an area of pinkish tissue that supports the entire nail plate. The bed is enriched with many tiny blood vessels that feed and clean the tissue. The nail bed lies directly underneath the solid nail plate, starting at the matrix and ending at the free edge. Facial skin and nail bed tissue have many things in common. Both contain two types of tissue, dermis and epidermis ⒻⓉ. The **dermis** is the lower or "basement" layer of skin. The **epidermis** is the upper layer of skin—in the case of the nail plate, the epidermis tissue is the upper layer of the nail bed, closest to the nail plate.

The dermis contains many tiny blood vessels. These **blood vessels** have two basic functions:

1. To nourish the cells within the dermis by carrying the food and oxygen needed for growth and reproduction

2. To cleanse the tissue cells and carry away wastes, toxins, and carbon dioxide

There are many types of epidermis found on the body. The epidermis under the nail plate is different from the epidermis of the hands or fingers. It more closely resembles the inside lining of the mouth. This very special type of epidermis is called **bed epithelium** (bed epp-uh-THEEL-ee-um). It exists only underneath the nail plate. The bed epithelium is a sticky tissue that adheres tightly to the bottom of the nail plate. As the plate grows toward the free edge, the bed epithelium separates from the dermis, allowing the nail plate to slide over the dermis, which is anchored firmly to the underlying structures of the finger *(FT)*. The dermis has grooves running from the lunula to the free edge, and the cells of the epithelium fill these grooves as the nail plate slides along, keeping the nail plate on track and attached to the nail bed (Figure 1–6).

The dermis has many ridges and groovelike channels running from the lunula to just before the free edge *(FT)*. The soft bed epithelium slides into these channels, creating tiny rails. These rails fit into the equally tiny grooves like a railroad car and track (Figure 1–6 and Color Plate 2). The dermis is anchored firmly in place by many attachments to the bone underneath. Besides keeping the nail plate "on track," the dermis grooves also hold the rails in place. This neat trick of nature keeps the plate from falling off the nail bed, while giving it mobility.

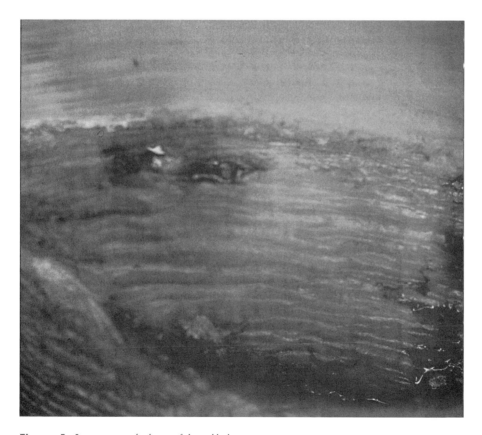

Figure 1–6 *Grooves in the dermis of the nail bed*

CONFUSED

Most clients don't know their nail bed from their nail plate or, even worse, think they're the same thing! These two parts of the fingernail are very different. It is common to confuse these terms, so you should take the time to teach all of your clients the difference between them.

The nail bed is made of soft tissues, rich with blood vessels. The bed supports the entire length of the plate as it grows. The nail plate is a hard keratin structure that protects the underlying bed. In short, the plate is the covering and the bed is the base. Together they make a perfect match!

The Solehorn

The bed epithelium remains attached to the underside of the nail plate until long after it grows past the fingertip. This thin epithelium can be seen by closely examining the underside of the free edge. It has the appearance of a thin layer of cloudy, yellowish tissue. This tissue is called the **solehorn** ⓕⓣ or *solehorn cuticle* (Figure 1–7 and Color Plate 3). The solehorn usually sloughs away by itself or may be removed during a manicure.

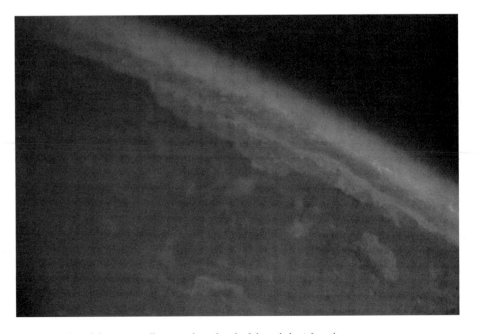

Figure 1-7 *Solehorn tissue adhering to the underside of the nail plate's free edge*

The Onychodermal Band

At the point where the bed epithelium passes off the nail bed to become the sole-horn, part of this delicate tissue becomes bunched up and squeezed more tightly together into a small zone called the **onychodermal band** ⓕⓣ (ON-ih-koh-DER-muhl band) (see Figure 1–8 and Color Plate 4). This narrow band of bunched-up tissue creates a protective seal under the free edge of the nail plate. This feature of the nail unit is often missed and can be seen only with careful observation. Look for the grayish, glassy-looking narrow zone under the nail plate. This protective band of tissue stretches across the entire width of the nail plate bordering the white free edge. The onychodermal band prevents infectious organisms and contaminants from getting underneath. If this seal is broken, the nail plate may lift away from the nail bed and dramatically increase the risk of infection. The onychodermal band also marks the place where the nail plate detaches from the bed to form the unsupported, free edge. This is an area of great importance to the health of the nail unit, so it must be treated with care. Manicuring this area should be done with caution and proper attention.

The Hyponychium

The farthest or most distal edge of the nail unit is the **hyponychium** ⓕⓣ. It is found under the free edge of the nail plate. The hyponychium is composed of

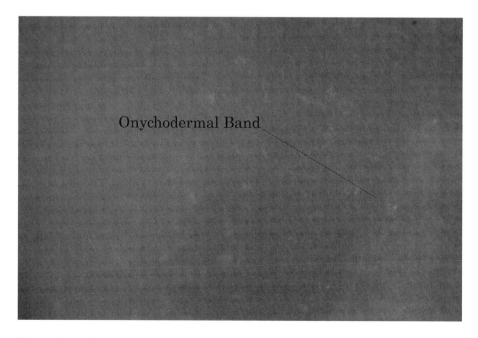

Figure 1-8 *The onychodermal band*

living epidermis tissue. In this case, the epidermis is more similar to normal skin and does not resemble the bed epithelium. This tissue is tougher and more resistant to abrasion, cuts, chemicals, etc. The hyponychium forms a watertight seal that prevents bacteria, fungi, viruses, etc. from attacking the nail bed. Care should also be taken to protect the hyponychium. Damage to this area can breach the seal created by the onychodermal band. As you have already learned, this can lead to serious infection that may even result in the loss of the nail plate *(FT)*. The hyponychium is an important nail bed guardian seal. It is the fourth guardian and its job is to protect the nail bed from pathogens under the free edge.

BLOOD AND NERVE SUPPLY FOR THE NAIL

A rich supply of nutrients and oxygen is delivered to the nail unit by the blood. **Arteries** carry blood from the heart to many parts of the body, including the fingernail. Two separate arteries supply each nail unit, one on each side of the finger *(FT)*. These bright red arteries pass through the lateral nail fold (the sidewall guardian seals) and then run deep into the dermis tissue of the nail bed. Many small branches carry blood from these main fingernail arteries to other parts of the nail unit. These tiny branches are called **capillaries** *(FT)*. It is the capillaries that give the nail bed its pinkish color. The capillaries carry blood to the nail bed dermis tissue, resulting in its healthy pink appearance *(FT)*. These capillaries do not reach into the nail plate. Therefore, the nail plate receives no blood or nutrients *(FT)*. Blood is drained away from the nail unit by **veins,** which collect blood from the capillaries and return it to the heart. The nail unit has two veins. Each lateral nail fold has its own vein. These veins carry blood and waste products away from the nail bed *(FT)*. Figure 1–9 shows the complex system of veins, arteries, and capillaries found in the hands and fingers.

Nerves provide the sensations of touch, pain, and warmth *(FT)*. They also move the muscles in the fingers and hands. The nerves end near the skin's surface. The nerve endings are very sensitive. Some of these **nerve endings** are highly sensitive to pain, some to pressure, and others to heat. The **nerve fibers** carry the sensations from the endings all the way to the brain for processing. The nail bed contains very few heat-sensitive nerve endings. Most of the nerve endings in the bed are sensitive only to pressure and pain. Using files with coarse abrasive or using aggressive filing techniques on the natural nail plate can overheat the nail plate. Excessive levels of heat can then activate the pain-sensitive nerve endings in the nail bed and cause a sensation that is often described as "heat spike." Overly aggressive filing techniques can friction-burn the nail bed, which can result in nail bed damage. You will learn more about avoiding this type of injury in Chapter 7.

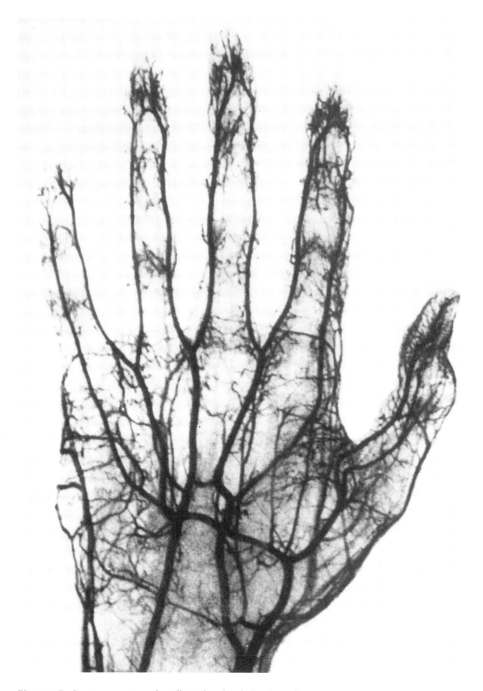

Figure 1-9 *Veins, arteries, and capillaries found in the hands and fingers*

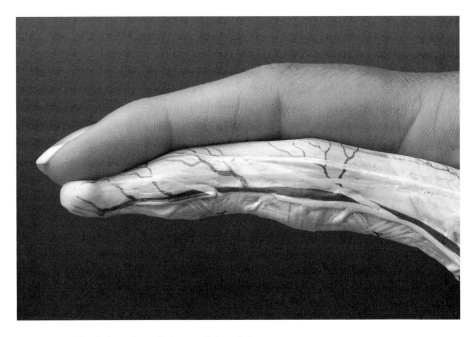

Figure 1-10 *The bone shapes the finger and the nail plate*

THE BONE

One of the purposes of the nail plate and bed is to protect the fingertip bones, or distal **phalanges** (FT) (fuh-LAN-jeez). This bone, the distal phalange, determines the overall length, shape, curvature, and spread of the nail unit, as shown in Figure 1–10. It gives strength and support to the dermis, which is firmly attached to the bone by tough, durable collagen fibers. Since the bone affects the curvature of the matrix, it also has a great influence on the curvature of the nail plate itself.

In the next chapter, you will learn how various parts of the nail unit work in harmony to grow healthy fingernail plates.

FAST TRACK (FT)

(FT) There are four guardian seals to keep out infectious agents and chemicals. Guardian seals are the cuticle, the hyponychium, and the two lateral nail folds.

(FT) *Proximal* means "nearest."

(FT) The skin on either side of the nail plate is called the lateral nail fold.

(FT) *Lateral* means "to the side."

FT The eponychium is the skin that lies directly on top of the newly developing nail plate.

FT The cuticle is dead tissue shed from the underside of the eponychium.

FT The matrix's size and shape determine the thickness and width of the plate.

FT The nail plate growing beyond the fingertip is called the free edge or the distal nail plate.

FT *Distal* means "farthest."

FT The lunula is the opaque area at the base (proximal end) of the nail plate.

FT The lunula determines the shape of the nail plate's free edge.

FT The nail bed is made of several types of tissue, dermis, epidermis, and bed epithelium.

FT Bed epithelium allows the nail plate to slide along the nail bed.

FT The dermis contains groovelike channels that guide nail plate growth.

FT Bed epithelium grows past the free edge and becomes the solehorn.

FT The onychodermal band is caused by the bunching up of the bed epithelium.

FT The hyponychium is the most distal (farthest) edge of the nail unit.

FT A damaged hyponychium can lead to infection and nail plate separation.

FT Two arteries supply each nail unit; one runs along each side of the finger.

FT Many small capillaries carry blood from the arteries to the nail unit.

FT The blood in the capillaries gives the nail bed its pinkish color.

FT The nail plate itself receives no blood or nutrients.

FT Blood is drained away from the nail unit by veins in each lateral nail fold.

FT Nerves in the nail unit provide touch, pain, and warmth sensations.

FT The nail plate and bed protect the bone in the fingertip (distal phalange).

Review Questions

1. What is the definition of *proximal*, *lateral*, and *distal*?
2. Which finger has the narrowest matrix?
3. If a person was born with _____ nails, their matrix must be shorter than normal.

4. List 10 parts of the nail unit.

5. _____ carry blood and nutrients from the heart to the nail unit, while _____ carry blood and waste products away from the nail unit.

6. Name the guardians of the nail.

7. Why is the onychodermal band important, and what does it protect?

8. What chemical substance is the nail plate composed of, and where else on the body is it found?

9. How are sensations such as pain relayed to the brain?

10. If the nail plate is firmly attached to the nail bed, how can it move when it grows?

11. Which two nail anatomy terms are commonly misused and sometimes used interchangeably even though they are completely different?

12. Where does the cuticle come from?

13. The fingernail plate is approximately _____ cell layers thick.

14. The nerve endings in the nail bed can detect _____ and _____ very well but cannot detect _____ very well.

15. Name the tissue that adheres to the bottom of the nail plate.

Chapter 2

Nail Growth and Function

Objective

In the last chapter, you learned about the various parts of the nail unit. Now you will see how these parts function. The nail unit is like an orchestra, with many instruments working together in concert to create something beautiful. The same is true of the fingernail. You will learn about the physical properties of the nail plate, as well as the effects of moisture, oil, and solvents.

NAIL PLATE GROWTH

How fast does the nail plate grow? This is a difficult question to answer. Many factors affect the growth rate. For example, the nail plates on each finger grow at different rates (see Figure 2–1). Nail plates also grow more slowly at night and during the winter. On the average, the normal thumbnail will grow about 1/10 inch per month or 1½ inches (3.8 cm) per year. It takes about five or six months to completely replace the entire nail plate and one to two months for new nail plate to grow out from the matrix to just past the eponychium. The toenail grows much more slowly. Toenails take about a year or longer to replace. The left thumbnail usually grows slightly faster than the right. The nail plate on the middle finger grows the fastest, followed by the nail plates on the pointer and ring fingers, which grow at almost the same rate. The thumb is the next slowest, but the slowest of all is the little finger, which grows about 1¼ inches per year. As a rule, the longer the finger, the faster the nail plate will grow.

Here are some interesting nail growth facts:

- Nail plates grow about 20 percent faster in the summer.
- Normally men's nail plates grow faster than women's, especially on the dominant hand.
- Nail plates grow fastest during pregnancy (see Figure 2–2).

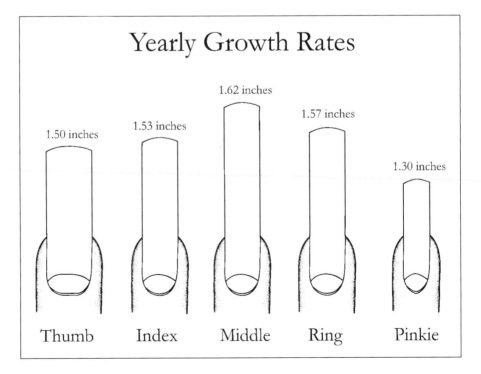

Figure 2-1 *Yearly growth rate of fingernails*

- Nail plate growth increases by about 3.5 percent between the fourth and eighth months of pregnancy.

- From the ninth month until after delivery, nail growth rate increases by a whopping 20 percent.

- Age also affects the nail growth rate, which peaks between the ages of 10 and 14 years and slowly declines after age 20.

- Nail biting, accidental damage, or loss causes nail plates to grow faster.

- Many factors cause slow growth of nail plates, such as being immobilized or paralyzed, poor circulation, malnutrition, lactation, serious infections, psoriasis, and certain medications.

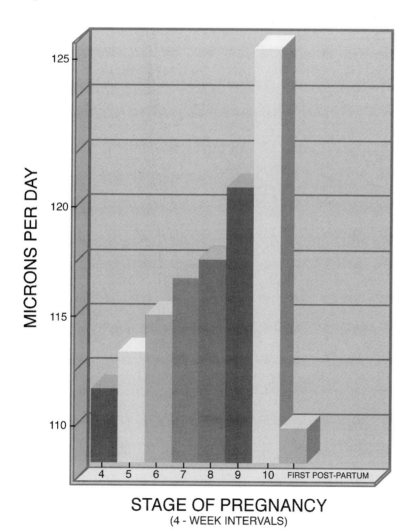

Figure 2-2 *Rate of nail growth during pregnancy*

Nutrition and Nail Growth

Nothing you can eat will make healthy nail plates become stronger than normal, but poor nutrition can certainly make them weaker. There are many scientific studies showing that malnutrition and even severe dieting make nail plates thin and/or weak. Poor nutrition may contribute to nail plate splitting and can dramatically slow nail growth. It can also affect hair growth (and other parts of the body) as well. One well-known myth says calcium makes nails stronger. In fact, studies show that the natural nail plate contains less than 0.1 percent calcium. It is unlikely that calcium is important to maintaining healthy nail plates. Eating calcium-rich foods or taking calcium supplements probably does nothing positive for the nail plate, either. Applying products containing calcium to the top surface of the nail plate is even less likely to have a positive benefit.

To date, no conclusive scientific studies have linked vitamin supplements, gelatin drinks, or special foods to faster growth of healthy nails. Studies on horses and sheep have found nutritional links to hoof and wool growth, but these are quite different from human fingernails. Each of these is made of keratin, but so are a bird's feather and a rhino's horn. There is no firm proof that particular supplements or foods work in humans. Someday scientists will develop a true nail growth formula. But when they do, it will be big news in the medical world and will be reported in a prestigious medical journal. You won't first hear about this new "miracle product" in the tabloids or on a TV shopping network. Personally, I think it's just a matter of time before science learns to regulate the growth of the nail plate. Until then, good nutrition is a great way to maintain normal nail health. Eating right and exercising regularly will keep your entire body healthy, including your nails. Neither the latest "secrets of the stars" nor vitamin supplements will make your nails as healthy as eating right and getting plenty of exercise. That's the best nail beauty secret known. Cosmetic creams, oils, and lotions that say they are "nail growth accelerators" are making false and misleading claims. It is illegal to make such statements about cosmetics, which are designed for beautifying only. No cosmetic product may legally claim that it changes or alters any function of the body—only FDA-approved drugs can make these types of claims.

The Role of Proper Circulation

The nail plate doesn't just grow from the matrix—it needs help with this task. To start, a constant supply of blood is necessary. The arteries supply the blood, which carries nutrients to tiny capillaries in the matrix. Capillaries are like long, one-way streets winding through tissue, carrying blood to the cells. The matrix has two arteries, so it has two sources of blood. If one of them becomes damaged or injured, the other will maintain the blood flow. There are also two different types of capillaries. One type carries fresh blood to deliver oxygen and important nutrients to matrix cells in the bed. The other type of capillary drains away the blood that carries waste products from these cells.

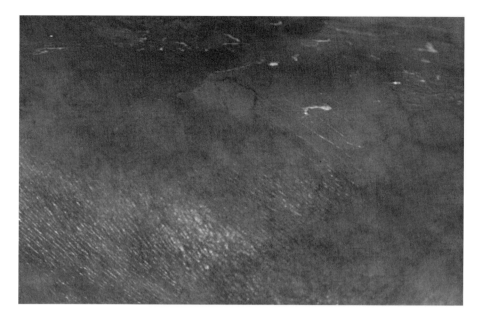

Figure 2–3 *Capillaries in the nail fold*

Capillaries are essential to our health. They are spread throughout our bodies and are found in all parts of the nail unit. In Figure 2–3 and Color Plate 5 you can see the capillaries in the lateral sidewall. The capillaries collect wastes from the tissues and carry them into the veins. The impure blood flows through the kidney and liver, where it is purified again and returned to the heart. The heart pumps the blood to the arteries and recirculates it throughout the body, 24 hours a day. Every cell in the body benefits from this efficient recycling method. This is how the matrix is fed and cleaned. You can see why proper circulation is a key part of maintaining a healthy nail unit.

WHAT ARE CELLS AND WHY DO WE NEED THEM?

Each organ in the body is made up of cells. The kidney has millions of kidney cells, the heart is made of heart cells, and so on. Biologists define cells as the smallest and simplest unit capable of being alive Ⓕⓣ. Cells are too tiny to be seen by the eye. Most cells in the body are 4/10,000 of an inch in diameter, about one-tenth the diameter of a single human hair.

This may surprise you, but cells in the nail unit are remarkably similar to cells found in other parts of the body. Even bacteria and plant cells share many common features with our body's cells. All cells bring in water and food so they can live and reproduce. They consume oxygen and nutrients and then excrete whatever waste is left over. In animals, the waste is transported back through the cell walls, where it makes its way to the outward-bound capillaries and eventually to the veins for removal.

THE BUILDING BLOCKS OF NATURE

The matrix is much like the dermis of the skin. Both are made up of special cells that are locked firmly in place by collagen fibers. In other words, matrix cells never become part of the nail plate. Instead, they are the incubators for the new cells (FT). As the newly formed nail plate cells begin to mature, they separate from the matrix. As more plate cells are made, the new cells push the older cells toward the eponychium and lunula. This is the process we call growth of the natural nail.

The plate cells are made of a type of protein called keratin. Like all protein, keratin is composed of amino acids. Amino acids are called the "building blocks of life" because they link together to create most of the tissues and organs found in the body. An amino acid molecule is a very small chemical that is about 13,000 times smaller than a cell. Amino acids link together into long strings or chains to form proteins (FT). The keratin found in the nail plate, like the keratin in hair and skin, is made from long chains of amino acids (FT).

If hair, skin, and nails all contain keratin, why are they so different? The reason is simple. There are many kinds of amino acids. Different arrangements of amino acids make different types of proteins. Amino acids are like letters of the alphabet. A limited number of letters (amino acids) can be used to spell an almost unlimited number of words (proteins). Since there are 20 amino acids, you can see why so many different proteins are found in the body. These amino acids link together in long chains called **polypeptides.** Proteins are made of one or more of these polypeptide chains. Interestingly, the shape of the protein depends on the amino acids used to make the polypeptide chain. Depending on the sequences of amino acids, the protein will fold together in complex patterns. In this way, the body makes many different and unique proteins to perform special tasks or functions in the body. Our nail plates are the perfect example!

Cross-linked for Strength and Durability

A protein can be thought of as a long rope made of amino acids. Imagine two long ropes lying side by side. Tie short pieces of rope between the two long ropes and you'll have a rope ladder. Tie several rope ladders together with these short pieces of rope and you now have a net! The ropes, ladders, and net are all made from the same material, but they are certainly very different, especially in how they function.

Protein chains can also be tied together like a rope ladder. The rungs or steps on the protein ladder are called **cross-links.** The cross-links are made from **cysteine** (SIS-teen), a type of amino acid. Cysteine contains sulfur and forms the **sulfur cross-links** in hair that make it curly. Figure 2–4 illustrates how cross-links

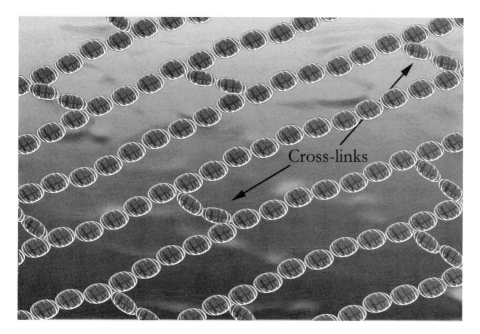

Cross-links

Figure 2-4 *Cross-linked versus non-cross-linked protein strands*

between molecules of different protein chains can reinforce those chains. Nail plates and hair are the most highly cross-linked tissues in the body. Very curly hair has many more cross-links than straight hair. In fact, breaking and re-forming these sulfur cross-links is the basis for permanent waving. These cross-links also make protein less likely to absorb substances that can cause stains. This is why naturally curly hair, which has more cross-links than straight hair, is more difficult to artificially color. Cross-links are very strong chemical bonds that are very difficult to break. This is one reason why they have greater strength, durability, and stain resistance. Both hair and nails are highly cross-linked, but nail plates have far more cross-links than hair. The combined strength of the millions of cross-links between molecules of cysteine contributes greatly to nail plate durability (FT). (However, you will learn in later chapters that excessive cross-linking can cause nail plates to become brittle. More is not always better!) Some types of advanced artificial nail enhancements copy nature and use cross-links to make their products stronger. As you can see, cross-links are a very important concept in nail structure and product chemistry.

HOW DOES THE NAIL PLATE GROW?

As keratin cells are pushed from the matrix they begin to change. They slowly lose their plump, round shape and begin to flatten, as shown in Figure 2–5. When they flatten, the inside of the cell breaks apart and loses its whitish color. The

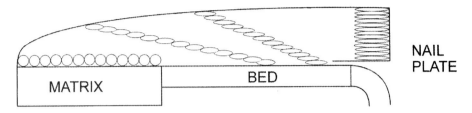

Figure 2-5 *Keratin nail cells flatten as they move away from the matrix*

cells become thin and transparent. They also become much more compact. So as the cells mature and travel toward the free edge, they pack together more tightly and the nail plate becomes harder and denser. Near the eponychium, the nail plate is softer and more flexible, while the reverse is true at the free edge. The free edge is made of the oldest, flattest, and hardest nail cells (FT).

It is very important to treat the lunula area with care. The nail plate over the lunula is thinner and softer. Also, the matrix is located in this region. From the last chapter, you will recall that the eponychium tissue and cuticle create a barrier against bacteria and other microscopic invaders. This seal must not be broken or harmed. Always use caution with any procedure involving this area of the nail unit. Damage here can permanently injure the nail. Sharp implements or a rapidly spinning electric file bit can tear through this thinner, softer nail plate and cause serious problems for clients.

For many years, it was believed that part of the nail plate grew up from the nail bed. As you learned in Chapter 1, this is incorrect. Almost every cell in the nail plate comes from the matrix (FT). One exception is the thin layer of bed epithelium that adheres to the bottom of the nail plate.

Travel Restrictions Apply

It might seem odd at first, but nail plate thickness is completely determined by the length of the matrix area (FT). You can see the reason for this by examining Figure 2–6.

The longest row of cells ends up being the tallest stack of cells. So, the longest row of cells in the matrix will produce the thickest part of the nail plate. The average fingernail plate has about 100 layers of stacked cells. The toenail can contain up to 150 layers. Each plate contains millions of cells packed into dense layers.

Look closely at Figure 2–6 and you see some interesting things about nail plate growth. The cells produced near the back of the matrix always end up on top of the nail plate. The cells from the lunula make up the bottom of the nail plate. The cells in the back of the matrix have the farthest to travel before emerging from under the eponychium. It takes about two months for the cells at the back of the matrix to reach a point directly over the lunula. Therefore, the

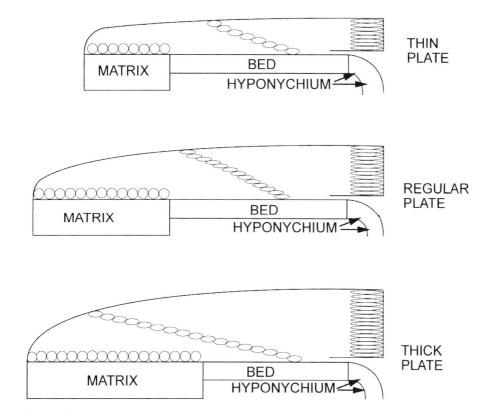

Figure 2-6 *The longer the matrix, the thicker the nail plate*

cells on top of the nail plate over the lunula are two months older that those on the bottom of the plate in that same spot. This also means that at the free edge, the top layer of nail plate is about two months older than the bottom layer. This helps explain why nail plates tend to peel at the top surface, rather than from underneath.

INVESTIGATION: NAIL PLATE

Analysis of nail clippings shows that besides the sulfur in amino acids, the plate contains many other chemicals. Some of these are iron, aluminum, copper, silver, gold, titanium, phosphorus, zinc, sodium, and calcium. Each of these is found in extremely low concentrations. Sulfur constitutes about 5 percent of the nail plate. Sodium is 3½ times more abundant than calcium in nail plates. Obviously, eating lots of table salt (sodium chloride) won't make nails stronger either!

DON'T THINK SO!

A common myth says that the extra weight of artificial nail enhancements makes the nail plate grow thinner. Supposedly, this happens because the nail bed "feels the extra weight." This is pretty unlikely since:

- The length of the nail matrix determines plate thickness.
- There is no way for the matrix to "feel" any extra weight on the nail bed.
- The nail bed doesn't make keratin cells, so it can't affect the plate's thickness.

This myth doesn't fit the facts and makes no sense. How do such myths spread? Because they sound reasonable to most people. Most people don't understand how the nail plate grows, so they are easily fooled. This is how knowledge can empower you as a nail technician. With knowledge, you won't be so easily fooled.

WHAT DO WE WANT OUR NAILS TO BE?

When talking about nails, many people use words such as *strong, hard, tough, flexible,* or *brittle,* but do we really know what these terms mean? What's the difference between them? Some may think their meanings are obvious, but are they? Usually clients don't really understand these terms and often misuse them. A thorough understanding of these terms will help you make the right choices for your client's nails and save you lots of time because you won't have to do unnecessary repairs.

Materials scientists are people who study the properties of many types of substances. They are very interested in what happens when you bend, twist, stretch, rub, or crush different types of materials. They study everything from concrete and steel to diamonds and granite to bones, wood, and rubber. All of these are very different materials, but they have some things in common. All materials share some important properties. Materials scientists seek to understand these properties. These unique scientists dedicate their lives to learning why things break, split, melt, evaporate, discolor, dissolve, or break down. Their quest is to learn more about the properties of all materials.

For any solid substance there are five important properties that you must understand. These five properties are extremely important to nail plates, and later you will learn that they are highly important to artificial nails. Let's take a look into the world of materials science and find out why these properties are so important.

1. **Strength** is the ability to resist breaking under a heavy load ⒻⓉ. A bridge must be strong to hold all the crossing cars. In this case, the cars are the

load. Tree branches must be strong to resist the load created by a heavy wind. Arms must be strong to pick up heavy loads. Nail plates need to be strong because we use them like tools. All the bending, picking, prying, scratching, and clawing we do with our nails is proof of their strength. But strength isn't the only property that nails must possess. Steel is very strong, but we don't want our nails to be like steel! They would be too hard and inflexible, and we would have to be careful not to poke out our own eyes. Besides, it is possible for nail plates to be too strong. Nail plates are designed to break rather than let more serious damage occur. If the nail did not break, the matrix might be damaged or even destroyed by a hard blow. Nail strength must be in balance with other important properties.

2. **Hardness** measures a surface's resistance to being scratched or dented (FT). Hardness is a property of the material's surface, even though some incorrectly use this word when they really mean strength. Diamond is the hardest known substance. Diamond can easily scratch glass, topaz, or quartz. But none of these materials can scratch the surface of a diamond. Their surfaces are much softer than diamond. The nail plate seems soft by comparison, but the hardness of its surface is still very important. When nail plates are softer than normal, they are more easily scratched or stained. Softer plates have a tendency to peel or become pitted. Healthy nail plates need to be hard, but not too hard. When nail plates become too hard, they are more susceptible to shattering and splitting. For example, overuse of nail hardening products may cause nail plates to become excessively hard, which leads to other types of damage. Some clients want their nails to be as hard as possible, but they really wouldn't be happy if they got their wish. If you had the choice, which would you rather your nails be like—hard as rubber or hard as glass? Rubber is not nearly as hard as glass, but most people would rather have their nails be more flexible, like rubber. Harder isn't always better!

3. **Flexibility** allows a substance to bend (FT). Flexible materials bend to absorb a strong force or impact. Substances that resist bending will often suffer damaging cracks or breaks when impacted or when they bear a heavy load. Bones are a great example. Young children's bones are highly flexible, but they lose flexibility as they age. Elderly people's bones have lost most of their flexibility and are brittle and easily broken. In nails, sudden breaking, cracking, or fracturing is a sign of **brittleness** (FT). Normally, nail plates are highly flexible and will usually bend before reaching the breaking point. You will learn in Chapter 4 that age, diet, health, and many other factors can influence nail plate flexibility and brittleness. Repeated or long-term exposure to harsh cleaners and solvents can also make nail plates brittle and less flexible. Flexibility is also sometimes confused with strength, though they are quite different. Many things are very flexible but have very little strength, and the reverse is also true. Aluminum can pop tops are an excellent example: they are very flexible, but bend them a few times and they will snap off. Factors in the environment—heat, cold, sunlight, moisture, and wear—can also affect flexibility.

4. **Toughness** is a balance of strength and flexibility (FT). When these two important properties are in balance, the result is a tough material with **durability.** Nylon fishing line and the plastic rings that hold together a six-pack

of soda are examples of extremely tough materials (see Figure 2–7). These substances will stretch a great deal before eventually breaking, but they never get brittle or fracture. Hair and nail plates are also very tough materials. This is their most important property! What goes wrong when nails become brittle, snap, or split too easily? If either strength or flexibility gets out of balance, then toughness is lost! Nail plates that are too flexible will lose strength. The reverse holds true. Nail plates can become too strong and lose flexibility. Either way the nail plate will lose its inherent toughness and resistance to breakage. These two properties are closely linked. Nails must have both! Tough, healthy nails have the best of both worlds.

5. **Wear resistance** is the ability to resist abrasion or rubbing ⒡ . This is an important property for the nail plate. Even hard surfaces can be worn away by certain abrasives. Most nail files have a layer of silicon carbide glued to a hard backing or dense foam base. **Silicon carbide** is a crystalline mineral that is inexpensive and nearly as hard as diamond. On a scale of 1 to 10, diamonds have a hardness of 10, while black silicon carbide is a 9. Silicon carbide is nearly perfect as a material for nail files. **Aluminum oxide** is another abrasive used on files. This abrasive is white and a little softer—on the same scale it has a 7.5 hardness. Files made with silicon carbide are more aggressive and have a greater potential to be damaging ⒡ , while the same grit aluminum oxide is noticeably less aggressive.

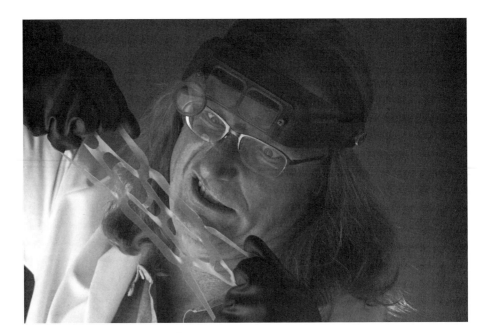

Figure 2-7 *Very tough materials are both strong and flexible*

TROUBLE-FREE TROUBLESHOOTING

Trouble! Nobody likes it, nobody wants it, and nail technicians get it. They're called problem nails. They cost time and money. Certain clients seem to have more trouble than others. It's a reality that every nail technician has to face. Luckily, there are always reasons for these nagging problems. Finding the reasons is the key to finding the solutions.

This is why it is so important for nail technicians to understand the meanings of terms such as *toughness, brittleness, durability, wear resistance, hardness,* and *strength.* They aren't just words—they are concepts that can help you understand many nail problems. These concepts will help troubleshoot the most perplexing problems and give you answers to your client's most challenging questions. If you learn about these important properties and use your knowledge, it will save you time, frustration, and lots and lots of money.

Abrasive files can quickly wear away the nail plate, scratching away the surface keratin cells. Large particles of abrasive on heavy-grit files create larger scratches, while the finer particles on small-grit files will create tinier scratches. This explains why heavy-grit abrasives can cause excessive thinning and damage to the nail plate. Heavy pressure can drive the scratches deeper. Under normal conditions the tough nail plate has very good wear resistance. The free edge can be worn down, but not very easily. (In later chapters you'll learn this isn't always true for artificial nails.)

THE STRUCTURE OF THE NAIL KERATIN

There are two basic types of keratin in the human nail, **crystalline** and **noncrystalline.** Crystalline substances have structures that are very orderly and (nearly) perfectly arranged. Quartz, sapphire, and topaz are crystals because their molecules are arranged in an orderly fashion. The tiny keratin fibers or fibrils inside the nail plate cell are an example of the crystalline type. The nail plate keratin fibrils themselves are made of dozens of individual protein chains. These chains are coiled and have a corkscrew appearance. These tiny coils lie side by side and are packed tightly into larger stacks to create crystalline keratin fibrils, as shown in Figure 2–8. These are so tiny that a bundle of 2,000 fibrils is as thick as a single human hair.

Each nail cell is filled with hundreds of keratin fibrils. These fibrils are embedded in the second type of keratin, noncrystalline (also called *amorphous*) keratin. A little less than one-half of the keratin in the nail plate cell is

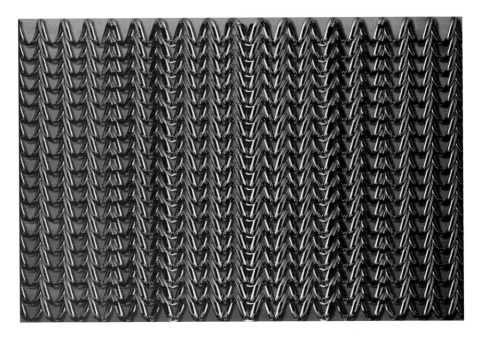

Figure 2-8 *Coiled protein chains stack into orderly bundles*

noncrystalline. In this type of keratin, the amino acid chains are randomly positioned and are not neatly stacked as they are in the fibrils. The crystalline fibrils are embedded in a sea of noncrystalline keratin, a gel-like substance. The noncrystalline keratin coats and protects the fibrils. It also helps regulate the passage of moisture and oil through the nail plate (FT).

How do oils and water move through the nail? **Diffusion** is the process that describes how liquids absorb or move through a solid (FT). When water and oil move through the nail plate, they obey the laws of diffusion. These laws state that a liquid substance will move away from places where its concentration is high into areas where its concentration is lower. You can see diffusion in action by dropping a cup of blue dye into a swimming pool. The dye will start out as a dark blue spot, but it will diffuse into the water until the pool is evenly colored. Oils and moisture are at a high concentration near the bed, so they diffuse by traveling toward the plate's surface, where the moisture escapes and the oil is washed away. That's why the concentrations of water and oil are always lower at the plate's surface. It is important to remember that water and oils will always diffuse from high to low concentration. Diffusion is one of the most important concepts in nature, and our bodies depend on it to survive. Throughout this book you will see a wide variety of examples that will demonstrate the importance of diffusion to many aspects of the nail industry.

Tough as Nails

We have seen that nail plates are a unique combination of strength and flexibility, but how is the proper balance achieved? Let's look at the most important ways.

1. Very strong chemical bonds join the amino acids into very strong chains. These protein chains usually contain somewhere between 5,000 and 100,000 amino acids. When equal thicknesses are compared, amino acid chains are stronger than steel! **Covalent bonds** (CO-vale-int bonds) are what link the amino acids together. These chemical bonds are the strongest type of chemical linkage Ⓕⓣ. Covalent bonds are found in many materials, not just keratin. Covalent bonds are found in muscle, hair, skin, lungs, and every other part of the body. In fact, they are extremely important to all living things. It is safe to say that without covalent bonds, humans, plants, and animals would not exist. The world would be like the moon. Covalent bonds account for everything from the amazing strength of spiderwebs to the extreme hardness of diamonds. You will learn more about covalent bonds in Chapter 7.

2. Sulfur cross-links are a special type of covalent bond created between two molecules of the amino acid cysteine found on separate protein chains. These two sulfur-containing amino acids can link protein chains together like rungs on a ladder. These links turn the single chains into an ultra-tough, netlike structure. Cross-links also make the surface of the nail more resistant to stains and the damaging effect of solvents, cleaners, etc. The high level of cysteine cross-linking in keratin is the primary source of its hardness, strength, and durability Ⓕⓣ.

3. Each cell in the nail plate must be connected to the surrounding cells or they would easily shed or flake away. What prevents this from happening? Nail cells are locked into a gigantic, interconnecting network (Figure 2–9) by **desmosomes** (DEZ-muh-soams), ringlike junctions that act like a tiny rivet between two nail cells. Each cell contains several of these permanent connections. The circular connection is hollow, but not empty. Desmosomes are filled with keratin fibrils, which further reinforce the connection between each cell. So you can see that the nail plate is a continuous, interconnected mass of keratin fibrils.

The cell wall is not always straight and smooth. Figure 2–10 shows that the cell wall can become contorted into knots. These knots also play an important role in holding cells together. Finally, the cells are embedded in a sticky substance that lies between the cells. Many other cells in the body also are adhered together using these methods.

While keratin is extremely important to the natural nail's flexibility, other substances found inside the plate play significant roles as well. The most influential of these is moisture. Nothing else has a more dramatic effect on the nail plate. Increasing moisture content instantly increases flexibility. The nail plate may appear solid, but it is not impenetrable. There are two ways for moisture to pass through the plate. One is for water molecules to pass through the microscopic spaces between the cells. The desmosomes form a tight junction point, but water

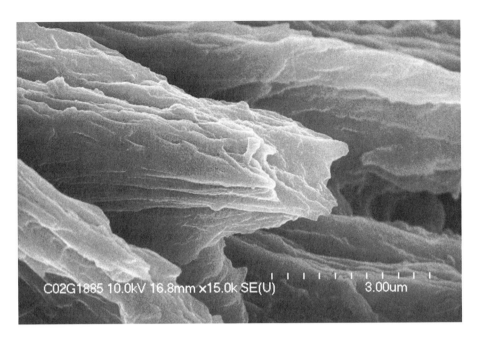

Figure 2-9 *High-magnification image showing a single layer of nail cells*

molecules are smaller than even an amino acid. These molecules easily pass between the cells. Of course, dodging around 100 layers of cells is certainly a long and winding road. It would be much shorter to pass directly through the cell wall and keratin fibrils. Moisture can travel through or between the cells. This explains why it moves so rapidly through the plate. If thickness is accounted for, water diffuses through the nail plate about 1,000 times faster than through skin! If you could shrink to the size of a water molecule, you could see why. The nail plate would seem like it was filled with small tunnels, as shown in Figure 2–11 and Color Plate 6. These tunnels connect with other tunnels, leading deeper into the plate. Water moves freely though these many millions of channels. There are many hollow, microscopic channels that allow the plate to absorb large quantities of water. In fact, a normal plate can hold almost one-third of its own weight in water.

A constant tide of water flows upward from the bed through the plate and quickly evaporates from the surface. While inside the plate, moisture acts as a lubricant and a shock absorber. How can moisture do this? Individual water molecules soak into the nail cells and keratin fibrils, coating them in sheaths of liquid lubricant. In this watery environment, the rigid amino acid chains become more relaxed. The higher the moisture content, the more relaxed these chains will become. In general, proteins relax by changing shape. When they relax, it is usually by unraveling, uncoiling, or unfolding into a simpler shape. Why is this

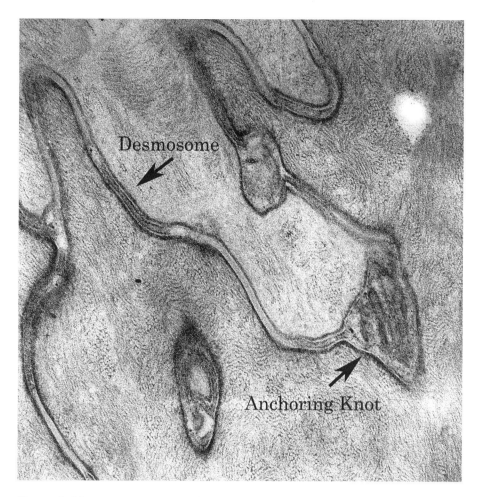

Figure 2-10 *Desmosomes are junctions between two nail cells, while anchoring knots help bind cells together*

important? Once relaxed, a protein chain has greater freedom of movement and is more flexible. To understand a keratin fibril, think of a guitar string. In many ways, they are similar. For instance, if the guitar string is loosened, it is less taut, more relaxed, and more flexible. So, the string is much less likely to break when played. Overtightening a guitar string increases the tension and makes the string more easily broken. The same is true for keratin. When keratin chains are less strained and relaxed, they are more flexible and less likely to be broken. Why? The chains get tougher when they're relaxed.

Normal nail plates contain about 18 percent water by weight. Flexibility is highest when the nail plate is totally saturated with water, at about 25 percent moisture. But too much moisture can weaken the plate and lead to damage. Nails that are constantly exposed to water can become soft and weak. On the other

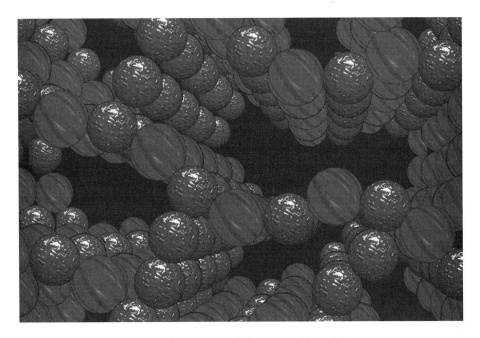

Figure 2-11 *A three-dimensional representation of the structure of the nail plate*

hand, too little moisture can leave the plate dry and brittle. Without question, the correct moisture level is vital to healthy nails. If the plate is suddenly hit or jammed, the extra flexibility lessens the force of the blow. Moisture acts just like the springs and shocks in your car to smooth the ride on a bumpy road. Moisture behaves like an internal shock absorber.

Other substances can also be absorbed into the plate. Liquids called plasticizers make solid materials softer or more flexible (FT). Leather conditioners and automobile seat and dashboard protectors are everyday examples of plasticizers. These products contain ingredients that soak into a solid substance to make it softer and more flexible. Approximately 5 percent of the nail plate's weight is from natural oils absorbed from the nail bed. These oils plasticize the nail plate, keeping it more flexible.

Oil and Moisture Balancing Act

Natural oils diffuse slowly upward from the nail bed into the nail plate and eventually are washed or worn off the top surface of the nail plate. These oils are composed of lipids, such as squalene (SKWA-leen) and cholesterol (ko-LESS-ter-awl). As noted previously, there is less oil in the nail plate than there is water—about 5 percent oil versus 18 percent moisture (FT). Of the two, moisture has a much great influence on flexibility and durability. Even so, these oils are very important to the nail health.

NOT GONNA HAPPEN

Some natural oil-based products are designed to soften skin as well as plasticize natural and artificial nails. They can perform this neat trick by being absorbed into the tiny spaces to increase flexibility and durability of the skin and nails. It is a myth that some oils can shrink cuticles. In fact, they do the opposite, which is why natural oil blends are used to soften the cuticles for easy and quick removal from the nail plate.

Oils don't mix with water, so how do both water and oil travel through the nail plate? It makes sense that oils and moisture would flow along different paths or channels. No one knows for sure, but many scientists believe there are special channels in the nail plate designed for oils. Here is how they would explain this phenomenon. Water can penetrate into the nail cell, through its outer wall, many times faster than oil. Oils can't readily penetrate the cell walls as easily. Since the cell walls block oil, the oil must travel a longer route, slipping though the spaces between individual nail cells.

Like moisture, oils have a plasticizing effect and can noticeably increase flexibility of the plate, especially with dry, brittle nails. How? Oils can increase the amount of moisture in the nail plate. When applied and absorbed into the nail surface, oils will slow down the passage of water through the nail plate. Oils block and temporarily seal the moisture channels. This can be especially useful for very dry nail plates. Oils slow water evaporation from the nail plate, which increases moisture content. The result is less brittle, more flexible nail plates, and all because the moisture content of the nail plate is increased. In theory, oils also have a lubricating effect between the cells as they diffuse around the junctions between the cells.

Oils will also be absorbed into the nail plate to plasticize it, but much more slowly than water. Just as oils are absorbed more slowly into the nail plate, it is also more difficult for the oils to escape. Therefore, oils stay in the plate for a very long time and can exert a dramatic long-term influence on the durability of the natural nail plate.

Solvent and Surfactant Effects

Anything that dries out or dehydrates the nail plate will also lower flexibility and toughness. Certain solvents can strip both oil and moisture from the nail plate. Removing these valuable plasticizers causes the nail surface to become much harder as well. Excessive use can lead to brittle nail plates or give the nail a dry or whitish appearance.

Artificial nail removers and nail polish removers contain solvents that can overly dry the nail plate, especially with repeated use. Acetone (ASS-a-tone) is a very common and safe salon solvent; ethyl acetate (EH-thul ASS-a-tate) and methyl ethyl ketone (MEH-thul EH-thul KEY-tone) are the non-acetone solvents used to remove polish. All three of these solvents will remove water and oils from the nail plate. Damage to the nail plate becomes more likely if these solvents are used excessively, that is, more than once a week. Proper use of these solvents is unlikely to cause damage. When used infrequently, the drying is a temporary effect that quickly corrects itself. Why is the drying effect only temporary? Remember that water and oil are constantly flowing upward and evaporating from the surface. The steady flow of moisture into the plate helps to maintain the proper balance.

Surfactant is a fancy word for detergents, cleaners, soaps, washes, and so on. Surfactants are ingredients that cleanse away oils and contaminants. Every time you wash your hands, surfactants remove oils from your skin and nails. Excessive hand washing can strip away protective oils and cause dryness (FT). Clients with overly dry nails or skin should avoid excessive hand washing and should use conditioning oils or lotions regularly.

FAST TRACK (FT)

(FT) Cells are the smallest and simplest living unit capable of being alive.

(FT) The matrix is an incubator that grows the cells of the nail plate.

(FT) Amino acids linked together into long strings or chains are called proteins.

(FT) The free edge is made of the oldest, flattest, and hardest nail cells.

(FT) Nail plate keratin is a protein made from long chains of amino acids.

(FT) Almost every cell in the nail plate comes from the matrix.

(FT) Nail plate thickness is determined by the length of the matrix area.

(FT) The length of the matrix determines the thickness of the natural nail plate.

(FT) Strength is the ability of the nail plate to withstand a heavy load.

(FT) Hardness measures the nail plate's resistance to being scratched or dented.

(FT) Flexibility determines how much the nail plate will bend.

(FT) Brittleness determines how easily the plate will break, crack, or fracture.

(FT) Toughness is a balance of strength and flexibility.

(FT) Wear resistance is the ability to resist abrasion or rubbing.

(FT) Silicon carbide abrasives are more aggressive than aluminum oxide abrasives.

FT Noncrystalline keratin helps regulate the passage of moisture and oil through the nail plate.

FT Diffusion determines how liquids flow through the nail plate.

FT Covalent bonds are the strongest type of chemical linkage.

FT The high level of cysteine cross-linking in keratin is the primary source of its hardness, strength, and durability.

FT Plasticizers make solid materials softer or more flexible.

FT The natural nail normally contains about 5 percent oils and 18 percent water by weight.

FT Surfactants found in hand washes, shampoos, and so on can cause excessive dryness of nails and skin by stripping away excessive amounts of natural oils.

Review Questions

1. Toenails grow _____ as fast as fingernails.

2. The natural nail plate contains less than _____ percent calcium.

3. _____ is a surface's resistance to being scratched or dented.

4. Which abrasive material is nearly as hard as diamond?

5. Diffusion is the process that describes how liquids _____.

6. _____ are the strongest type of chemical linkage.

7. _____ are a special type of covalent bond created between two molecules of cysteine found on separate protein chains.

8. Water diffuses through the nail plate about _____ times faster than through skin.

9. The nail plate contains about _____ percent oil and _____ percent water.

10. Oils have a _____ effect and can noticeably increase flexibility of the plate.

11. Why do nails tend to peel at the top of the free edge, rather than underneath?

12. It is much better for nails to be _____, rather than hard.

13. Besides oils, water, and keratin, name five other substances that are found inside the nail plate.

14. The hollow junctions between nail cells that rivet them together are called _____.

15. Nail enhancement or polish removers can _____ the skin.

Chapter

3

Understanding the Hand

Objective

In this chapter you will learn about the hand and wrist. You will also discover the many important interactions and synergies that exist between each part of the hand and finger—how blood vessels, nerves, tendons, ligaments, bone, and tissue all work together to benefit the whole. Finally, you'll also learn about one of the most common types of salon injuries and how to prevent it from occurring.

YOUR SHOCK-ABSORBING TOOL

Today's nail technician does a lot more than just nails. Modern nail technicians use their hands to provide a broad spectrum of services, so a deeper working knowledge of the hand is useful and necessary. The hand is one of our power tools. It is constantly used and abused, but we always expect it to perform properly. Understanding this tool is an important step toward helping both you and your clients maintain healthy hands and wrists. In Figure 3–1 and Color Plate 7 you will see a basic overview of the hand's complex structure.

FUNCTION OF THE HAND

Muscles flex and extend the fingers, turn the wrist, and provide power and grip *(FT)*. The long bands extending from the wrist to each finger are muscles. Without these, we would have no ability to extend or contract our fingers. There are several types of muscles in the human body: cardiac muscles (found in the heart), smooth muscles (found in the blood vessels and internal organs), and skeletal muscles. Cardiac and smooth muscles are called **involuntary muscles,** since they are not under our voluntary control. Skeletal muscle is made up of thousands of cylindrical muscle fibers bound together by special types of connective tissue *(FT)*.

    The muscles in the hand are primarily skeletal muscles, which are attached by tendons directly to the bones *(FT)*. Contraction or inward pulling of these muscles is under **voluntary control.** Triceps and biceps are examples of skeletal muscles in the upper arm. The triceps is a special type of muscle called an **extensor.** This type of muscle allows the arm to straighten or extend *(FT)*. But what if we want to bend our arm or lift something? For that we need a different type of muscle. **Flexor** muscles are needed to flex or bend a joint *(FT)*. The biceps is an example of a flexor muscle, since it bends the arm at the elbow joint. Flexor and extensor work as a matched team. When muscles work together in this way, they are called an **antagonistic pair.** The triceps and biceps are a perfect example, since one muscle straightens the arm while the other bends it. You will discover that it is important to keep such teams of muscles working together and in balance with each other *(FT)*.

Food, Form, and Motion

Blood vessels (shown in red, Color Plate 7) are called arteries. They carry oxygen and nutrients into the hand, fingers, and nail beds. Veins (shown in yellow, Color Plate 7) carry waste and carbon dioxide away from the tissue. Without them, the cells that make up the hand could not survive. Nerves are what give our brain its voluntary control over the skeletal muscles. Bones give the hand and fingers their structure (shape) and supporting framework. Bone is linked to bone by specialized tissues called **ligaments** *(FT)*. Our hand bones could not stand up to the daily rigors and abuse without rugged protection. Fatty tissues surround each bone and

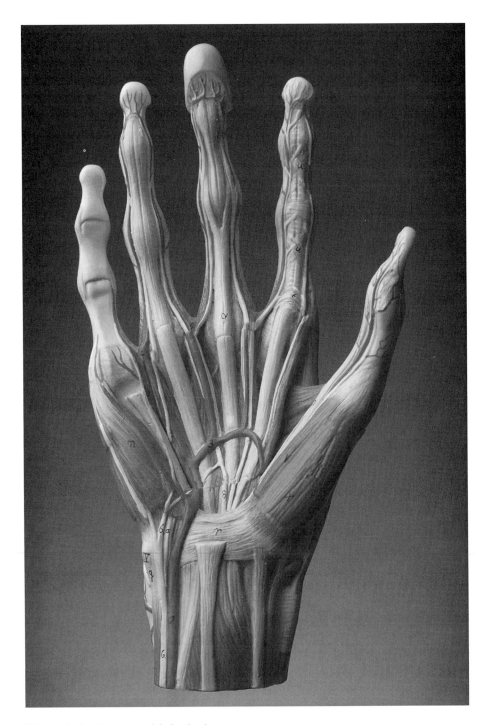

Figure 3-1 The structure of the hand and wrist

absorb much of the shock and impact experienced by the hand. But there's a limit to this protection. Excessive shock and impact can lead to trauma and permanent damage of the hand or its parts, including the nail.

The Function of the Skin

The skin covers the hand by stretching over the underlying bone and other structures. Since the hand must be able to flex, the skin must also be highly flexible as well. Much of this amazing flexibility comes from the arrangement of deeper tissues over the joints, as well as the skin folds. Furrows and creases in the palm and across the back of the hand allow the skin to stretch so that the hand may freely open and close. Notice that these furrows are deepest over the joints. This is because of their greater need for movement. Faint lines in the skin also crisscross the backs of the hands. The lines are unique, just as every person's fingerprints are unique.

There are three layers of tissue on the hands. The epidermis is the top, translucent layer (*translucent* means that light can only partially pass through it). It does not contain any blood vessels. The epidermis does contain pores, tiny openings in the surface of the skin that allow moisture and oils to escape from the lower layers. The epidermis is the layer that is shed when we exfoliate the skin. The second, middle layer is called the dermis or "true skin." This highly elastic, collagen-rich layer contains blood vessels, hair roots, sweat glands, and nerves. Below this lies the third layer, **subcutaneous fat.** It contains large blood vessels and nerves and is made primarily of fat-filled cells called **adipose cells.** The subcutaneous fat is attached to the dermis by connective tissue and serves as a smooth cushion for the muscles and bone. The **basal layer** is actually the bottom layer of the epidermis and sits directly on top of the dermis. New skin cells are created in the basal layer. In this bottommost part of the epidermis, a dark pigment called melanin is scattered through the tissue, coloring and protecting our skin from **ultraviolet (UV) light.**

Function of the Tendons and Ligaments

Muscles are linked to the bone by thick, inflexible bands of fibrous tissue called **tendons** (*FT*) . The largest ligament in the hand is a wide band that practically encircles the wrist. This ligament can be seen in the wrist in Figure 3–1. This ligament creates the infamous carpal tunnel, which causes many nail technicians unnecessary pain and distress. Tendons, found inside the carpal tunnel, are wrapped in a membrane of very soft tissue (*FT*) . When these tissues become inflamed and swollen, a painful condition called **tendonitis** can develop (*FT*) . Typically, this type of inflammation is created by cumulative trauma or repeated injury to the area. **Cumulative trauma disorders (CTDs)** usually involve inflammation of these tissues, as you will see below (*FT*) .

UNDERSTANDING CTDS

Cumulative trauma disorders or CTDs (also known as repetitive motion or repetitive strain disorders) are the fastest-growing type of occupational injury. The term *CTD* refers to several different conditions. Each can cause painful and crippling illness that may become permanent, if not properly treated. **Carpal tunnel syndrome** is the most common type of CTD. Carpal tunnel syndrome is a problem for many nail technicians. The carpal tunnel is a small passage underneath the ligament encircling the wrist, as described above. The carpal tunnel houses the tendons and nerves running from the fingers into the arm. Repetitive motions can injure this area and create pressure on the nerves.

Repetitive motions such as typing or filing nails almost always cause this type of injury. Constant vibration from tools can also cause or aggravate the condition. Although the nerve is pinched in the wrist, pain and numbness often spread into the arm and fingers. If ignored, CTDs usually become worse and are sometimes disabling. Continued injury can permanently damage the nerves. Of course, other things besides repetitive motion and vibrations may cause or aggravate CTDs. For example, sitting or working in the same position, repetitive awkward reaching, stretching, and twisting all can cause injury, not just to the hand and wrist but also to the neck and shoulder. Symptoms include

- Pain
- Numbness
- Aching
- Stiffness
- Tingling
- Weakness
- Swelling

If you experience any of these symptoms, pay closer attention to how you work. It isn't too difficult to figure out which motions are causing the pain. Even so, it can be difficult to solve the problem without proper advice. It would be wise to seek medical attention immediately. Take action before it is too late to correct the problem. This is why it is so important to recognize these symptoms. Early attention can reverse the injury and prevent further damage.

What Should I Do?

There are many things nail technicians can do to avoid CTDs:

- Always sit in a natural, unstrained position.
- Change positions often.
- Take frequent stretch breaks, even if they are only for a few seconds.
- Avoid using vibrating hand tools.

- Wear gloves that fit well.
- Hold your wrists straight and avoid bending them while filing or using a brush.
- Avoid hunching over the client's nails.
- Stop working and stretch or shake out your hands periodically, if only for a few seconds.
- Develop a regular routine for exercising and stretching arms, wrists, and hands.

An easy and effective exercise is to press your hand on a flat surface while stretching your fingers and wrist for five seconds. Exercises are great, but if you develop symptoms, you should see a doctor. Your doctor will see your problem objectively and make great recommendations that you might not have considered. Remember, the problem won't go away by itself. You must avoid further trauma to the injured area and give the body a chance to heal. CTDs are easy to prevent and correct. Don't take chances with your hands. You'll need them!

Dealing with Carpal Tunnel Disorder and Tendonitis

Nail technicians depend on their hands and use them for extended periods. This can lead to repetitive strain injuries of the muscles and can cause carpal tunnel syndrome and tendonitis. Usually the neck and shoulders are also involved. The results are headaches or upper back stiffness.

Tendonitis starts as microscopic tears in the muscles *(FT)*. These tears are caused by excessive use and fatigue and can lead to chronic (long-term) inflammation. This is how all cases of carpal tunnel syndrome get started—people ignore this inflammation. Inflammation prevents muscles from receiving an adequate supply of oxygen, which causes lactic acid to accumulate, further increasing inflammation *(FT)*. Symptoms often become more frequent and may eventually develop into a **chronic inflammatory pain cycle**—not a good thing! When your livelihood is dependent on your hands, wrists, and shoulders, these injuries can be both threatening and painful.

What can you do about it? Lots! That's the good news! There are some easy steps that are great for prevention and can also help alleviate existing symptoms. Jana Wright is an expert in body mechanics and has a bachelor of science degree in exercise physiology from California State University, Fullerton. She examined common tasks performed each day by nail technicians and came up with the following recommendations. If you follow her advice, you will be on the road to a long, successful, and pain-free career.

1. Sitting in a relaxed position will help alleviate strain, especially on your wrists. Avoid sitting in any uncomfortable position that puts you out of balance or restricts your movement. Tables that are too low or high can put pressure on the wrists and may lead to inflammation and pain *(FT)*. Reaching too far across the table creates another out-of-balance situation that often translates into

shoulder, neck, and/or upper back pain or headaches. Sitting in a twisted position can worsen these problems and may lead to injury of the lower back.

2. Use ice therapy when the area develops warmth, redness or swelling (FT). Applying ice in a bag cools the affected area and reduces inflammation (but avoid leaving the ice on too long, which can lead to freezing). You can also try a therapeutic liniment.

3. There are many commercially available splints that are comfortable enough to wear at night. Wearing a splint while you sleep can help maintain proper blood circulation and let you get a good night's sleep.

4. Wrist exercises are very useful (FT). Since excessive use caused the syndrome, it sounds contradictory to say that exercise helps. But it's true—exercise can alleviate some early-stage symptoms of carpal tunnel syndrome. When you are working on a client's hands or feet, the wrist will rely on the flexor muscles to keep it in a flexed position. So nail professionals should strengthen and develop the other half of the antagonistic pair, the extensor muscles in the wrist and hand. The extensor (top of the wrist) and flexor (bottom of the wrist) muscles must be continuously stretched and conditioned and kept in proper balance if muscles are to remain resilient and able to resist daily rigors.

5. Stretching exercises are important and will help eliminate tendon irritation (FT). While working, your wrist is constantly contracting. To prevent repetitive injuries from occurring, stop every thirty minutes and stretch your hands and wrists. You'll be amazed at how beneficial this will be. Stretching and strengthening the muscles can also help prevent these problems.

6. Acupuncture can also be very useful for pain caused by chronic inflammation. This type of therapy may help increase blood flow and improve healing to the affected areas.

7. Massage works wonders! Remember the healing power of touch. Avoid massaging areas that are swollen, red, or visibly inflamed, but mild kneading and squeezing on tender areas can provide great results.

8. Finally, when you are experiencing this type of chronic inflammation, overwork is usually part of the problem. If possible, take a short leave of absence and deal with the issue. That may be all you need, and it's a great excuse for a vacation!

FAST TRACK (FT)

(FT) Muscles flex and extend the fingers.

(FT) Skeletal muscle is made up of thousands of cylindrical muscle fibers bound together by special types of connective tissue.

(FT) The muscles in the hand are primarily skeletal muscles.

(FT) Extensor muscles extend and straighten.

(FT) Flexor muscles flex or bend.

(FT) Together flexor and extensor muscles create an antagonistic pair.

(FT) Muscles in an antagonistic pair must work together and be in balance.

(FT) Bone is linked to bone by specialized tissues called ligaments.

(FT) Muscles are linked to the bone by fibrous tissue called tendons.

(FT) Tendons are wrapped in a soft membrane-like tissue.

(FT) Tendonitis is inflammation of the membrane surrounding the tendon.

(FT) Cumulative trauma disorders usually involve tissue inflammation.

(FT) Tendonitis starts as microscopic muscle tears caused by fatigue.

(FT) Inflammation prevents muscles from receiving sufficient oxygen, which further increases inflammation.

(FT) Avoid nail tables that are too low or too high, as they put pressure on the wrists.

(FT) Ice therapy is a great treatment for these types of inflammation.

(FT) Wrist exercises are very useful to prevent and alleviate inflammation.

(FT) Stretching exercises are important and will help eliminate tendon irritation.

Review Questions

1. The triceps is an example of an _____ muscle, since it allows the arm to be straightened or extended.

2. The biceps is an example of a _____ muscle, one needed to flex or bend a joint.

3. When two muscles work as a matched team to extend and contract, they are called an _____ pair.

4. Define tendonitis.

5. Name the three main layers of tissue on the hand.

6. In what part of the epidermis are new skin cells created?

7. Which layer is called the "true skin"?

8. Which type of muscle do we have in our hands?

9. Fat-filled cells are also called _____ cells.

10. The carpal tunnel is created by a wide _____ that nearly encircles the wrist.

11. Carpal tunnel syndrome is always preceded by which disorder?

12. What is the best therapy for tendonitis?

13. Muscles usually become torn by _____.

14. Name seven symptoms of cumulative trauma disorders.

15. How often is it recommended to stop and stretch to prevent cumulative trauma disorders?

Chapter

4

Trauma and Damage

Objective

In Chapter 2 you learned about the normal, healthy nail. Using your new understanding of the normal nail will make it easier to understand problem nails. In this chapter you will learn about nails that are damaged and injured and what you can do to help these clients.

EYES ARE A WINDOW TO THE WORLD

If you're observant, you'll find it easy to recognize problems and help your clients get proper information. In some cases the solutions are simple; at other times the causes are unknown and there may be no solution. Natural nails can provide a wealth of information to the trained observer. But even experts can misdiagnose nail diseases and conditions. This chapter is not meant to make you an expert in nail disorders. Only qualified medical professionals can properly diagnose most health-related nail conditions. But as a nail professional, you can help your clients understand common nail disorders.

DON'T RUB ME WRONG

Overfiling is one of the most common causes of nail damage in the salon *FT*. Even though there are a little more than 1 million nail cells in your pinkie, the nail plate is only 100 cell layers thick *FT*. A heavy hand with a coarse abrasive (60 to 120 grit) or an electric file can quickly remove half the layers. This leaves the nail plate overly thin and weak, creating many additional problems for both clients and nail technicians. For example, using electric files incorrectly on the natural nail can overly thin the nail plate. Ideally, nail techs should use 180- to 240-grit abrasives *FT*. But remember, in careless hands even a 180-grit file can create considerable damage to the nail plate. Using even coarser files on the natural nail is unwise and potentially dangerous to the nail. A good rule to remember: *the lower the grit, the easier it is to create serious damage FT*. Heavy abrasives and electric files should be used cautiously and with a light touch.

Thin nail plates are too flexible. This can have a negative effect on adhesion for both nail polish and artificial enhancements. Nail treatments such as polish, base coats, and topcoats don't adhere well to these types of nails. Thin nail plates also allow some ingredients to pass more easily through the nail plate. You'll learn in Chapter 12 that this can contribute to allergic reactions or lead to other serious nail problems.

In general, nail professionals tend to overfile the nail plate. The old myth is that you need to really rough up the nail to make the product stick. This may sound reasonable—after all, we sand wood to make paint stick. But who would strip away half of the wood? No one, of course! We remove only the topmost surface. So why strip away many layers of the natural nail? Early nail products had poor adhesion, and lifting was far more common. Today's advanced products are designed specifically for improved keratin adhesion, so heavy filing is no longer needed or desired!

A better way is to remove only the top few layers of cells, then thoroughly clean the nail plate, taking the time to use proper preparation procedures. This will keep the nail thicker and in the long run healthier. Only the shine—the uppermost surface of the nail, which is saturated with oils that cause the surface to reflect light—needs to be filed away. One of the most important things you can learn as a nail technician is that only the very topmost four or five layers need to be removed to create good product adhesion ⒻⓉ. This is about 5 percent of the plate's thickness. This will leave 95 percent of the thickness of the nail plate intact. If the nail is visibly thinned—that is, if a ledge exists between the filed plate and new growth—then overfiling has probably occurred. When clients remove artificial nails, they shouldn't notice that their nails are any thinner.

PINCHING

Nail technicians often apply artificial nail coatings to the natural nail. When properly applied, artificial nails do not harm the natural nail surface. But if improperly applied, damage may occur. To improve the natural curvature of the nail plate (C curve), technicians sometimes pinch the sidewalls of the artificial nail before the product has fully hardened. This technique will alter the curvature, but the process can cause serious nail damage. As the sidewalls are pushed inward, the center portion of the artificial nail is pushed up. This pulls up on the center of the plate's free edge. This constant upward force can tear the seal between the nail plate and the nail bed, causing them to separate. The pinching forces can also damage the surface of the natural nail, as seen in Figure 4–1 and Color Plate 8. Notice the white spots that appear under the nail plate, showing where the nail plate has separated from the nail bed.

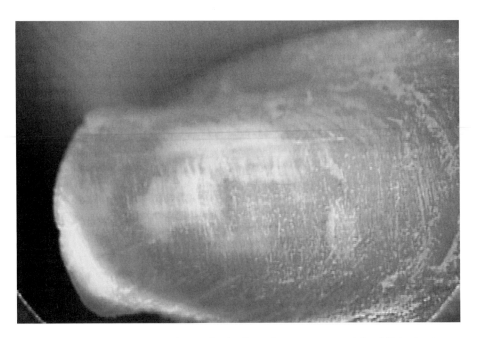

Figure 4-1 *Damage created by pinching artificial nails into dramatic curvatures before fully hardened*

The pinching technique started in artificial nail competitions. But competition nails are not designed to meet real-world demands and generally are removed (or break) in a few days. When this technique is used on a client's nails, serious problems can occur. Never pinch or force the nail plate into a more dramatic curvature. It is much better to build the curvature with a wooden dowel or sculptured nail form during product application. This will avoid putting excessive stress on the nail plate and nail bed.

IMPACT

Sudden impacts or jams are another common type of nail damage. If the injury is in the matrix area, serious or permanent damage could result. If the injury destroys part of the matrix, keratin cells will not be produced in that area. This will have a visible effect on nail plate growth, as you can see in Figure 4–2 and Color Plate 9.

If a small part of the matrix stops growing new nail cells, the keratin plate will develop a thinner area as it grows out. This can create a groove in the plate. The greater the damage, the wider or deeper the groove will be. Often the groove widens as it grows toward the end of the plate.

TRAUMA DRAMA

Each of the conditions seen in Figure 4–3 was caused by some type of physical trauma.

Injured Matrix

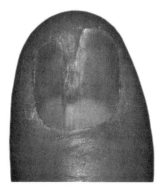

Figure 4-2 *Permanent split caused by damage in the matrix area*

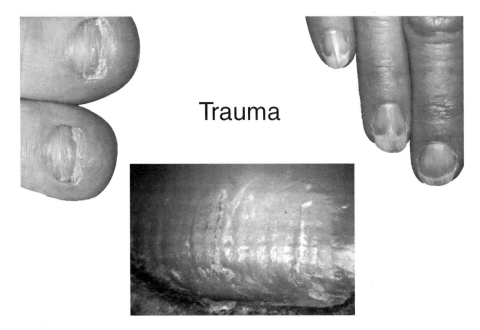

Trauma

Figure 4-3 *Three examples of trauma-induced injury*

Runner's Toenails

The toenails (upper left) were damaged by a shoe that fit too tightly. This is an example of how the nail plate flows and deforms under pressure. This runner wore shoes that were too tight in the toe box area and pushed against the toenails. The pressure on the toe caused the nail plate to separate from the bed, and a minor infection then occurred under the plate. How does this occur? After the plate lifts, common bacteria or fungi inside the shoe may get into the soft tissue under the plate, creating an infection. Improperly fitted shoes can exert enough pressure to cause such injuries. Runners and long-distance walkers or hikers often forget that the feet can swell one or two sizes. Feet also swell from standing all day on a hard floor. Whenever shoes might be worn under conditions where swelling may be an issue, always allow some extra room in the toe area.

Onycholysis

Pressure can cause damage in other ways. The medical term for the condition seen in this photo (upper right) is **onycholysis** (AH-nih-koe-LIE-sis). *Onycho-* is the Latin term for nail. So any words containing this term probably have something to do with finger- or toenails.

Onycholysis is commonly caused by trauma or abuse to the nail ⒻⓉ. It is often seen in nail salons as a result of aggressive filing techniques, although other types of trauma can cause this problem. People who use their nails as tools have a high incidence of onycholysis. In this condition, the nail plate and bed separate, forming a small space under the nail plate. To review what you learned in Chapter 1, there is a system of rails and grooves that allow the nail plate to slide across the nail bed (refer to Figure 1–6). The rails are created by specialized tissue called bed epithelium, which attaches to the underside of the nail plate and flows into grooves found in the nail bed, as discussed in Chapter 1. Any trauma that causes damage to the soft tissue under the free edge can break the hyponychium, one of the four guardian seals. When the hyponychium is broken, the delicate tissue of the bed epithelium is easily torn.

If the nail is snagged on a piece of clothing or some other objects, the tear can spread further. The zipperlike tearing effect enlarges the gap under the nail plate. Further trauma will prevent healing, so keep the nails short in length to prevent accidents. The condition will not quickly go away, nor will the plate just stick back to the nail bed. The nail must grow out normally over time. Tell the client to keep the area clean and dry and to avoid putting unnecessary upward pressure on the fingernail, to prevent further separation. Also, warn the client not to stick any objects under the nail when cleaning. A pharmacist can recommend an ointment to coat the underside of the nails to block out contaminants and help prevent infection. As new plate grows, the open gap will grow smaller until the plate and bed are rejoined.

Wavy Nail Plates

Habit tic is caused by the nervous, habitual rubbing of the nail plate. This plate (bottom) was deformed by a plumber who constantly rubbed the corner of his nail. This constant and repeated pressure can distort the surface of the nail plate. In Chapter 2 you learned that the nail plate is not completely solid. It is actually a "flowable" solid, much like a glacier is a flowable sheet of ice (FT). The "waves" in the nail seen in this example show how easily the plate is permanently deformed under constant pressure. Usually people with this condition have an uncontrolled urge to flick or stroke the nail plate with their other fingers. The surface waviness shows how the plate flows under repeated or constant force.

SPOTS AND WHITENING

The nail bed contains many small blood vessels or capillaries. When damage occurs in the bed, a small amount of blood oozes out, forming a red spot under the plate. Eventually tiny clots form and the bleeding stops. The red color is from the iron found in the blood. The stain can have lasting power, surviving until it grows past the free edge. These spots are called **splinter hemorrhages** (refer to Figure 7-3). Often they're caused by some type of hard impact or other physical trauma (damage) to the nail bed (FT). As the blood seeps into the tissue of the nail bed, note how it follows the rail pattern described in Chapter 1.

Leukonychia (LOO-koh-NIH-kee-uh) is defined as any condition that causes abnormal whitening of the nail plate Ⓕ⌢Ⓣ. *Leuk-* comes from the Latin for white. **Leukonychia spots** are large groups of whitish nail cells trapped inside the plate. These spots are generally caused by injuries to the matrix area. For example, spots found in the cuticle area are from one-month-old injuries, since that is about how long it takes the spot to grow past the eponychium. White areas are rich in nail cells that didn't flatten normally and turn transparent. In Figure 4–4, the leading spot has grown almost to the free edge, so the original injury must have occurred about three or four months earlier. Notice the other leukonychia spots trailing behind, indicating that more recent injuries have occurred. It's apparent that the owner of this nail frequently traumatizes this finger.

Two other types of nail plate whitening can occur. In **true leukonychia** (Figure 4–4), the nail plate looks as though it was painted with white nail polish. This condition also begins in the matrix. After leaving the matrix, these cells do not become translucent. The plate may turn completely white or may only have a solid white band running the entire length of the nail. This condition is rarely seen; it can be inherited and may be seen at birth or in young children. Other causes are internal disorders such as hepatitis, heavy metal poisoning, or zinc deficiency. It can also occur in postmenopausal women. True leukonychia is an excellent example of how internal body conditions can show up as symptoms in the nail plate.

Pseudoleukonychia

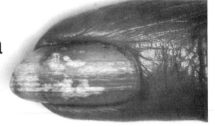

True Leukonychia

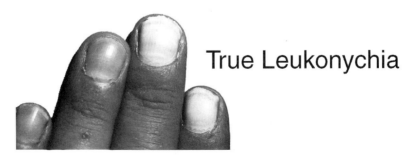

Figure 4-4 *True leukonychia and pseudoleukonychia*

External factors can also cause whitening. For instance, stripping oils and moisture from the nail plate can cause a condition called **pseudoleukonychia,** or false leukonychia *(FT)* (see Figure 4–4 and Color Plate 10). In this condition surface layers develop a dried-out, white, or flaky appearance that easily files away with a 180- or 240-grit abrasive. False leukonychia can be treated with a penetrating, oil-based nail conditioner. Because the surface whitening is caused by a lack of moisture and oil, rubbing penetrating oil into the plate will cause most of the whiteness to disappear. The oil will also cause moisture to build up inside and rehydrate the plate.

Nail polish remover can cause pseudoleukonychia if used excessively. Excessive use of many solvents can remove necessary oil and moisture from the nail plate. Clients who remove their nail color more often than once a week are more prone to this condition. Educate your clients and warn them about this issue. Acetone is a very safe and useful remover, but diluted acetone (one part water for every ten parts acetone) will quickly remove the color while preventing excessive drying *(FT)*. Also, adding a drop or two of penetrating nail oil to the diluted acetone will help replenish the lost oils in the plate and surrounding skin. Many solvents and aggressive cleaning solutions can strip oils and moisture from the nail plate. Solvents can also strip away the adhesive proteins responsible for holding together the layers of the nail plate.

Prolonged and repeated exposure to water may also cause splits and cracks in the plate *(FT)*. Splitting, peeling, and breakage can be caused by too much moisture in the nail plate. Hands that are in water a lot are often plagued by skin and nail problems; cosmetologists, waitresses, bartenders, florists, and frequent hand washers fall into this category. Excessive water in the nail plates leads to oversoftening of the nails. The extra water can cause them to swell and then contract when they dry. Repeated swelling and contracting of the plates may lead to peeling or splitting of the free edge.

Some creams and lotions can prevent nail plates from drying out. Oils can't moisturize the nail plate, because only water can be moisturizing. But the nail plate can absorb oil to seal the surface and prevent water evaporation. As water

WICKED WATER

As harmless as water seems, excessive exposure can damage the natural nail. Water is one of the most powerful solvents known. In fact, water is often called the universal solvent, since it can dissolve more substances than any other solvent. Frequent exposure to water can have a dramatic effect on the nails, especially if combined with cleaners, washes, soaps, shampoos, or detergents. These work with water to strip essential oils from the nail plate. To combat excessive exposure, use high-quality hand lotion, cream, or penetrating nail oil.

builds up inside the nail plate, dryness is eliminated. Also, oil-based lotions or creams will help clients who have their hands in water all the time, as oils seal the skin and nail plates and help increase water repellency. Gloves offer even better protection against water's damaging effects.

Nipping nail enhancements from the nail plate can also cause pseudoleukonychia. For this reason it is best to save the nail plates and avoid nipping. Nipping pulls chunks of keratin from the surface of the nail plate, leaving them pitted and whitish due to the separation of the cell layers.

FRICTION BURNS, A LOT

Excessive heat can burn the sensitive tissue of the nail bed (FT). Bed epithelium is delicate and easily damaged by friction burns created by electric files, coarse abrasives, and heavy-handed filing or excessive buffing. Once the damage has been done, onycholysis and secondary infections of the nail bed may result. Research shows that the nail bed can't feel heat very well. In fact, clients can't feel heat until the temperature rises to about 118°F (47°C). At these high temperatures, the nail bed is more likely to be damaged.

STAINS AND DISCOLORATION

The nail plate can absorb many discoloring substances. For example, nicotine from cigarettes held in the fingers is slowly absorbed into the oil channels of the nail plate. As it accumulates, the intensity of the stain increases, turning the plate brown. Other substances can cause discoloration as well. In Figure 4–5 and Color Plate 11, the nail in the upper right corner was exposed to a phenolic-based disinfectant solution. When the exposure discontinued, the nail plate began to grow out normally. The nail plate on the left is stained by a metal cleaning agent. Certain **dyes** can deeply stain the nail plate. Early nail color formulations used high concentrations of staining dyes. Today, high-quality, professional nail polishes use low levels of dye and use only those that don't permanently stain the nail plate. However, some inexpensive brands cut corners and use large amounts of dyes to reduce the cost, making them more likely to discolor the plate.

Many things can cause the nail plate to change color. Table 4–1 lists just a few examples.

In general, nail discoloration is caused by dyes, damage, drugs, disease, injury, or illness. Some topcoats can cause yellow or light brown stains when applied directly to the bare natural nail. Base coats do more than improve nail polish adhesion—they help seal and protect the plate from staining. Base coats will also help prevent staining of artificial nails. Normally, the plate is resistant to stains, but damaged or injured nail plates are more absorbent. Stains are absorbed more deeply into cracks, splits, or pits in the plate. Certain drugs can affect the matrix cells and discolor the nail plate. Diseases of the nail or illness somewhere else in the body may also cause the nail matrix cells to produce

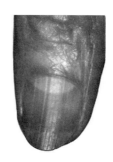

Environmental

Discoloration

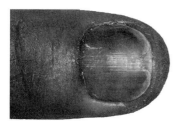

Figure 4–5 *Natural nail discoloration*

discolored nail plates. For example, psoriasis often leads to nail plates that are pitted, are more porous, and stain more easily.

DON'T STARVE YOUR NAILS

Nothing you can eat will make healthy, normal nail plates stronger (FT). But poor nutrition can certainly make them weaker. Malnutrition or severe dieting can leave nail plates thin and/or weak or cause depression lines across the width of

Table 4–1 *Some causes for discoloration of the nail plate*

Brown	Henna, mercury, malnutrition, dyes, glutaraldehyde, iodine, nicotine, radiation therapy, infections, hydroquinone, tetracycline, pregnancy
Gray	Formaldehyde, silver, malaria
Black	Silver nitrate, chlorhexidine, hair dyes, infections, drugs, blood under the plate
Yellow	Tetracycline, weed killer, infections, hydroquinone, excess vitamin D, psoriasis, disinfectants
Green	Chlorophyll and derivatives, chlorhexidine, infections
Blue	Metal cleaner, ink, fluoride, tetracycline
Pink to red	Carbon monoxide poisoning (cherry red), cardiac failure, lichen planus, blood under the plate

the natural nail. Poor nutrition may contribute to splitting as well. Poor nutrition can also make nail growth slow down dramatically! The hair and other parts of the body will be similarly affected.

It is a myth that calcium is needed for nail health, as discussed in Chapter 2. The calcium content of the nail plate is less than 0.1 percent. Most of the calcium found in nail plates is probably on the surface and comes from hand washing. In short, it is extremely unlikely that calcium is needed to maintain the health of the nail plate. So eating calcium-rich foods or taking calcium supplements will have no positive effect on the nail plate. Also, applying calcium to the top surface of the nail plate will have no benefit for the nail plate.

BRITTLE AND WEAK

So far we have discussed many things that can make nail plates weak or brittle. But what's the difference between these two terms? We discussed key concepts in Chapter 2 that would be helpful to review:

- Hardness measures the difficulty of scratching the surface of the nail.
- Brittleness causes the plate to crack or shatter when a force is applied.
- Weakness occurs when there is an overall loss of nail plate strength.
- Toughness is the nail plate's ability to resist cracks and breaks and comes from the right combination of strength and flexibility.
- Strength gives the nails the ability to resist a force or stress.

Brittle nails don't have the toughness they should. Brittle nails usually crack or shatter because they have lost flexibility and/or strength. Brittle nails often result when the nail plate's moisture/oil balance gets out of whack *(FT)*. As a rule, weak nails don't shatter, but instead will make clean breaks. In general, weak nails benefit from being reinforced with a strong, protective coating. And brittle nails need more oil! Excessive amounts of water can be harmful to brittle nails. Water swells the plate, causing tiny cracks to enlarge. Water manicures—soaking the plate for more than two minutes in warm, soapy water—are a terrible way to treat brittle nails!

Nails often break in specific patterns, depending on impact. Some of these patterns are discussed below and shown in Figure 4–6.

Serrations

Serrations (suh-RAY-shuns) are a sign of a weak free edge *(FT)*. Excessive force on the free edge—such as drumming fingers on a desktop, typing on a keyboard, or using the nail as a tool—creates this kind of damage.

Delamination

Delamination occurs when nails are overexposed to solvents or AHA (glycolic acid) *(FT)*. Delamination is the separation of the natural nail plate into thin

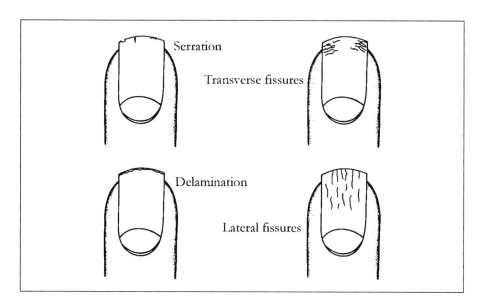

Figure 4-6 *Symptoms of brittle and weak nails*

sheets or layers. Soaking brittle nail plates in water or exposing nails to other solvents can lead to delamination. Frequent nail polish changes should be avoided. Changing nail color more than once a week can strip the plate of oils and lead to dryness. This is often seen in elderly clients, since their nails grow much more slowly.

Transverse and Lateral Fissures

Transverse fissures and **lateral fissures** usually occur when the nail is sharply bent. Transverse fissures are caused when the nail plate is nearly bent and small cracks form in the stress area. Lateral fissures are often caused when the free edge is sharply impacted.

FAST TRACK Ⓕⓣ

- Ⓕⓣ Overfiling is one of the most common causes of nail damage in the salon.
- Ⓕⓣ The fingernail nail plate is only 100 cell layers thick.
- Ⓕⓣ Use only 180- to 240-grit files to prepare the nail plate.
- Ⓕⓣ The lower the grit of the abrasive, the easier it is to create nail damage.
- Ⓕⓣ Only the very top four or five layers of plate need be removed to create good adhesion.
- Ⓕⓣ Onycholysis is commonly caused by trauma or abuse to the nail.

(FT)   Habit tic shows that the nail plate is a flowable solid.

(FT)   Splinter hemorrhages are spots of blood under the plate often caused by impact or other trauma.

(FT)   Leukonychia is a condition that causes abnormal whitening of the nail plate.

(FT)   Pseudoleukonychia is often a sign of dry nail plates.

(FT)   Diluted nail polish remover can help prevent pseudoleukonychia.

(FT)   Prolonged or repeated exposure to solvents (including water) may cause plate splits and cracks.

(FT)   Friction burns can seriously damage the nail bed.

(FT)   Nothing you can eat will make healthy, normal nail plates become stronger.

(FT)   Brittle nails may result as the nail plate's moisture/oil balance gets out of whack.

(FT)   Serrations are a sign of a weak free edge.

(FT)   Delamination occurs when nails are overexposed to solvents.

Review Questions

1. Under most circumstances, nail techs should use _____- to _____-grit abrasives.

2. If the delicate tissue between the bed and plate is friction-burned by an abrasive, what nail condition could result?

3. Other than injury or illness, name four main causes of nail discoloration.

4. Toughness is the nail plate's ability to _____ cracks and breaks.

5. What nail products can cause pseudoleukonychia and why?

6. _____ is a condition that causes the nail plate to grow with an abnormally white appearance.

7. What common natural dye can stain your nail plates brown?

8. How can damage to the nail bed cause brown spots under the nail plate?

9. Can oils moisturize the nail plate?

10. How can excessive washing of your hands dry out nail plates?

11. *Onycho-* is Latin for _____.

12. The calcium content of the nail is _____.

13. *Leuk-* comes from the Latin word for _____.

14. Carbon monoxide poisoning causes nail beds to turn _____.

15. Where is bed epithelium found and what does it do?

Chapter 5

The Abnormal Nail

Objective

In Chapters 1 through 3 we learned about the normal nail. Using your new understanding of the normal nail will make it easier to understand abnormal nails. While only a qualified medical doctor can provide a diagnosis of a specific medical condition, by learning how to recognize nails that are infected, deformed, or otherwise unhealthy, you can educate your clients and help them keep their nails healthy.

NAIL PLATE INFECTIONS: THE REAL STORY

There are three main types of nail plate infections: those found on top of the plate, those found underneath the plate, and those found inside the plate. The first two are usually caused by bacteria, while the third is usually caused by a fungus.

Bacterial Infections

Infections found on the surface of the nail plate are almost always caused by bacteria *(FT)*. Bacteria are one-celled, living organisms *(FT)*. Bacterial infections are most often green in color from the waste products created by the bacteria *(FT)*.

Bacterial infections result when large numbers of bacteria are trapped between a nail coating and the plate. The coating causes oil and moisture to build up inside the nail plate. The extra moisture and oil allow the bacteria to thrive and multiply, since bacteria feed on the oil and need water to live. This type of infection can occur if the nail plate is not properly cleansed and prepared before an artificial nail is applied. Bacterial infections can also occur under nail polish, but not as commonly.

As a bacterial colony grows, the bacteria produce an extremely dark stain that should not be removed by filing. These stains resist fading and can last for months after the infection is gone. This can fool nail technicians and clients into thinking the infection is still active.

Infections can grow under the nail plate if it separates from the bed. Once a separation occurs, bacteria can infect the delicate tissues. These are more serious infections and usually require a doctor's care. If the infection is creating redness and swelling or significant pain or discharging fluid, no services should be provided until a doctor has examined the nails. An example of a bacterial nail infection is shown in Figure 5–1, on the left, and in Color Plate 12.

Fungal Infections

Infections inside the nail plate are usually caused by a fungus. Fungi are not the same as bacteria; in fact, the fungi that cause skin and nail infections are parasitic, plantlike organisms related to mushrooms and yeast. These infections are relatively rare on fingernails and are most often found on the toenails, since shoes provide the ideal growth environment for fungi *(FT)*. Fungi prefer the dark and love warmth and moisture. The feet and shoes provide an ideal home for fungi. Unlike bacteria, a fungus eats the keratin that makes up the nail plate. It can digest both skin and nail plate. When this happens, the nail plate will break apart and swell, especially when exposed to moisture.

Overall, the vast majority of the fingernail nail infections seen in the salon are caused by bacteria—possibly as much as 95 percent. Dermatologists report that roughly half of the infections they see are fungal, but dermatologists see the most difficult cases that don't go away on their own. Most clients never see a doctor for bacterial infections of the nail plate, since they usually go away on their

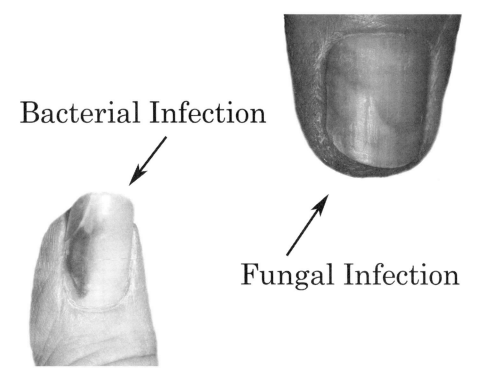

Bacterial Infection

Fungal Infection

Figure 5-1 *Examples of bacterial and fungal nail infections*

own or grow off with the nail. The only way for a doctor to determine if a fungal infection exists on the nail plate is to obtain a culture of the infection and submit it to a laboratory for proper analysis. Figure 5–1, on the right, shows a typical fungal infection of the nail plate.

DON'T KNOCK BACTERIA

Bacteria are often misunderstood. We see them only as the causes of diseases in humans and animals. But bacteria can do good—in fact, most bacteria do exactly that. Bacteria usually live in a balanced symbiosis with humans—for example, inside the intestinal tract, where they help to digest our food. They also help plant roots convert soil nitrogen into nutrients the plant can use. Bacteria put the tang in yogurt and the sourness in sourdough bread. They also do us a huge favor by breaking down dead organic matter, such as leaves and wastes. Bacteria are known for their extreme flexibility and their capacity to rapidly grow and reproduce. The oldest fossils known, nearly 3.5 billion years old, are fossils of bacterialike organisms. Bacteria have been around for a long time and aren't going away—it's best to understand them so that we can live in harmony.

Preventing and dealing with nail infections is a very important topic and will be vital to your professional success. In Chapters 12 and 13, you will learn how to keep infections from occurring.

FUNGAL INFECTIONS OF THE FEET

Athlete's foot or **tinea pedis** (TIN-ee-uh PEH-dis) is the most common type of skin infection on the feet. It is a fungal infection that often occurs on the bottom of the feet but usually is found in the webs between the toes. The most common forms of this infection are called the **moccasin** form and the **interdigital** form (*FT*).

Moccasin Form

This condition gets its name because it covers the entire bottom of the foot. Usually the skin is scaly with a dry appearance. If the skin is just dry, moisturizers and emollients will improve its appearance. But if these are ineffective and the skin still looks dry, there's a good chance that the client has this condition. In mild cases, the foot may have small, scaly rings. Oftentimes only one foot becomes infected.

Interdigital

Feet with this condition are scaly and itchy with skin that is splitting between the toes. This is the most common type of skin fungal infection worldwide. The infection can spread to other nearby parts of the foot, but it does not always do so. The infection often has a reddish border extending beyond the white scales. The red area will increase in size as the infection spreads. The web between the fourth and little toes is most commonly affected by this form of athlete's foot, but often every web between the toes is affected.

Chronic fungal foot infections last more than six months, as seen in Figure 5–2 and Color Plate 13. Sometimes such infections last for many years. Chronic infections can be controlled, but oftentimes they cannot be cured—even after months of taking expensive oral medication! For this reason, physicians sometimes are hesitant to treat them and will recommend the use of over-the-counter antifungal medication to control these skin problems, unless the infection is painful or poses other serious problems. In most cases, frequent pedicures can help. Exfoliating the flaking tissue can dramatically improve skin condition and may make taking oral prescription medication unnecessary.

It is safe to pedicure feet with mild athlete's foot or other minor fungal infection (*FT*). The pedicure may actually help the body rid itself of the fungus. With proper care and treatment these conditions will eventually disappear and the skin will return to normal. However, performing salon services on infected feet is prohibited by many states' regulations. This is because infections may be spread by improperly cleaned and disinfected implements. It is best to refer these cases to a podiatrist for treatment.

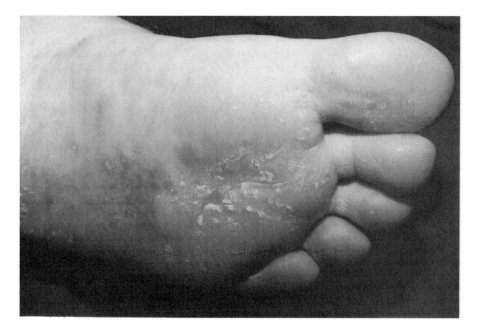

Figure 5–2 *Most athlete's foot infections come from floors and carpets, especially in hotels, health clubs and gyms, swimming pools, and other places where many people walk barefoot*

You have learned that fungal infections are more likely to occur on the feet because they are in a warm, moist environment and out of the sunlight. This is why these infections rarely occur on the hands. But what if there are no obvious symptoms of a fungal infection and a nail technician performs a pedicure on an infected foot? Can the infection spread to the hands or other clients? If normal salon hygiene practices are followed, this is extremely unlikely to occur. Clean

BEWARE OF ANTIFUNGAL CLAIMS

Over-the-counter topical antifungal medications are effective only on soft tissue and have virtually no effect on nail plate infections. These medications easily penetrate the skin but can't penetrate the nail plate or get into the matrix. The nail plate is much denser and much more difficult to penetrate than the skin. This explains why the FDA forbids companies from claiming that nonprescription antifungal treatments can be used for the nail plate. Some companies avoid the FDA ruling and get away with selling bogus treatments by carefully instructing users to apply the product to the skin surrounding the nail plate. Don't be fooled! These products won't work for clients with a true fungal infection.

salons and implements, along with proper disinfection, can easily prevent the spread of infections. This is why you must avoid using implements and files on another client before properly cleaning and disinfecting them. Taking these steps will help avoid spreading infections. You will learn more about proper disinfection and preventing infections in Chapters 12 and 13.

WARTS WILL LOVE YOU FOR CUTTING

Damaged tissue is an open window into the skin, allowing **pathogens** (disease-causing microscopic organisms) to enter the damaged tissue and begin to multiply. Figure 5–3 and Color Plate 14 show the finger of a small child who persistently chewed his finger. Eventually, the broken skin became infected with a virus that causes warts. Some organisms, especially those that cause skin infections such as warts, are **opportunistic pathogens** (FT). This means they take advantage of damaged, broken, irritated, or abraded tissue. Normally, the pathogen would not cause an infection, but damaged skin loses much of its ability to ward off infection—another good reason to keep skin healthy! Similar infections can occur when the living tissue around the nail plate is intentionally cut.

Each time you cut the eponychium (part of the guardian seal) it will cause the living tissue to grow back thicker and harder. If you stop, the tissue will return to normal in a month or so. Clients don't realize that cutting the living

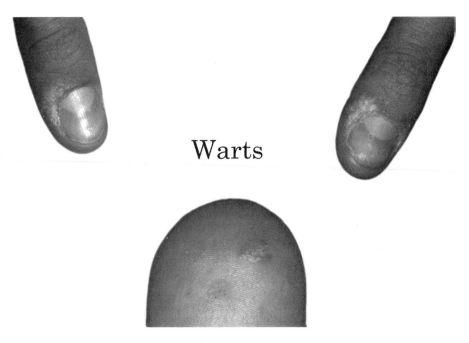

Figure 5–3 *Warts around the nail plate and on the fingertip*

tissue creates the hard skin. Instead of cutting, keep the eponychium softened with high-quality oil or lotion designed to soften skin. This will restore the damaged skin to health and provide maximum protection. Cutting living tissue creates the same damage as biting and can allow viral warts to invade the skin (FT). Clients want the best for their nails, so if they insist on cutting away this tissue, explain the risks and show them the benefits of keeping the skin around the nails healthy and intact. In short, it's fine to carefully trim a little tag of dead skin, but never rip or cut into living tissue (Figure 5–4). This is what state boards are

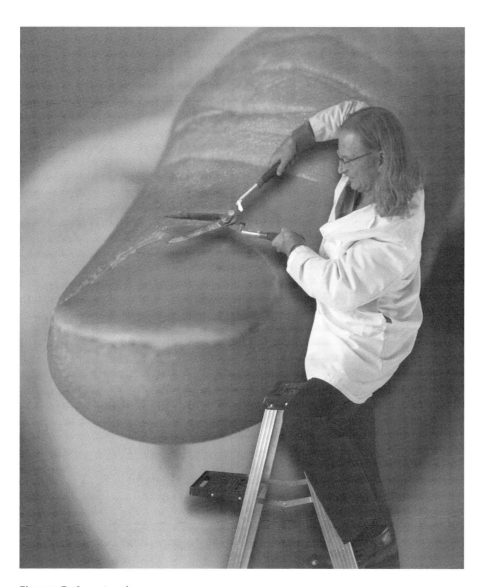

Figure 5-4 *Don't cut living tissue*

HEY, GET SOME TREATMENT!

Warts are contagious. Nippers, pushers, abrasives, and so on can transmit them. If you spot a wart anywhere on the finger or foot, advise the client to seek treatment by a qualified medical professional. Cysts and paronychia are also conditions that should not be ignored. Advise the client to deal with them promptly to avoid more serious complications.

trying to tell you when they require no cutting of the so-called cuticle. Some boards may use the wrong terminology, but even so, avoid cutting living tissue!

The same caution also applies to foot or hand calluses, even though those consist of dead skin. Calluses are designed to protect the underlying living tissue from repeated friction or pressure. A callus should never be removed, only smoothed down. Removing them can cause skin blisters and potentially may lead to more serious problems.

WILL THE REAL PTERYGIUM PLEASE STAND UP?

Pterygium (ter-RIJ-ee-um) is not the cuticle and they have nothing in common. Unlike the cuticle, pterygium is living tissue. Pterygium is defined in medical books as any abnormal, winglike structure of skin. According to Dr. Mix, a well-known podiatrist and author, "Pterygium as it relates to the nail is the abnormal adherence of the normal skin to the nail plate and is usually caused by injury." Sometimes the term *true pterygium* is used, suggesting that there is another kind of pterygium, but there is only one kind, so adding the word *true* is unnecessary.

Pterygium can be found in many places on the body, including the eye. It is seen on the nail plate, but only as an abnormal condition. When the eponychium or hyponychium becomes severely injured or damaged, pterygium may develop. Never confuse pterygium with the cuticle—they are very different *(FT)*.

There are two types of nail pterygium: **inverse pterygium** and **dorsal pterygium.** The inverse type of pterygium is shown underneath the free edge of the nail plate in Figure 5–5 and Color Plate 15.

This condition is seen when skin on the tip of the finger remains attached to the underside of the nail plate. As the plate grows away from the fingertip, the attached skin is stretched and pulled. This condition can be painful and can bleed if cut. The condition can be inherited, but it is almost always a result of trauma or allergic reaction *(FT)*. Slamming the fingers in a car door or aggressively cleaning or manicuring under the nail plate are examples of trauma that can cause this disorder. Allergic reactions to formaldehyde-containing nail hardeners can also cause pterygium, as can repeated applications of monomer liquids, UV gels, or acid-based nail primers to the skin near the underside of the nail plate.

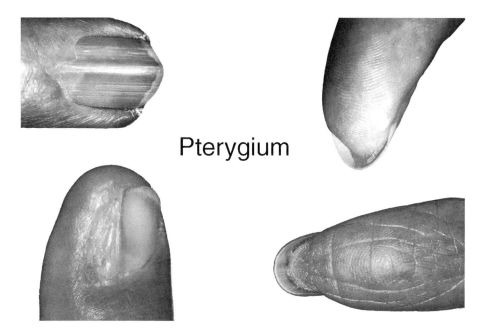

Pterygium

Figure 5–5 *Pterygium is an abnormal winglike growth of skin; the term pterygium should never be used to describe the cuticle or any other normal growth of skin*

Pterygium on the top surface of the plate is called *dorsal pterygium. Dorsal* means "top side"—that's why the fin on a dolphin's back is called the dorsal fin. This type of pterygium can be inherited, but only rarely. The dorsal type is more likely to be caused by severe trauma, such as warts, burns, lichen planus (the most common cause), and blood circulation disorders. **Lichen planus** (LYE-kin PLAY-nus) is a recurring skin inflammation that forms small, itchy lesions on the wrists, arms, and elsewhere. Experts believe this condition causes the underside of the eponychium to become fused to the matrix. This prevents normal nail plate growth. The skin is slowly stretched and dragged along the bed, as shown in Figure 5–5.

Clients with either type of pterygium should talk to their doctor. In the case of inverse pterygium, avoid exposing the client's skin to monomer and discontinue using formaldehyde-containing nail hardeners until the condition is resolved.

LUMPS AND BUMPS

A cyst is a large, soft lump under the skin. The pressure they create can cause pain in the nearest finger joint. Mucus-filled or **mucoid cysts** (MYOO-koyd cysts) are often found under the eponychium. Cysts can put a great deal of pressure on the matrix, as well. You can see in Figure 5–6 and Color Plate 16 how the plate's growth pattern has been dramatically altered. The pressure on the matrix caused thinning of the nail plate, creating the appearance of parallel ridges in the plate. Left untreated, cysts may cause permanent damage to the matrix and lead to plate deformity.

Paronychia (payr-uh-NICK-ee-yuh) closely resembles the appearance of cysts. Both can cause redness, swelling, and tenderness of the eponychium and/or lateral sidewalls *(FT)*. Mucoid cysts can appear for apparently no reason, while paronychia result from bacterial infections. They are caused by the same bacteria that lead to "greenies" under enhancements.

Paronychial infections may become chronic if left untreated. **Chronic paronychia** is most often seen in women between the ages of 20 and 40. The infections are often associated with common household chores, such as doing laundry or changing diapers. Thumb sucking in children can also lead to these infections. Chronic infection may weaken natural defenses and increase the risks of developing a fungal infection of the nail or may permanently deform the nail plate.

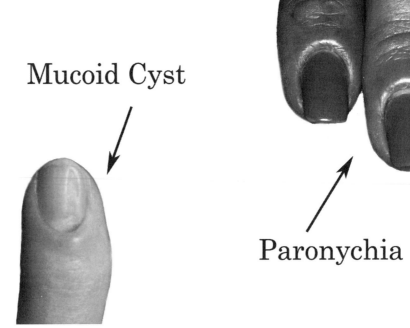

Mucoid Cyst

Paronychia

Figure 5-6 *Cysts and paronychia*

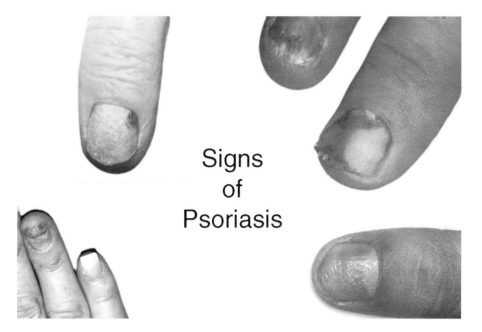

Figure 5-7 *Signs of psoriasis*

PSORIASIS ON THE NAILS?

One of the most common skin diseases in the world is **psoriasis** (suh-RYE-uh-sis). In a very large percentage of cases, symptoms of psoriasis are seen in the nail plates. Up to 90 percent of all people with psoriasis will experience a mild to serious nail disorder sometime during their lives *(FT)*. Clients may show no signs of psoriasis anywhere else on their body except the nail plates, so it is important to know the basic symptoms. Psoriasis often causes tiny pits or severe roughness on the surface of the plate, as well as yellowish to reddish patches called **salmon patches.** Usually the pits are randomly scattered across the plate. Sometimes they form straight lines running from the eponychium toward the free edge. The fingernails are more likely to be affected than the toenails. Pits occur because the surface cells are weakly bonded and fall out in small chunks. Splinter hemorrhages are often seen as well. Figure 5–7 and Color Plate 17 show the various ways psoriasis can affect nails.

Clients with significant signs of psoriasis should talk to their doctor. Clients with psoriasis should avoid all nail trauma, such as soft tissue cuts or friction burns to the bed *(FT)*. These can result in tissue scarring or loss of the nail plate. Take great care with these clients and be very careful to avoid trauma! For many of these clients it may be best to keep their nails short to prevent accidents and injury.

SPLITS AND RIDGES

Splits

The nail plate is very tough and will resist splitting. Even so, some types of damage can create temporary splits. These splits eventually grow past the free edge. If the nail continues to split as it grows, this may be a sign of permanent damage to the matrix. If a small section of the matrix is permanently injured or destroyed, it will not add to the thickness of the nail plate. This will create a thin, weak strip running the entire length of the nail plate, as seen in Chapter 4, Figure 4–2.

As we learned earlier, the length and width of the matrix determine the thickness and width of the nail plate. The same holds true for damage to sections of the matrix—the width of the damaged area determines the width of the split. Because the damage runs to the entire thickness of the nail plate, the split will separate the plate in the two. If a strip of damaged matrix runs from the front to back, the nail plate will grow as two separate plates. If the body ever repairs the matrix, the split will eventually grow off the free edge. But if the plate has been split for more than a year it is unlikely to return to normal.

Age-Related Ridges

As we age, our nail plates begin to change. Small ridges begin to appear on the plate's surface ⓕⓣ. It's normal to find narrow ridges running from the free edge to the eponychium, especially in older clients. These ridges can be lightly buffed to reduce their appearance, but take care not to overthin the nail plate. Ridge-filling base coats can also help create a smoother appearance. Other normal signs of aging are brittleness and slower growth. These two may be related. As nail growth begins to slow, the nail plate takes longer to reach the free edge, so the plate is exposed to more abuse before the free edge is clipped or filed.

Beaded Ridges

Ridges with a "beaded" appearance (Figure 5–8 and Color Plate 18) are often associated with circulatory problems in the nail matrix or in other parts of the body ⓕⓣ. High blood pressure, heart disease, blood clots, gangrene, and other blood circulation problems may create beading.

BEAU'S LINES

Beau's lines are depressions or valleys stretching across the width of the nail plate (Figure 5–8 and Color Plate 18). They happen when nail plate growth is temporarily slowed or halted. In extreme cases, the plate depression can extend completely through the nail, causing the nail plate to be shed. Beau's lines are usually a result of severe, short-term illness, such as pneumonia, a heart attack, a drug reaction, or a severe fever lasting several days or more ⓕⓣ. Usually all the nails

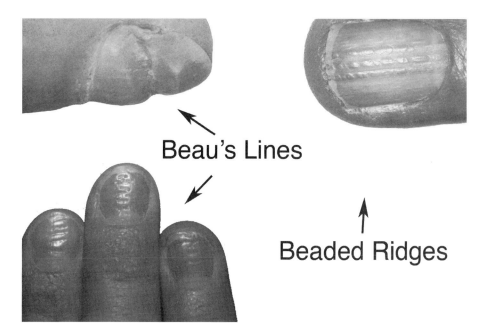

Beau's Lines

Beaded Ridges

Figure 5-8 *Beau's lines and beaded ridges*

(including toenails) are involved, on either one or both hands, but in some cases only a few nail plates will be affected.

SPOON NAILS

Normal nail plates are concave to almost flat. But sometimes the plate develops a large upward curvature. The common name for this condition is **spoon nails** (Figure 5–9, right). "Ski jump" nails are a mild form of spoon nails. These nail plates are different from nails with a normal curvature. That difference is the reason for their extreme flexibility. They contain fewer sulfur cross-links, so the nails become more flexible and weaker. They are usually thinner as well. Overfiling thins the plate and can worsen the condition, so avoid this!

OUCH!

It is not uncommon to find deep, wavy lines across the width of the big toe. When they appear on the big toe only, it is probably not a Beau's line. These wavy lines are often trauma-related and usually are caused by shoes that are too small. The impact on the toenail by the shoe causes these wavy lines—more evidence that the nail plate is a flowable solid.

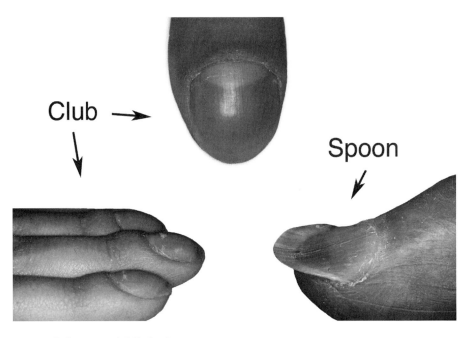

Figure 5-9 *Spoon and clubbed nails*

Overexposure to solvents can soften or corrode the nail plate and lead to spoon nails (FT). Spoon nails can also be a symptom of psoriasis, lichen planus, or iron deficiency. Finally, spoon nails is a condition that may be inherited and is often seen in both mother and daughter.

CLUBS FOR NAILS

Clubbing results in nail plates with an extreme degree of curvature (Figure 5–9). This condition was first reported by Hippocrates, the father of medicine, in 400 BC. You can see that the fingertips appear enlarged or swollen in extreme cases. Usually the condition is painless. A doctor should see painful club nails, since this could be an indication of a more serious condition. Clubbing may be inherited, but it is normally caused by heart disease, lung disease, chronic hepatitis, liver disease, malnutrition, or poisoning by mercury, arsenic, or alcohol (FT). Up to 80 percent of cases of clubbing are related to lung disorders and related illnesses. Clubbed nails can be a symptom of chronic bronchitis, but usually only after ten years or more. It is believed that these changes happen when blood vessels in the nail bed become enlarged and swollen.[1] If only one fingernail is

---

[1]Currie, A. E., & Gallagher, P. J. (1988). The pathology of clubbing: Vascular changes in the nail bed, *British Journal of Diseases of the Chest, 82,* 382–385.

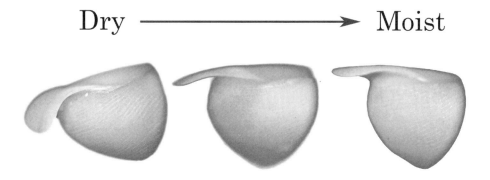

Figure 5-10 *Changes in parrot beak nails after being soaked in warm, soapy water for 10 minutes and 20 minutes*

clubbed, then trauma is the likely culprit. When this is the case, white leukonychia spots will often be seen on a traumatized fingernail.

PARROTS IN THE SALON

Extreme curvatures in the opposite direction of spoon nails are called **parrot beak nails.** When exposed to water or solvents, parrot beak nails behave differently than spoon nails. Soak these nails in warm, soapy water and they will straighten. Soaking in hot oil will not change the shape of the nail as dramatically (Figure 5–10).

When dry, these nails are usually rigid and don't easily bend. In previous chapters, you learned about the amazing effect that water has on the nail plate. Parrot beak nails provide a perfect example of how water affects the flexibility and shape of the nail plate. It's not known why the nail plate grows this way. But we do know why water affects flexibility. As you learned previously, water lubricates the keratin chains. This allows the chains to slip and slide past each other.

ARTIFICIAL NAILS VERSUS MANICURES

An important question is whether nails affected by any of the conditions discussed in this chapter can be safely enhanced with artificial nails. Table 5–1 lists each condition along with general guidelines and some suggestions.

Table 5-1 A brief list of guidelines in suggestions for enhancing problem nails

Onycholysis	If no infection is present, protective overlays are better than extending the length of the nail. Nails should be kept short until the condition is resolved. Okay to manicure if care is taken.
Leukonychia	Okay to enhance. Okay to manicure.
Discoloration	If no signs of infection or disease are present, discolored nails can be enhanced. Okay to manicure.
Brittle nails	Carefully applied and correctly maintained enhancements can protect and strengthen brittle nails. File lightly and keep extensions short. Okay to manicure. Use hot oil soaks and avoid water.
Overfiled	Correctly applied and correctly maintained enhancements can protect and strengthen weak or thin nails. Avoid additional filing and keep extensions short. Okay to manicure.
Warts	Recommend that the client see a physician to have the wart treated before servicing.
Infections	Recommend that the client see a physician to treat the infection before servicing.
Pterygium	Recommend that the client see a physician before servicing.
Paronychia	Recommend that the client see a physician to treat the infection before servicing.
Cysts	Recommend that the client see a physician for treatment, before servicing.
Psoriasis	Client should see a physician before applying enhancements or manicuring. Trauma could lead to nail shedding and scarring of the eponychium or lateral sidewalls.
Splits	Enhancement overlays can seal splits and prevent them from worsening. They may also seal the split until it grows past the free edge. Do not apply artificial enhancements if the nail bed is exposed or if there is significant damage (for example, if the finger has been smashed with a hammer). Okay to manicure.
Ridges	Okay to enhance. Okay to manicure.
Beaded ridges	Recommend that the client see a physician before enhancing or manicuring.
Beau's lines	Okay to enhance or manicure if the condition is minor and the nail bed is not exposed. Otherwise, recommend that the client see a physician.
Spoon nails	Okay to enhance or manicure. Use care to avoid thinning the nail plate.
Club nails	Recommend that the client see a physician before enhancing. Okay to manicure.
Parrot beak nails	Okay to enhance and okay to manicure.
Not sure	Play it safe and recommend the client see a physician if there is any doubt.

FAST TRACK (FT)

(FT) Most fingernail infections are caused by bacteria.

(FT) Bacteria are one-celled living organisms.

(FT) Bacterial infections on the surface of the nail plate are usually green in color.

(FT) Fungal infections are usually found on the toes and are rare on fingers.

(FT) The most common forms of athlete's foot are the moccasin form and the interdigital form.

(FT) It is safe to do pedicures on feet with athlete's foot or other mild fungal infections.

(FT) Skin infection pathogens are opportunistic and often grow in injured skin.

(FT) Warts can be spread whenever the skin is cut.

(FT) Pterygium is an abnormal skin growth—don't confuse it with the cuticle.

(FT) Inverse pterygium can be caused by trauma or allergic reaction.

(FT) Paronychia is a bacterial infection that occurs under soft tissues around the nail plate.

(FT) Almost 90 percent of people with psoriasis experience mild to serious nail disorders.

(FT) Clients with psoriasis should avoid nail trauma, such as soft tissue cuts or friction burns to the bed.

(FT) Unbeaded ridges on the nail plate are a normal sign of aging.

(FT) Beaded ridges on the plate are often associated with circulatory problems.

(FT) Spoon nails have extreme flexibility and are usually very thin.

(FT) Beau's lines indicate a past serious medical condition or illness.

(FT) Solvents overexposure can damage the nail plate and lead to spoon nails.

(FT) Clubbed nails may be inherited or caused by a wide range of ailments.

Review Questions

1. What government department prohibits the marketing of nonprescription products to treat fungus on the nail plate?

2. Fungus eats _____ and bacteria eats _____ on the nail plate.

3. Interdigital fungal infections are found where on the feet?

4. What percentage of people with psoriasis have moderate to serious nail problems at some point during their lives?

5. If your client had been seriously ill three months ago, what symptoms would you expect to see in the nail?

6. What nail condition could be caused by exposure to solvents or is inherited and can be seen in both mother and daughter?

7. What nail products can cause pseudoleukonychia and why?

8. _____ is a condition that causes the nail plate to grow with an abnormally white appearance.

9. What is the world's most common type of fungal foot infection?

10. What effect do hot oil soaks have on parrot beak nails?

11. What type of foot infection covers the entire bottom of the foot and has a scaly, dry appearance?

12. Warts are an example of pathogens that are _____. In other words, they take advantage of damaged, broken, or abraded skin to start infections.

13. Which cause most fingernail infections, bacteria or fungus?

14. *Dorsal* means _____.

15. What is lichen planus?

Chapter 6

The Principles of Nail Product Chemistry

Objective

In this chapter you will learn about chemicals and study their many forms. Then you will study the various ways that chemicals can change or interact with each other. Finally, you'll explore some of the myths and misunderstandings about chemicals and learn about using them safely.

WHY LEARN CHEMISTRY?

It may seem like there is no reason for a nail technician to understand chemistry. Actually, the opposite is true. A good nail technician must have a basic understanding of chemistry. Why? A little chemical knowledge goes a long way. You don't need to be a chemist to see the benefits of understanding your products. Nail technicians make their living from chemistry. Mixing liquid and powder to create artificial nails is chemistry. Curing gel enhancements under UV light is chemistry. Spraying a catalyst on a wrap resin to speed curing is chemistry. Even applying a base coat, polish, and topcoat involves chemistry. If you don't understand some basic chemistry, how can you hope to solve problems when they occur? Learning a little about chemistry will save you money and time. You'll have fewer problems and fewer service breakdowns and you'll be better able to answer your clients' questions. There are a lot of good reasons for learning the chemistry of nails!

JUST WHAT IS A CHEMICAL?

Most people believe that all chemicals are dangerous and toxic. This is completely false! How could it be true? Everything around you is made of chemicals. Your chair, the air, this book, all of your food and vitamins, even your skin—they are all chemicals. In fact, everything you can see or touch, except light and electricity, is a chemical (FT). Typically, the word *chemical* is used only in a negative way. We forget that just about everything around us is a chemical and that everything is made of chemicals.

Nail plates are 100 percent chemicals. In Chapter 1, we learned that the nail plate is mostly protein. Proteins are made from amino acids. Amino acids are composed of the basic chemicals or **elements** carbon, nitrogen, oxygen, hydrogen, and sulfur. There are 88 naturally occurring elements (others have been created in the laboratory), but these five are considered to be the basic building blocks of life, as you will learn in the next section. Sulfur is the chemical responsible for the sulfur cross-links that make nail plates strong, hair curly, and skin resilient. Nail plates also contain traces of iron, aluminum, zinc, copper, silver, and gold. All matter is made of chemicals. Almost everything is matter.

YOU GOT YOUR PICK: MATTER OR ENERGY?

Everything that exists in the world can be divided into two categories. That's because everything is either matter or energy—no exceptions! (FT) It's one or the other. **Matter** is anything that takes up space or occupies an area. If it takes up space, then it's matter. For instance, this book occupies or fills a space. A book that is 8 × 4 × 2 inches occupies space. So you can be sure that it's made of matter. Most things take up space, so most things are made of matter. Even microscopic viruses take up a tiny amount of space.

Light doesn't take up any space. Neither do radio waves, microwaves, or X-rays. These are not made of matter—they are energy. **Energy** has no substance and is not made of matter. But energy can affect matter in many ways. Energy is the only thing that is not made of chemicals. Everything else in the universe is a chemical!

MOLECULES OF LIFE

Water is a chemical made from two parts hydrogen and one part oxygen. Chemical shorthand for this combination is H_2O. Two hydrogens combine with one oxygen to create one molecule of water. A molecule is the simplest form of a chemical substance and is the basis of life ⒻⓉ. All living things are made of molecules. Substances that can't be broken down any further are called elements ⒻⓉ. If a water molecule was broken down any further, it wouldn't be water anymore. It would revert back to its basic components of hydrogen and oxygen. Of course, molecules are far too small to be seen. A single droplet of water contains a trillion water molecules. If a glass of water were enlarged to the size of the Earth, water molecules would only be the size of volleyballs. Now that's petite-sized!

MATTER, MATTER EVERYWHERE!

Matter comes in several forms. Matter can be a solid, liquid, or gas! Most substances exist naturally in only one or two forms, but water has a rare property. It can naturally exist in all three forms. It can be frozen into a solid, melted to a liquid, and evaporated into a vapor. **Vapors** are created when liquids evaporate into the air ⒻⓉ. When a liquid changes into a gas, it's called **vaporization** ⒻⓉ. For example, the evaporation of water makes water vapor. The evaporation of dry ice makes the dense, white carbon dioxide vapor that bubbles out of Halloween drinks. Dry ice changes from a solid directly into a vapor, without becoming a liquid. Like most things, dry ice exists in only two forms. Both dry ice and water vapors can be cooled back into the solid state. Some liquids must be heated before they will evaporate. Others will quickly form vapors, especially on a warm day. Liquids that easily evaporate at room temperature must be kept in closed containers to prevent them from escaping into the air. This is true for all **volatile** or quickly evaporating liquids.

Many salon products contain volatile ingredients. Nail polish is a perfect example. Some ingredients in polish will evaporate quickly. This is why nail polish thickens over time. The polish hasn't just "gone bad." Instead, some of the ingredients have evaporated. Obviously, keeping the cap tightly sealed will prevent vapors from escaping. Keeping the threads on the neck of the bottle free of polish will ensure a tighter seal and also help prevent evaporation.

Increasing the temperature of a volatile liquid will speed up evaporation. For example, blow dryers evaporate water from hair with hot air. On warm days, volatile ingredients in your products will escape even more quickly. Storing products in a cool location, out of direct sunlight, and closed tightly will keep them in top condition and lengthen their shelf life. Avoid keeping products in the refrigerator. If products are cold upon opening, moisture can condense inside the bottles, much the way frost forms on a windowpane or water condenses on the outside of a glass of ice tea.

Fumes are tiny solid particles suspended in gases (*FT*). Examples of fumes are car exhaust, smoke from chimneys, and welding fumes. Fumes are not found in the salon. No salon product releases fumes. This word is frequently misused and should not be confused with salon vapors or odors.

VAPORS AND SMELLS IN A NUTSHELL

Odors are caused by vapors in the air. These vapors touch sensitive nerves in the nose lining. The nerves send messages to the brain. The messages report the vapor's odor so that the brain can identify it. For example, the nerves may detect chemical vapors from a lemon and send a "lemon signal" to the brain. The brain determines whether it likes the odor or not and decides what to do. This is how we smell, in a nutshell.

Our noses are extremely sensitive odor detectors. But every vapor is different. Some vapors are noticeable in very low amounts or concentrations. Other vapors must be highly concentrated before we smell them. Odors can be deceiving. A strong smell can occur for three different reasons. It could be that (1) there are a lot of vapor molecules in the air, (2) the nerves responsible for smell are hypersensitive to the vapor, or (3) a person may have an aversion to the smell, even in extremely low amounts.

Some vapors have a very strong smell even if there is only 1 molecule of the vaporized substance mixed with 1 million air molecules, or 1 ppm. This is how vapors are measured in the air: *parts of vaporized substance per every one million parts of air.* You will see this written as **parts per million** or **ppm** (*FT*). For example, 20 molecules of a vaporized substance in 1 million molecules of air is 20 ppm. Now imagine trying to find one pink straw in a haystack of one million red straws! Your nose can do it with vapors. That's how sensitive the nose is to certain vapors. But some molecules are more difficult to smell. Their odors will be weak, even at very high concentrations. That's why it is practically impossible for the nose to tell how much vapor is in the salon's air (*FT*). A certain chemical may smell very strong at 2 ppm, and others may have a weak smell even at 1,000 ppm. When vapors are difficult to smell they are sometimes called **odorless.** If you don't smell anything, does that mean there is no vapor in the air? Probably not! It could very well be that you just can't smell the vapors.

Quickly evaporating liquids produce large amounts of vapor. A few chemicals used in the salon have odors that some find offensive. Many believe that "smelly" chemicals must be dangerous. This is quite wrong! A bad smell merely means that your brain does not like the odor. It does not mean the chemical is more toxic or dangerous. Also, the odor may smell terrible even though there are

Fact: The amount of vapor that escapes into the air is not determined by the odor. It is determined by how quickly the liquid evaporates.

hardly any vapor molecules in the air—say, 1 ppm. Some people develop a condition called **smell aversion.** In other words, they dislike a particular smell so much that they can't tolerate it even at low concentrations. Others may think that the same odor is acceptable or has a weak smell. But the person with the smell aversion may feel faint, weak, nauseous, or dizzy, among other symptoms, even when others are bothered not nearly as much by the odor. Smell aversions can develop with any type of odor, even sweet or floral scents. In this case, the odor may make the person feel ill, even though it's perfectly safe to breathe. You will learn much more about vapors, odors, mists, dusts, and how to control them in the salon's air in Chapters 14 and 15.

PHYSICAL AND CHEMICAL CHANGES

When water freezes or thaws it undergoes a **physical change.** In other words, only the physical appearance is different—it still is water. When a lump of sugar is crushed into powder or dissolved in water it is physically changed. It is still sugar, but now it has a different appearance. If you evaporate a sugar-water mixture, you will find sugar in the bottom of the container. Of course it is sugar, not something different. In each case, the chemical simply changes form or appearance. It is not chemically altered into a new substance.

Matter can be chemically changed as well. For example, burning sugar produces a black tarry substance. It's not sugar anymore! It has undergone a **chemical change.** Chemical molecules are like a Tinkertoy set. Their parts can be arranged and rearranged into an almost unlimited number of combinations. Petroleum can be chemically converted into vitamin C. Acetone can be changed into water or oxygen. Paper can be made into sugar. The possibilities are endless. In medieval times, alchemists searched in vain for ways to turn lead into gold. Today, even this is possible. Why isn't it done? It costs more to do it than the gold is worth!

IT'S A CHEMICAL REACTION

Molecules like to change. If you give them a reason to change, they usually will. In chemistry, a reaction occurs when two or more molecules interact and something happens ⒡. If a new molecule is created, this interaction is called a **chemical reaction.** Many things can cause chemical reactions. But chemical reactions require energy to make them happen. Most chemical reactions get this energy from heat or light. Heat and light are types of energy. Plants use light energy to cause many chemical reactions in their leaves. These chemical reactions make food for the plant and create oxygen. Cooking uses heat energy to cause chemical reactions in food. For example, egg whites are liquidy and clear when raw but become firm and white when heated because the egg protein undergoes a chemical reaction as well as undergoing a physical change. Increasing the temperature usually causes chemical reactions to happen more quickly. This is why food cooks faster at higher temperatures. In general, a chemical reaction will happen twice as fast if the temperature is raised by just 10°F (6°C). A major part of a nail technician's work is to cause chemical reactions to occur on the nail plate. For instance, artificial nail enhancements use either heat or light energy to create the finished product (FT).

ACIDS, BASES, AND pH

Scientists created the **pH scale** (Figure 6–1) to measure the amount of acid or base in water mixtures. A substance must contain water before it can have a pH (FT). Products that contain no water have no pH. The pH scale goes from 0 to 14. Distilled water is right in the middle at 7. It is considered to have a neutral pH. **Acids** are found between 0 and 7 (FT). **Bases** (alkaline substances) are between 7 and 14 (FT). Our skin has a wide range of pH values, usually between 4.5 and 6.5, depending on the type of skin. So by nature our skin is slightly acidic.

It is commonly believe that acids are dangerous substances. This is false. Lemon juice, vinegar, and saliva are examples of safe acids. Substances become dangerous only if they are too low in pH. For example, glycolic acid skin peels often have a pH below 3.0. If the pH of the acid peel was changed to 6.0, it would lose its effect on skin. The same is true for alkaline substances (bases). If the pH of a substance is above 10, it may be damaging to skin. **Corrosives** are substances

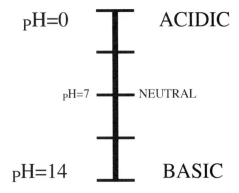

Figure 6-1 *The pH scale*

Table 6-1 A table of common substances and their pH values

pH	Substance
0	Battery acid
1	Stomach acid
2	Lemon juice, vinegar
3	Orange juice, soda, apples
4	Tomato juice, acid rain
5	Black coffee, softened drinking water
6	Saliva, milk, egg yolks
7	Pure water
8	Ocean water, blood, liquid hand soap
9	Baking soda, borax
10	Stomach antacids, clothing detergents
11	Ammonia, bar hand soaps
12	Cuticle removers, phenolic-based disinfectants
13	Household bleach, oven cleaners
14	Liquid drain cleaner, lye

that can cause serious and sometimes irreversible damage to skin. Corrosives can be low-pH acids or high-pH bases, but they're usually found at the extreme ends of the pH scale. Acid-based nail primers, acid skin peels, high-volume hydrogen peroxide, bleach, phenolic-based disinfectants, and cuticle and callus removers are examples of corrosives that are found in salons. Table 6–1 shows the pH of some common substances.

A CATALYST FOR CHANGE

A **catalyst** changes the rate at which a chemical reaction occurs ⓕⓣ. In other words, catalysts make chemical reactions go faster or slower. Trillions of chemical reactions occur in our bodies every day. Most of these happen because of catalysts. Different chemical reactions require different catalysts. A specific catalyst will usually work for only a few types of chemical reactions, much the way a key will open only certain locks. That is why so many different catalysts exist. Catalysts are very important chemical tools. Many chemical reactions happen very slowly. For instance, graphite (pencil lead) will slowly change into diamond, but it takes many thousands of years. Obviously, a graphite-to-diamond catalyst would be an important discovery if it is ever found.

In nail products, catalysts are used to make chemical reactions happen more quickly. Reactions that normally take days will happen in a fraction of a second with the right catalyst. Some chemical reactions used to make overlays and sculptured nails would take several months to happen without the proper catalysts. Obviously, that's a whole lot longer than clients are willing to sit at your station!

The important role that catalysts play in professional nail products will be discussed in later chapters. For now, it's just important that you know what they are and how they work.

SOLVENTS AND SOLUTES

A solvent is anything that dissolves another substance (FT). Solvents are usually liquid. The substance being dissolved is called a **solute** (FT). As a general rule, most solutes are solids. Sugar dissolving in water is an example of a solute dissolving in a solvent. But liquids and gases can be solutes too. Oxygen dissolves in water. This is how fish breathe. Their gills extract the oxygen from water. Water is an incredibly good solvent. In fact, water is called the universal solvent because it will dissolve more substances than any other known solvent. Other examples of safe and powerful solvents used in the nail industry are toluene and acetone.

Acetone is frequently used to remove nail polish and to dissolve artificial nail enhancements and other types of **coating.** It is one of the safest solvents used in nail salons. When used as a polish remover, acetone dissolves old polish (the solute). Acetone works quickly because it is a good solvent. A poor solvent dissolves solutes very slowly. The better the solvent, the faster it will dissolve the solute. But sometimes a solvent can be too good! In Chapter 4, you learned that putting a small amount of water in polish remover prevents skin dryness. Why is that? Water is a poor solvent for skin oils, while acetone is a good skin oil solvent. A small amount of water helps balance acetone's strength, making it a slightly poorer solvent. Therefore, it will strip away less skin oil. The more water there is in acetone, the less oil it will remove from skin. Water is also a poor solvent for nail polish. Otherwise, washing your hands would remove the polish. Putting water in polish remover will make it a slightly slower polish remover, but it will also be easier on the skin. But if you put in too much water, it won't work at all.

Solvents dissolve only a certain amount of solute before they become **saturated.** In other words, a saturated solvent cannot dissolve any more solute

COMMON AND FRIENDLY

Toluene has been used since the 1930s to dissolve ingredients in nail polish. Toluene keeps nail polish in a liquid form until applied. When the solvent evaporates, the polish dries to a hard finish.

Studies show that the average amount of toluene found in salon air is about 200 times lower than the federally established safe limit. Even poorly ventilated salons generally have less than 1 ppm toluene vapors in the air, which is still 100 times below the federal safe limit. Clearly, toluene is a safe solvent for use in nail salons.

(*FT*), much the way a sponge becomes saturated with water and won't absorb any more. Saturated solvents are very ineffective. Using a saturated solvent is a waste of time and needlessly exposes the client's skin to the substance. Always use fresh solvents. Fresh, clean solvents work much faster. Never reuse solvents on the next client. Time is money, and reusing solvents is a waste of both!

Warming solvents will also make them faster-acting. This is especially true when removing artificial nail enhancements. Most removers require 30 to 40 minutes to loosen the product at room temperature. Warming the solvent to 104°F (40°C; Jacuzzi temperature) will shorten the soak-off time by 10 to 15 minutes. Warming solvents should be done with great care and caution! Many solvents are highly flammable, including acetone and alcohol. To safely warm the solvents, place a partially filled plastic bottle containing the solvent under hot running water (Figure 6–2). *Never* warm solvents on a stove, in a microwave

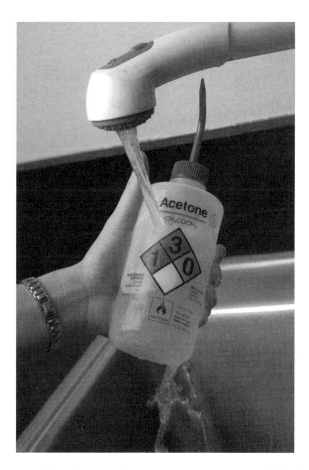

Figure 6–2 *Warming solvents by running hot water over an appropriate, properly labeled container is much safer than using hot plates, stoves, microwaves, hair dryers, and so on*

NICE AND EASY

An easy way to warm solvents is by using the body's own natural heat. Artificial nails can be removed more quickly by using this simple technique:

1. Soak a cotton ball with product remover (solvent).

2. Place the saturated cotton ball on the artificial nail.

3. Wrap the cotton ball and finger with tinfoil.

The body's heat will warm the solvent to near 98°F (37° C) and will dramatically speed product removal.

oven, or with an open flame. Most salon solvents are far too flammable and may catch fire. Also, loosen the cap so that pressure doesn't build up in the bottle, causing it to crack or burst open. Finally, cover the dish and hand with a damp cloth while soaking to reduce vapors in the air. The product manufacturer should be able to provide additional safe handling information. Be sure to read, understand, and follow all manufacturer's instructions before using any solvents.

Solvents are usually very volatile. Volatile liquids are more likely to escape into the salon air. They may increase the risk of accidental fire or lower the quality of your breathing air if not handled properly. Fortunately, solvents are easy to use safely. Remember, always use and dispose of solvents as directed by the manufacturer's instructions and other information. In later chapters, you will learn more about working safely with solvents.

IS ACETONE SAFE?

Why do so some nail technicians avoid acetone? Probably because they've heard untrue things about this beneficial substance. What is the truth about acetone? Acetone is one of the most important solvents in the world. Except for water itself, acetone is one of the safest solvents that nail technicians use!

Myth: Acetone Is Absorbed Through the Skin, So It Is Dangerous

Many chemicals can be absorbed through the skin. Sometimes this can cause harm, but not always! Skin creams, for example, are designed to penetrate the skin. They are not considered dangerous. Just because a chemical is absorbed through the skin doesn't mean it must be unsafe. In the case of acetone, it is almost impossible for dangerous amounts to penetrate the skin. Unless you soak your fingers every day in a bowl of acetone for long periods, it is very unlikely to cause serious harm or damage. This is why acetone is safe to use in salons. It is pretty hard to become overexposed to acetone in the salon.

Myth: Acetone Damages the Liver or Kidneys and Causes Cancer

Acetone does *not* cause cancer! Under normal salon use conditions, it is not considered to be dangerous to the liver, kidneys, or blood. The only way it could cause these types of problems is if massive long-term overexposure occurs—the kind of overexposure that's extremely unlikely in the salon. Many other industries use large amounts of acetone without serious complications. Nail technicians need not worry about suffering internal injury from acetone.

Myth: It Is Risky to Inhale Too Much Acetone

It is risky to breathe too much of anything except air. But nail technicians use relatively small amounts of acetone. It would be uncomfortable to stay in a room that had an unsafe amount of acetone in the air. The eyes would burn, and it would become difficult to breathe. At these high concentrations, acetone has excellent warning properties. In other words, you will know that you need better ventilation long before there's too much acetone in the air. It is practically impossible to breathe too much acetone in the salon.

Myth: The FDA Is Going to Ban Acetone

Nonsense! This is an utterly foolish myth. Acetone is considered to be an extremely safe and useful solvent. The FDA has never even considered banning this important chemical. This is a common myth about other chemicals in the nail industry. These rumors are almost always spread by uninformed individuals or someone who wants to create irrational fear and panic. It's common to hear that a certain chemical "causes cancer" or "is toxic" or "is going to be banned by the FDA." Be wary of such claims! They are usually designed to scare you, not inform you. Unscrupulous, greedy marketers will often use these types of claims to frighten you into using their products. Avoid buying anything from people who try to scare you into using their products. These are fear-based marketers and they rarely have your best interest in mind.

Myth: Acetone Will Dry Out and Damage the Natural Nail

Acetone can absorb some water from the natural nail plate, but so will the nonacetone solvents commonly used in salons. Even so, this is not an important issue. Normal moisture levels are restored quickly. This temporary change in the surface of the natural nail does not cause damage. In fact, pure acetone is often used to clean the nail plate and improve product adhesion.

Myth: Non-Acetone Polish Removers Are Safer

False! Sadly, many nail technicians choose non-acetone polish and product removers because they believe they are safer. Although non-acetone substitutes can also be used safely, none is safer than acetone. Non-acetone removers usually use either ethyl acetate or methyl ethyl ketone as the solvent. Neither is any safer than acetone.

RULES FOR WORKING SAFELY

There are many rules for working safely. Many of these rules will be discussed in much more detail in Chapters 11 and 14. Below are a few tips that will help you work safely with solvents.

- Always work in a well-ventilated area *FT* .
- Use a self-closing metal can for waste disposal.
- Empty each waste receptacle often.
- Always keep your hands clean and dry.
- Wear safety glasses to help prevent accidental eye exposure.
- Store and use all flammable substances away from flames and heat.
- Never use candles or smoke cigarettes near flammable products.
- Never store flammable products in your car trunk.
- Keep all products tightly closed and out of children's reach.
- Always read and follow manufacturer's instructions.

What's the best way to avoid falling victim to rumors and myths? It's called thinking critically. Unfortunately, this skill is not often taught in school, even though it's an important skill to possess. With this skill you can identify myths and expose misinformation. It's not a difficult skill to master if you know the basics. What is critical thinking? It's a way of think that uses your reasoning skills to decide what to believe or not to believe. Critical thinking helps uncover bias and prejudice. Critical thinking helps identify half-truths and deceptions. Critical thinkers distinguish between fact and opinion. They ask questions, make detailed observations, use properly defined terms, and make decisions based on sound logic and solid evidence. Critical thinking is a basic element of successful communication. Below is a list of some qualities that critical thinkers use to make decisions. Critical thinkers:

- Ask relevant questions
- Carefully examine the statements and arguments made by others
- Will admit when they lack understanding or don't have all the information

- Have a sense of curiosity and are interested in finding new solutions
- Will examine others' beliefs, assumptions, and opinions by weighing them against the known facts
- Listen carefully to others and provide feedback
- Don't make a judgment until all the facts have been gathered and considered
- Ask penetrating and thought-provoking questions while evaluating new ideas
- Understand their own personal thoughts and ideas about the topic
- Are open and willing to reassess their own views when given new or different evidence or information
- Are open-minded and willing to adapt when convinced the information or facts are correct

Be a critical thinker for life . . . and your life will be much more rewarding!

FAST TRACK Ⓕⓣ

Ⓕⓣ Everything you can see or touch, except light and electricity, is a chemical.

Ⓕⓣ Everything in the world is either matter or energy.

Ⓕⓣ A molecule is the smallest unit of a substance that still retains all of the properties of that substance.

Ⓕⓣ Substances that cannot be broken down any further are called elements.

Ⓕⓣ Vapors are formed when liquids evaporate into the air.

Ⓕⓣ Converting a liquid into a gas is called vaporization.

Ⓕⓣ Fumes are tiny solid particles suspended in gases.

Ⓕⓣ *Parts per million* or *ppm* is a measure of the number of molecules of a vaporized substance per million molecules of air.

Ⓕⓣ The nose cannot tell how much vapor is in the air.

Ⓕⓣ A chemical reaction occurs when a molecule changes its structure or composition.

Ⓕⓣ Nail enhancements can use either heat or light energy to create the finished product.

Ⓕⓣ A substance must contain water before it can have a pH.

Ⓕⓣ Acids are substances with a pH between 0 and 7.

Ⓕⓣ Bases are substances with a pH between 7 and 14.

FT A catalyst is a chemical that changes the rate of a chemical reaction.

FT A solvent dissolves another substance, which is called a solute.

FT Once a solvent is saturated with solute, it is no longer useful.

FT Always work in a well-ventilated area and keep products out of children's reach.

FT Use a self-closing, metal can to dispose of waste and empty often.

FT Wear safety glasses to help prevent eye damage.

FT Store all flammable substances away from flames and heat.

Review Questions

1. What is a chemical?
2. What is the difference between matter and energy?
3. What is a molecule?
4. What is the difference between vapors and fumes? Give an example of each.
5. What is the cause of all odors in the salon air?
6. Give three reasons that explain why some vapors smell stronger than others.
7. Define and give an example of a chemical change.
8. Define and give an example of a physical change.
9. What are catalysts? Why do you think they might be important to nail technicians?
10. Define solvents and solutes.
11. Why is it wasteful to use a saturated solvent?
12. What is an element and how many types of elements occur in nature? Why are they important?
13. What does *ppm* stand for? What is it used for?
14. What is a corrosive?
15. What types of products have no pH?

Chapter 7

Adhesives and Adhesion

Objective

In this chapter you will learn about the various physical and chemical forces that create good adhesion and how you can maximize their effectiveness. You'll learn about the many types of primers and adhesives, as well as the importance of properly preparing the natural nail to ensure maximum product adhesion.

WHY STUDY STICKINESS?

Clients want beautiful nails, but they expect problem-free nails. Who would want a gorgeous set of nails that started lifting from the nail plate after a few days? Any type of enhancement service breakdown is a waste of time for both the nail technician and the client. It's also a waste of money and creates dissatisfied customers. Clients don't want problems or excuses; they want solutions. But think about it—problems related to improper adhesion (lifting) are difficult to solve if you don't understand why they happen. Once you understand why things stick, you'll discover that lifting problems are easily prevented. Don't waste time fixing nails. The key to success is to understand the causes and to avoid the common pitfalls. If you do this, you'll make more money in less time and have happier clients. Sound good? Then read on!

ADHESION IS NEVER HAVING TO SAY YOU'RE SORRY

Adhesion is a force of nature that causes two surfaces to stick together (FT). What causes adhesion? To understand why things stick, we must know something about surfaces. The first thing to know is that a surface can be solid or liquid. You learned in the last chapter that matter is made of molecules. Therefore, molecules can be found at the surface of both liquids and solids. When two surfaces stick together, it is the surface molecules that interact with each other and cause adhesion (FT). In other words, adhesion is caused when the molecules on one surface are attracted to the molecules on another surface. The forces that draw and hold them together can be either physical or chemical. There are three types of interactions between the surface molecules:

1. *Entanglement*—the molecules become tangled together and can't separate very easily. Entanglement is how Velcro works. But in the case of nail products, the tangled molecules are invisible and many thousands of times smaller. Entanglement is a physical force that creates adhesion (FT).

2. *Attraction*—the molecules are pulled toward each other but never permanently link together. Socks held together by static cling is an example of an attraction. Static does not hold products to the natural nail; with nail products, the adhesion is created by chemical forces of attraction and entanglement.

3. *Reaction*—the molecules are drawn toward each other and link together with strong chemical bonds that are difficult to break. This reaction is a chemical force (FT).

In each case, the interactions will not occur unless the surfaces are compatible (FT). Paint sticks to canvas because it is compatible with the canvas's surface. The molecules of paint "like" the molecules of the canvas's surface. Therefore, they are attracted toward each other. Wet paint on canvas forms a liquid surface on top of a solid surface. Where the two surfaces meet is called the

interface. If the paint is not compatible with the solid surface, it will be repelled. The paint will bead up or refuse to stick. When surface molecules are not compatible, there is no adhesion.

The Teflon coating on pans creates a surface that repels foods. Putting cooking oil in a pan has the same effect as Teflon—the oil blocks adhesion and prevents food from sticking to the surface of the pan. In other words, the food is compatible with the surface of the pan but incompatible with the surface of the oil. There are many such examples of surfaces that repel each other. For instance, wax on a car hood repels water and causes it to bead up. Beading and streaking are signs that the solid surface is repelling the liquid ⒻⓉ. Oil, tar, and dirt are also repelled and won't stick to a freshly waxed car. This happens because the wax alters the surface. Now the surface is coated with molecules that repel water and debris. In general, clean, dry surfaces will always give better adhesion. A clean surface allows the liquid's molecules to get closer to the surface and to cover more of it. Both of these effects will increase the powerful attractive forces of adhesion. Liquids will not bead up on surfaces that are compatible and clean. Instead, they spread out and flatten, improving adhesion.

You've probably noticed as the wax wears off the car, a bead of water will begin to spread out and flatten into a sheet of water. This effect is called **wetting.** The wetting effect causes liquids to spread out and cover more of the surface, especially a clean, dry surface ⒻⓉ. Water soaks into a compatible surface and causes it to become wet, but other liquids can also wet surfaces. When it comes to adhesives, wetting creates better adhesion. How? If a liquid adhesive can better cover the surface and penetrate more deeply, it will certainly be able to hold much more tightly (Figure 7–1). In general, the better an adhesive or nail enhancement product can wet the surface, the better the adhesion will be. A liquid will wet a surface if it is compatible and not repelled by the surface.

Wetting agents are special ingredients found in many types of products. Wetting agents are designed to make liquids more compatible with a solid surface and less likely to be repelled ⒻⓉ. Automatic dishwashing detergents use wetting agents to keep water from beading and spotting glass. Laundry detergents use wetting agents to help the detergent soak deeper into the fabric instead of being repelled by the surface. Wetting agents help clothing dyes soak in to give a deeper, darker color that resists fading when washed. Wetting agents are also mixed with plant food to improve soil penetration of fertilizers. Wetting agents are used widely around the globe in many thousands of applications. In the professional nail industry, wetting agents are used to improve the adhesion of artificial nail products and help nail cleansers remove oil and contaminants from the nail plate.

The small area between two adhered surfaces (interface) is called the **adhesive bond.** As long as this bond is intact, the surfaces will not come apart. Delamination occurs when the adhesive bond breaks and the two surfaces peel away from each other. Properly cleaning the solid surface and proper application techniques will help prevent delamination.

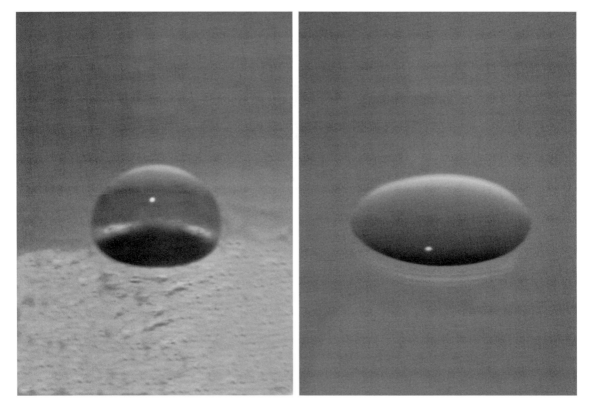

Figure 7-1 *Proper versus improper service wetting—the bead on the left is poorly wetting the surface, while the bead on the right shows better wetting because it has spread out to cover more of the surface*

ADHESIVES KEEP US TOGETHER

An **adhesive** is a chemical that causes two surfaces to stick together. There are many thousands of types of adhesives. Even our bodies create and use adhesives to hold many cells and tissues together. As another example, barnacles are shell-fish that make a natural adhesive that bonds them tightly to the bottom of ocean liners and cargo ships. Adhesives are usually liquids or gooey semisolids. Adhesives perform an important function. They allow incompatible surfaces to be joined together. For example, Scotch tape is a plastic strip coated with a sticky, semisolid adhesive. Without the adhesive coating, the plastic tape would not stick. The sticky adhesive layer acts as a "go-between." It firmly holds the tape to the paper surface. Adhesives are much like an anchor on a ship. One end of the anchor is attached to the ship; the other end is attached to the bottom of the ocean or river. This is how double-sided sticky tape works. Tape with adhesive on both sides can be sandwiched between two surfaces to hold them together.

Adhesives are usually designed specifically for use on certain surfaces. Wood, paper, cloth, ceramic, leather, stone, plastics, metal, and glass are just a few of the surfaces that can be held together with adhesives. Adhesive products are usually formulated to be compatible with a specific surface. If an adhesive was formulated to be compatible with both wood and glass, it could bond them together. It could also hold together two pieces of wood or two pieces of glass. It would not be a very good choice for holding together metal and wood. As with all professional tools, success depends on choosing and using the right adhesive for the job.

GLUES: EARLY TOOLS OF THE ANCIENTS

All glues are adhesives, but not all adhesives are glues. **Glues** are a type of adhesive made from plants or animal parts. Crude glues have been used for over 30,000 years. Ancient stone tools using tar-based glues show that adhesives were probably invented during the Stone Age. Egyptian carvings made 3,300 years ago show workmen gluing thin pieces of fine wood over cheaper pieces of wood (much like the furniture of today). They also used paste made from flour to hold together papyrus fibers to make fabrics. Egg whites were used as book glues and as binding agents for pigments in early art paints. Wood glues have been made of fish, horn, and even cheese. Around 1,500 years ago some North American Indian groups began using collagen adhesives to make archery bows. In the northwestern United States, the local Indians made a waterproof paste out of burned clamshells, salmon eggs, seal's blood, and fish skins. By the 18th century, animal and fish glue technology reached its peak.

Glues are still in use to this day, but only for special purposes. Animal glues are made from collagen, the primary protein of skin, bone, and muscle. When treated with hot water the collagen slowly becomes soluble, and the end result is either gelatin or glue. Casein comes from milk and is used as wood glue. Corn, wheat, potatoes, and rice are used to make cardboard and wallpaper glues. Gums are another type of glue that is usually extracted from tree sap.

During the 19th century new and more effective types of adhesives were introduced. Today, high-tech adhesives have largely replaced old-fashioned natural glues. This new breed of adhesive is not based on animal or vegetable sources and is vastly superior. Oftentimes the word *glue* is incorrectly used to describe professional nail adhesives. Glue is not a type of adhesive that is useful in salons. True glues are low in strength and do not adhere well to the nail plate. They also dissolve easily in warm water. Nail technicians use advanced adhesives designed specifically for professional salons, not glues. You will learn more about professional salon adhesives in later chapters.

PRIMERS MOVE TO PRIME TIME

If wetting agents make liquids more compatible with a solid surface, then what makes a solid surface more compatible with a liquid? **Primers** modify solid surfaces (i.e., the natural nail), making it easier for wetting to occur. Primers can modify the surface in other ways, and these modifications improve product adhesion (FI). Primers are used in many ways. Metal and wood often require primers to keep paint from peeling. Nail polish base coats are primers, too. Nail polish will resist chipping and peeling if a good base coat is used. Base coats adhere better than nail polish. They act as the "go-between" or "anchor" to improve adhesion.

Natural nail primers are sometimes required with artificial nail enhancements. These products are especially useful if the client has oily nail plates or skin, as well as thin or ski-jump nails. There are three main types of nail primers for artificial nails: **acid-based, non-acid,** and **acid-free.** The original primers used in the nail industry were the acid-based primers. Acid-based primers contain between 30 and 100 percent **methacrylic acid** (METH-uh-KRIH-lick acid). Nail technicians around the world have depended on these products to help ensure nail enhancements adhere, even on clients with oily, lift-prone natural nails. A drawback of methacrylic acid primers is that they can cause the enhancement product to yellow. If this type of primer touches the nail enhancement product during a rebalance, it can cause yellowing. If a fresh nail enhancement is applied over wet acid-based primers, yellowing is almost a certainty. For this reason, wet acid-based primers should never be allowed to touch artificial nail products.

But acid-based primers have another disadvantage. Methacrylic acid is highly corrosive to human skin. In Chapter 6, corrosives were defined as substances capable of destroying human tissue on contact. Exposure to corrosive materials can cause permanent, irreversible damage if not quickly treated. As you might expect, they can be very dangerous to the eyes. Over the years hundreds of children have suffered chemical burns in the home when they were accidentally exposed to these products. As a result, in 2001 the Consumer Products Safety Commission (CPSC) began requiring all products containing more than 5 percent methacrylic acid to be sold only in child-resistant packages.

Of course, acid-based primers can be used safely if the appropriate care is taken. This fact was confirmed by the **Cosmetic Ingredient Review (CIR)** expert panel in 1999. The panel, which is made up of independent experts—including doctors, dermatologists, and scientists—who work with the FDA and trade associations to determine the safety of cosmetic ingredients, determined that methacrylic acid is safe for use by trained professional nail technicians who have been taught how to safely handle these professional tools and to avoid skin contact. Of course, if used excessively, acid-based primers can cause problems. For example, if this primer runs into the soft tissues surrounding the nail plate, it can cause painful burns. Also, in Chapter 4 you learned that onycholysis is a condition where the nail plate separates from the nail bed. Several things can lead to this condition. One cause may be overexposure of the nail plate to these acid-based primers. If excessive amounts of methacrylic acid are used (i.e., triple priming), the acid can seep through thin nail plates and cause damage to the underlying nail bed. When it comes to these types of primers, less is more!

Non-acid primers actually do contain an acid, but not methacrylic acid. They are based on other, less corrosive acids. Non-acid primers will not burn skin if they come into contact with it. Even so, prolonged or repeated contact can still cause adverse skin reactions. As with all primers, skin contact must be avoided. Both acid-based primers and non-acid primers improve adhesion by creating many hydrogen bonds between the nail enhancement and natural nail. Hydrogen bonds are temporary bonds that create adhesion by means of the attraction between molecules (as described earlier in this chapter) (FT). Hydrogen bonds do not create permanent chemical linkages. They are the same kind of bond that holds temporary water curls in the hair.

If you were small enough to see a methacrylic acid molecule, you would discover something interesting. This molecule has two "arms." One arm of the molecule develops a hydrogen bond to the keratin surface. The other arm undergoes a chemical reaction and develops a different type of chemical bond, called a covalent bond, linking the primer molecule to the nail enhancement. Covalent bonds are the strongest chemical bonds and are much stronger than hydrogen bonds (FT). Covalent bonds are also longer-lasting. Covalent bonds are everywhere in nature. They make hair curly and give natural nails their strength, durability, and toughness.

Both acid-based and non-acid primers are designed to make the nail plate more compatible with the enhancement product. Even so, the nail enhancement may still lift. One reason is that the hydrogen bond is relatively weak and can be broken. The newer acid-free primers contain absolutely no acid components at all. These primers work in a different way. Both sides of their molecules create covalent bonds between the nail plate and enhancement. These primers do not rely on the weaker hydrogen bonding. Like non-acid primers, they are not corrosive to skin. Nor will they discolor artificial nail products. When used properly, acid-free primers' performance is equal to that of methacrylic acid-based primers and is superior to non-acid primers.

GET A CLEAN START

You can use the best products and application techniques and still have lifting. How can that happen? Nail coatings, such as artificial nail enhancement products, nail polish, tip adhesives, or nail hardeners, will adhere if the natural nail is properly prepared. As you learned in earlier chapters, the nail plate contains a high percentage of both water and oil. Both of these can cause lifting if they are found on the surface of the nail plate. The best way to ensure proper adhesion is to start with a clean, dry surface. Scrubbing the nail plate will remove surface oils and contaminants (such as from cigarette smoke) that interfere with proper adhesion (FT). Scrubbing also gets rid of the bacteria that can lead to infections. Skipping this important step is one of the biggest causes of nail infections. There are several high-quality professional hand and nail scrubs available through your nail product distributor. Both you and your client should use them before every service.

Temporary nail dehydrators are also extremely important tools for nail technicians. Surface moisture will interfere with the adhesive bond between the product and natural nail (FT). Surfaces must be dry before any nail coatings will adhere. Even if you thoroughly dry the nails after scrubbing, the surface of the plate will be covered with an invisible, ultra-thin layer of moisture. This moisture layer must be removed to ensure proper adhesion. This is especially important for artificial nail enhancement products. Nail dehydrators eliminate surface moisture for up to 30 minutes. Moisture will then move up through the nail and rehydrate the nail surface, but this will not affect the nail enhancement's adhesion after the product has hardened.

Since nail polish has much poorer adhesion than artificial nail enhancement products, moisture has a much greater effect on it. Moisture travels upward from the nail bed through the nail plate, but nail polish slows down its evaporation from the nail plate. As moisture builds up underneath the nail polish, the pressure it creates can have a major impact on adhesion. It is believed that the pressure from the moisture, called "back pressure," can literally push the coating from the nail plate, much the way a jack lifts a car. You learned in Chapters 4 and 5 that water manicures can contribute to nail polish lifting. Although water is the culprit in both cases, lifting happens for very different reasons. When water saturates the nail plate, the problem isn't pressure but shape. The nail plates can soak up water and change their shape; some clients' nails undergo a greater change in shape than others'. If the polish dries before the nail reverts back to its original shape, the polish can crack and peel away.

GO FIGURE!

Suppose for a moment that you have a client whose natural nail plates change shape after water manicures. The nails start with a nice curve but end up flat! She insists that you give her a water manicure and won't believe that's the reason her polish cracks so quickly. She wants you to change polish lines instead! You remember that temporary nail dehydrators are important for artificial nail enhancement adhesion and wonder if they will keep her polish from cracking.

They won't. Nail dehydrators designed for use with nail enhancement products will only pull moisture from the very uppermost layers of the natural nail. Since her nails will not fully revert to their normal shape until all excess moisture is gone, a surface dehydrator will have very little effect. These products cannot dehydrate the nail enough to make the plate revert to its original shape. Nature will just have to take its course.

OUCH! NO ROUGH STUFF, IF YOU PLEASE

One of the most dangerous misconceptions in the professional salon industry is that products don't stick unless you "rough up the nail." This is absolutely false and very harmful for clients as well as your business. Nail adhesives and coatings always work better if the nail plate is clean and dry. Roughing up the nail with heavy abrasives or electric files is one way to remove oils and dirt, but it is the wrong way!

Heavy abrasives strip off much of the natural nail plate, leaving it thin, weak, and damaged (FT). This technique weakens the base or supporting structure for the nail enhancement. When artificial nails are removed, clients will quickly discover the damage and thinning caused by overfiling. Often, they will mistakenly assume this is proof that nail enhancement products cause the nail to become thin. Of course, this is a complete myth. Artificial nails do not thin or weaken the natural nail. Abrasives and heavy-handed filing are usually responsible. Coarse abrasives or heavy filing can also damage the nail bed, leading to nail plate separation from the nail bed (onycholysis) and possibly an infection.

Overfiling is a leading cause of nail technician and client problems (FT). Aggressive filing techniques are responsible for:

- Overly thin nail plates
- Increased risks of allergic reactions and infection
- Client's nails aching with pain
- Promoting nail infections
- Nail plate loss
- Product lifting and breakage
- A black eye for the entire nail industry

Roughing up the plate causes dangerous and excessive thinning of the natural nail. This must be avoided at all costs! It makes no sense to improve enhancement adhesion by destroying the natural nail. That's not the job of the professional nail technician. Artificial nails are called "enhancements" for a good reason. Artificial nails are not designed to be replacements for the nail plate. They should enhance and add beauty to the hand and fingers.

Overfiling the natural nail plate is a bad trade! In exchange for better adhesion, the artificial enhancements become more likely to lift, crack, and break. There is less nail plate to support the artificial enhancement. Thin nail plates are more flexible, and the extra flexibility allows the enhancement to bend too easily. This creates invisible, hairline fractures that eventually lead to breakage. Figure 7–2 shows a typical microscopic surface crack. This tiny crack is less than 1/100th of the width of a human hair and would normally go completely unnoticed, but cracks spread. This crack can widen and grow longer each time the nail is hit or bumped. Eventually, the crack will become visible to the client as a break in the artificial nail.

CAN I SHAG YOUR NAILS?

Imagine pouring a small amount of adhesive onto a linoleum floor and some into a deep pile carpet. After the adhesive dried, which would be easier to clean up? The dried adhesive would peel easily from the smooth floor, but it would be a nightmare to clean the carpet.

Aggressive filing techniques on the natural nail can give the keratin a shag-carpet-like surface. Adhesion is achieved because the enhancement product can harden into the damaged nail surface. Luckily, with the right products and techniques, it's not necessary to damage or destroy the nail plate to get good adhesion.

Lastly, thinning the nail plate makes it easier for ingredients to soak through the nail plate and into the nail bed. This can increase the risks of allergic reactions and chemical burns to the nail bed. There is much more to learn about allergic reaction causes and prevention, but that will have to wait until Chapter 12.

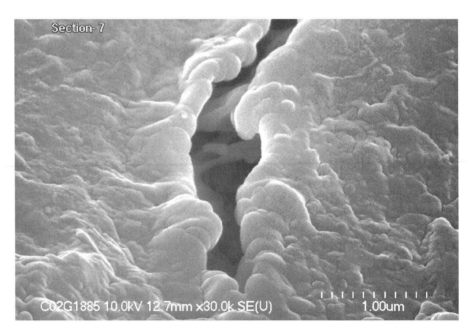

Figure 7-2 *Microscopic crack on the surface of the natural nail. This nearly invisible crack is about 1/100th of the width of a human hair*

Figure 7-3 *Nail bed hemorrhaging (bleeding) under the nail plate can be caused by aggressive filing techniques*

HOT TIME IN THE SALON

It's very easy to seriously injure the natural nail with an abrasive. How? Heat is the culprit! Heat is created by friction when two surfaces rub together. Rubbing the hands together creates enough heat to make them feel very warm. Imagine how much heat an aggressive filing technique can generate. When the heat becomes excessive, it can literally burn the nail bed with temperatures as high as 145°F (63°C). Friction burns on the nail bed can lead to all sorts of problems. Some examples of aggressive filing techniques are:

- Using abrasive files harsher than 180 grit on the natural nail
- Using too much pressure or downward force on the board while filing
- Using an electric file on the top surface of the natural nail[1]
- Excessive pressure or use of a three-way or chamois buffer

Each of these has a great potential to overthin the nail and possibly injure the nail plate or bed (Figure 7–3). A light touch with a 180-grit file or higher is

---

[1]Improperly using an electric file on the natural nail is a leading cause of client injury. This is an advanced technique that should be used only by skilled and experienced nail technicians who have received the proper formal training and understand how to avoid damaging clients' nails. This is not a suitable technique for students or beginners.

the best way to protect the health of the natural nail. Also, be careful not to focus your filing on any one area for too long. This can also create sufficient heat to burn the nail bed tissues.

Need to rough up the nail plate to get good adhesion? Then something is wrong! Many nail technicians have great success without roughing up the nail plate. How do they do it? The answer is simple: they take the time to properly prepare the nail plates and use correct application techniques and high-quality products. Lifting problems are always traced back to one of these three areas: improper preparation, incorrect application, and poor-quality products. So if you excel in proper nail preparation, you'll be spending much less time doing repairs.

SAFELY USING ELECTRIC FILES

Electric files can be useful tools, but only if they are used by licensed and trained nail professionals who understand how to safely and correctly handle these devices. Just because you can buy an electric file doesn't mean you can or should operate one! Nail technicians should not use electric files without the proper training. These devices operate at high speeds, generate large amounts of heat, and can cause serious nail damage and injuries if used incorrectly *(FT)*. For more information on electric file training courses, you should contact the **Association of Electric File Manufacturers (AEFM)** at their Web site, www.aefm.org. Make sure you get proper training before using these devices on clients. The AEFM can help you find basic electric file training courses, as well as advanced courses for those who wish to further develop their skills. For further information, see the useful checklist in Chapter 17 entitled "Dos and Don'ts for Safe Electric File Use" by Nancy King, AEFM director.

Nail products are not all alike. Some are more compatible with the nail plate. The same is true for application techniques. Heavy filing can compensate for low-quality products or improper preparation or application. But overfiling is not a solution—it's a problem! In fact, this is one of the bigger problems in the professional nail industry. Overfiling is a crutch that will eventually lead to failure. Remember, professional products require skill in order to use them correctly. If you are sloppy or use improper techniques, you can expect to have problems. Remember, when quality products are properly applied to a well-prepared surface, it is not necessary to damage the nail plate to get good adhesion.

FAST TRACK *(FT)*

(FT) Adhesion is a force of nature that makes two surfaces stick together.

(FT) Adhesion is an interaction between molecules on different surfaces.

(FT) Entanglement is a type of adhesion created by tangled molecules.

(FT) A chemical reaction must occur to link molecules together with strong bonds.

(FT) Adhesion is more likely to occur when two surfaces are compatible.

(FT) Beading and streaking are signs that a solid surface is repelling a liquid.

(FT) Removing oils and moisture may overly dry and damage the nail's surface.

(FT) Wetting agents make liquids more compatible with solid surfaces.

(FT) Primers make solid surfaces more compatible with liquids.

(FT) Hydrogen bonds are temporary bonds that rely on attraction.

(FT) Covalent bonds form permanent bonds between molecules.

(FT) Surface oils and contaminants interfere with proper adhesion.

(FT) Surface moisture can interfere with the adhesive bond of nail coatings.

(FT) Heavy abrasives strip the natural nail plate, leaving it thin and weak.

(FT) Overfiling is a leading cause of nail technician and client problems.

(FT) Heavy abrasives or drills used at high speeds generate large amounts of heat and may cause serious damage.

Review Questions

1. What causes adhesion?

2. If two surfaces are not compatible they will _____ each other.

3. _____ are special ingredients that make liquids more compatible with solid surfaces.

4. _____ are special ingredients that make solid surfaces more compatible with liquids.

5. What is the area between two adhered surfaces called?

6. Define delamination. How is it prevented?

7. An _____ is a chemical that causes two surfaces to stick together.

8. List three types of artificial nail primer. Which are not corrosive?

9. Hydrogen bonds form _____ bonds, while covalent bonds form _____ bonds.

10. Is it necessary to rough up the nail plate to make high-quality, professional nail products adhere well to the nail plate? Explain why or why not.

11. What causes the heat generated during heavy filing of the natural nail?

12. Why do nail dehydrators improve adhesion?

13. Explain how moisture in the nail affects nail polish adhesion.

14. How long will the nail remain dry after nail dehydrators have been used?

15. Give two examples of an aggressive filing technique.

Chapter

8

Product Chemistry Essentials

Objective

In this chapter you will learn the essentials needed to understand the chemistry behind artificial nails, nail polish, and treatments. You will discover the difference between products that polymerize and those that rely on evaporation. With the knowledge you gain in this chapter, you will be better equipped to understand these important products and how to troubleshoot problems.

A PRETTY COAT FOR MY NAILS?

Nail technicians must perform many tasks. One of the most important of these is to apply coatings to the nail plate. *Coating* is a generic term for any products that cover the nail plate with a hard film. Some examples are nail polish, topcoats, base coats, treatments, artificial enhancements, and tip adhesives. All nail coatings can be divided into two categories: coatings that cure or polymerize and coatings that harden upon evaporation. Let's take a look at both and see how they work.

COATINGS THAT POLYMERIZE

Nail enhancements are a special type of coating used to provide artificial nail services. There are three basic types:

1. *Natural nail overlays* are coatings that cover only the nail plate.
2. *Tip and overlays* cover an artificial, preformed plastic tip and the natural nail plate.
3. A *sculptured nail* extends a coating beyond the free edge of the nail plate without the use of a preformed tip.

Many different types of products are used to perform these artificial nail enhancement services. They may seem quite different at first glance, but they have many things in common. For example, every product uses a chemical reaction called **polymerization.**

Monomers and Polymers: What's the Difference?

In Chapter 6 we learned that a molecule is the simplest form of a chemical substance. You also learned that molecules are like a Tinkertoy set. They can be arranged and rearranged into almost unlimited combinations. Molecules are rearranged by chemical reactions. Creating an artificial nail enhancement is a good example of a chemical reaction. Billions of molecules must react and join together to create a single sculptured nail ⓕⓣ. Some molecules link together into extremely long chains. These very long chains are called **polymers.** Polymers can be liquids, but they are usually solid. *Poly-* means "many" and *-mer* means "unit." In this case, the units are molecules. Therefore, polymers are many molecules joined together. The polymers used to make artificial nail powders are a perfect example. Each individual bead contains many thousands of different polymer chains. Each chain contains between 3,000 and 10,000 molecules. Chemical reactions that create polymers are called polymerizations ⓕⓣ. Sometimes the term **cure** or *curing* is used, but these terms all have the same meaning. There are many different types of polymers. Teflon, nylon, and plastics are polymers. But even hair, paper, and wood are polymers. In Chapter 2, we learned that amino acids are molecules that link together into long chains called proteins. Proteins are also polymers. Nail plates are made of a polymer protein called keratin.

Many molecules hook together to make a long polymer chain. By itself, just one of these molecules is called a **monomer.** *Mono-* means "one." Therefore, a monomer is a molecule that can join with others to create polymer chains Ⓕ. If only one type of monomer is used, then the polymer will consist of a long chain of these monomers. When a polymer is made from only one monomer, it is called a homopolymer Ⓕ. If two different types of monomers are used, then the polymer chain will consist of two different types of monomer. Polymers made from two different types of monomers are called **copolymers** Ⓕ.

Many different types of monomers are used to create nail enhancements. Nail technicians use tip adhesives, wrap resins, liquid/powder systems, UV gels, and no-light gels. These product types may seem very different, but they all use monomers in their formulation.

The Great Monomer Race

Have you ever wondered how monomers turn into polymers? Monomers are like track runners mingling around the starting line, patiently waiting for the race to begin, walking back and forth past each other but never bumping into or brushing against each other. Their race starts only when the proper signal is given. Once the signal is given, nothing can stop them until they reach the finish line. Monomers are like that, too. They need a signal to start their race toward becoming part of a polymer chain. Until that signal is given, they mingle around the container. They are waiting for the **initiator** molecule to signal the start of polymerization Ⓕ.

In the first step, the initiator molecule absorbs some extra energy and forms a chemical bond with a monomer. The energetic initiator molecule is in an excited state and wants to relax, so it gives a jolt of energy to the monomer. But monomers prefer the quiet life. They don't appreciate too much excitement, so they immediately try to get rid of the extra energy. The only way to do that is by attaching themselves to the tail end of another monomer and passing the extra energy on to their newest partner. The second monomer doesn't like the energy either, so it uses the same trick and attaches firmly to a passing monomer's tail. As the game of tag continues, the chain of monomers gets longer and longer and longer. Sooner or later the polymer chain won't be able to find any more monomers and the chain reaction will come to an end. We can watch this great race from start to finish, right on the nail plate. Of course, monomers are far too small to see. Even so, you'll soon discover that you can see them in action.

And They're Off!

Nail product monomers have the appearance of thin, free-flowing liquids. They are like this because the molecules are free to roam anywhere in the container, unhindered. But once the energized initiators begin the reaction, monomer chains sprout up everywhere. They begin to grow longer, rapidly adding new monomers to the end of their chains. Soon the many long strings of monomers start getting in each other's way, becoming tangled and knotted. Eventually, they can no longer move freely and the polymer becomes a mass of microscopic strings. It may look solid and even feel solid enough to file with an abrasive, but the chemical reaction is not finished. It will take days, weeks, or months before the chains reach their ultimate lengths. How long it takes will depend on many factors, including the ratio of monomer to polymer as well as the type of monomer and initiator used.

Now imagine for a moment that you were small enough to watch this with your eyes. What would happen if there weren't enough monomers to make long polymer chains? Many stunted, short chains of monomers would develop. They are so short that it would take many of them linked together to make a polymer. What would the short chains be like? Would they be solid or liquid?

Oligomers are short chains of monomers (FT). *Oligo-* means "few." Oligomer chains usually contain between 5 and 500 monomers. Oligomer chains are too long to flow freely like monomers, but they are too short to become a solid mass. Oligomers exist between these two states. They are usually very thick and have a stringy, gel-like appearance. You will learn in Chapter 10 that UV gels are made of oligomers. Even though their appearance is different from that of monomers, oligomers will react in the same way as monomers to form polymer chains. They pass energy to the next oligomer by linking together in a head-to-tail fashion.

Would You Like Your Polymer Simple or Cross-linked?

Once the growing chain contains around 500 monomers, a **simple polymer** is formed and begins to harden. As they continue to lengthen and polymerize, the polymer chains become intertwined and harden into a tangled mass of chains. The chains are now locked into place, much like a very dense undergrowth of vines in the rain forest. But soak the polymer in the right solvents and the entire mass will unravel!

Recall from Chapter 6 that solvents have the ability to dissolve other substances (solutes) (FT). Acetone provides the perfect example of how this works. Tip adhesives and wrap resins (which are actually monomers) will form simple polymers that harden into tangled masses. Soaking in acetone will cause them to unravel and dissolve, making removal a quick and easy task. Other solvents will also dissolve these polymers, but not as safely or efficiently. Even soaking in water for a few days will cause some simple polymers to begin to break down. This is why nail polish removers (solvents) can weaken wrap-type artificial nails and tip adhesives. These solvents seep into tiny nooks and crannies on the surface and are absorbed. As more and more solvent is absorbed, the polymer swells and microscopic cracks form on the surface. These tiny cracks may grow later and lead to breakage when stress is put on the nail.

Figure 8–1 shows a highly magnified photograph of a crack caused by solvents. This crack is 1/10th the thickness of a human hair. Even though it is small, it can quickly grow larger if the polymer is flexed or stressed. Many things can

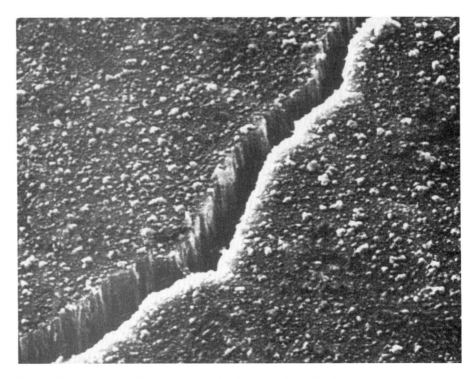

Figure 8-1 *Highly magnified microscopic crack in the surface of a simple polymer*

cause cracks to grow. Even a rapid and dramatic change in temperature can enlarge cracks. For example, taking bare hands from a warm salon into the cold of winter can damage enhancements and cause service breakdown. Why? The rapid change in temperature can cause small, invisible cracks to grow in size, becoming large visible cracks or lifted areas. This is why gloves are highly recommended for artificial nail wearers in cold climates.

Polymer chains can also be unraveled by force. Products with simple polymer chains are easily damaged by sharp impacts or sudden stresses. Strength and durability are not their strong points. Dyes and other substances can also get lodged between the tangled chains. Nail polishes, marker ink, and foods are some of the things that can be absorbed and cause unsightly stains on the surface.

To overcome these problems, many types of nail enhancement products use a very special type of monomer called a **cross-linker.** A cross-linker is a monomer that can join different polymer chains together. Cross-linkers are monomers with two or three extra "arms." Monomers and cross-linkers also will join together in a head-to-tail fashion. Once they become part of the polymer chain cross-linkers use their extra arms to either develop a new branch or join with other nearby chains. Each place where two chains are joined together is called a cross-link. Cross-links are like rungs on a ladder. Their job is to create strong, netlike polymer structures out of wimpy, stringlike polymers (FT). Cross-links can also join layers from any direction, even from above or below. This is what creates a three-dimensional structure of much greater strength and durability than simple polymer chains could ever hope to achieve (Figure 8–2 and Color Plate 19). Obviously, a cross-linked net is stronger than a bunch of tangled chains. Nets are less likely to break under sudden impacts or stresses. Besides increased durability, the cross-linking protects the surface from nail polish, ink, and dye stains. Cross-linked surfaces are also impervious to nail polish removers. The disadvantage is that cross-links make the artificial nails more resistant to all solvents, so removal becomes much more difficult.

IPNs: The Reinforcers

Polymer chains can be strengthened in many ways. Cross-linking is one important way. But too many cross-links make polymers brittle and more easily shattered, since this lowers flexibility and reduces toughness. A better way to reinforce and toughen is with interpenetrating polymer networks, or IPNs. Imagine weaving a strong polymer rope through the holes of the cross-linked net. The rope will add toughness to the net without causing brittleness. This is how IPNs work: they start as monomers, but they weave new and different chains through the polymer network. They do not become part of the cross-linked net. Instead, they reinforce it! IPNs were first used for high-tech aerospace polymers but now are found in certain nail enhancement products. Why? Remember from Chapter 2, a balance of strength and flexibility equals toughness. This technology is used

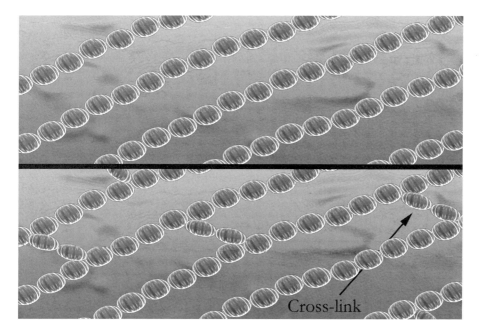

Figure 8-2 *Simple versus cross-linked polymers: the simple polymer chains appear in the upper half of the image, the cross-linked chains in the lower half*

to create nail enhancements with dramatically increased toughness and durability without sacrificing flexibility.

Energize Me!

Energy is the final key to understanding how monomers become polymers. Monomers need energy to become part of a polymer chain. This energy comes from the initiator molecule. Initiator molecules control everything. They are the starting gun that begins the monomer marathon. But where does the initiator molecule get this energy? What is the source? This is one of the most important questions in nail chemistry!

Different initiators use different kinds of energy. Initiators absorb and hold energy. In a sense, they are like batteries. Some initiators only absorb light energy. Other initiators only absorb heat energy. Light and heat are the only types of energy useful for making nail enhancement polymers. Products that require light will generally depend on ultraviolet (UV) light. All other artificial nail products use heat as their energy source, such as body heat, the heat from a table lamp, and room heat.

Light and Heat Are Energy?

If you have ever seen sunlight passing through a prism or watched a rainbow in the sky, then you know that sunlight is made of many colors. These colors are called the **visible spectrum** (FT). All light is a form of energy. We use this energy every day. Solar cells absorb light energy and transform it into electricity. Plants need light energy to grow. Clearly, sunlight is a powerful form of energy. Each color we see is a different level of energy (FT). That is why they look different to our eyes. Red has the lowest energy level of visible light. Violet has the highest energy level of visible light (FT). The next energy level above violet is called ultraviolet (FT). Levels higher than violet cannot be seen by the human eye, but some reptiles, amphibians, birds, and fish have ultraviolet vision. Even though we cannot see UV light, we can see its effects. For example, UV light will tan the skin and cause photographs to yellow. At the other end of the spectrum, the next lower level of light energy under the color red is called **infrared light** (FT). We can't see infrared light either, but we feel it. Infrared light is also called heat. Heat is a form of light that we cannot see. Its energy level is too low for the detectors in our eyes. But rattlesnakes can see infrared light and use it to hunt at night. Even though our eyes can't see it, the skin is sensitive to infrared light energy and can be burned at high intensities.

Understanding which type of energy an enhancement product needs for polymerization can solve many problems in a salon. For example, it is important to cover UV-light-curing products even when they are not near a UV gel light. Sunlight through a window and true-color lights contain enough UV light to start the polymerization process. The result? The composition of your product will change, lowering its quality and even causing it to harden in the container.

Also, it is easier to see why heat-curing monomers should never be left in a hot car or truck, a store window, or other warm area. The high heat can cause a small amount of product to prematurely polymerize in the container, thus lowering the quality of the product. This may go unnoticed, but it can still cause problems. Heat can cause the liquid monomer product to form a gooey gel at the bottom of the container, while remaining a liquid on top. If this product is used on clients anyway, expect a wide range of service breakdown issues to occur. See how a little knowledge goes a long way? Solving and avoiding problems is a lot easier if you understand the basics!

Which Is Which?

Products that use light energy are light-curing products. All other nail enhancement products are heat-curing products. Why don't they have to be heated? The answer is simple. They use the heat in the room and body heat to cause polymerization or curing. That's enough energy for them. You might not notice the heat in most rooms unless you had just come in from a snowstorm. But there is a tremendous amount of heat in the average room; otherwise we would freeze to death. Artificial nail enhancement products will cure best at room temperature, 68–77°F (20–25°C). The same is true for tip adhesives and wrap resins. Body heat is important as well. Your fingernail beds are approximately 97°F (36°C). That's pretty warm compared to room temperature. Sculpt on a plastic tip on a stick and you will see that the heat-curing products polymerize more slowly on the tip than when applied to a fingernail.

Some types of products require normal incandescent lightbulbs to harden. These are *not* light-curing monomers. They are using the extra heat released from the lightbulb to evaporate the solvents and speed drying. Even though a light is used, these products are still heat-curing. The same thing happens when these products are put under UV lamps. These lamps produce enough warmth to speed up solvent evaporation. But the UV light can discolor the topcoat. This "heat trick" will work with any type of topcoat or polish. Remember, just because the product will harden under UV light doesn't mean it's curing by UV light. The best way to tell if a product is truly UV-curing is by examining its ease of removal. True UV-curing products undergo cross-linking and will not be easily removed with any solvent. If the artificial nail enhancement can be removed in a few minutes with acetone or damaged within seconds by using polish remover, the product is not UV-curing.

See the Light

Rather than absorbing UV light, some initiators absorb blue and violet light. It is possible to cure some artificial nail products with blue and violet light. These products have some advantages, but there are two major drawbacks. The amount of UV light in the normal salon is very low, except near a sunlit window. But there is lots of blue and violet light in the salon. Just like photographic film, visible-light-curing products are extremely sensitive to room light. They prematurely polymerize more easily than UV gels when exposed to normal salon lighting. Too much light exposure can cause products to thicken in the container and can lead to many other quality-related problems. Therefore, if you use a visible-light-curing product, make certain to minimize exposure to all light. You can easily tell if a product uses visible light. The unit used to cure it puts out a very hot, bright white light, instead of the familiar soft blue light of a UV gel lamp. The intense heat generated by visible-light lamps is yet another drawback of this type of a system. Because of these issues, visible-light-curing products have not become a commercial success.

Catalysts Turn Initiators On

Although catalysts were discussed in Chapter 6, their role in product chemistry has not been completely explored. As you recall, catalysts are used in nail products to make chemical reactions happen more quickly. At the beginning of this chapter, initiators were compared to a starting gun. In many ways, catalysts are like a trigger on the gun. By themselves, initiators are fairly slow to excite monomers or oligomers. Catalysts "turn on" the initiator *FYI* . They make initiators work faster and more efficiently. Later, you will see that all artificial nail products need initiators, energy, and catalysts. If one of these is missing, chemical reactions will happen much more slowly or not at all.

Shrinkage

All polymers shrink when they are created. There are no exceptions for any artificial nail enhancements or tip adhesives. Monomers are so small they are invisible, even under the most powerful microscope. Still, scientists know many things about them. Monomers used to create artificial nails are some of the most researched and studied molecules on earth. They are used in thousands of other applications, including bone cement, dentures, contact lenses, airplane windows, and many household items. Scientists know that monomers normally don't touch each other. They bounce around the container at high speeds trying to avoid other monomers. They join only when the conditions are correct. When they do come together and link, the monomers embrace each other tightly. This explains why polymers shrink! Imagine watching a billion monomers suddenly coming closer together. The shrinkage would be very noticeable as the crowd of molecules moved inward and became more compact. That's what causes shrinkage. In fact, nail enhancement polymers shrink between 4 and 18 percent or more. Some types shrink more than others. Excessive shrinkage (above 12 percent) causes many problems; such as lifting, tip cracking, and other types of service breakdown.

Too much cross-linking causes excessive shrinkage as well. Overshrinkage may cause the product to lift in the center of the nail plate. When the enhancement pulls away in small pockets, it can have the appearance of small bubbles underneath the nail enhancement. As mentioned before, one way to increase the durability without increasing shrinkage is with IPNs. Because IPNs don't add extra cross-links to the net, they don't create shrinkage.

How can nail technicians control shrinkage? It is important to understand that the improper ratio of liquid monomer to polymer powder (too wet a consistency) causes excessive shrinkage. Using products at the correct ratio will lower shrinkage. Avoiding working with too wet a ratio is one of the biggest challenges that nail technicians face. Products must be used with a medium consistency, not wet! Other problems caused by shrinkage and incorrect product ratios will be discussed in later chapters.

Exothermic Reactions

When two monomers join and bond, an extremely tiny amount of heat is released. This is called an **exothermic reaction. Exothermic** means "heat-releasing" *FT* . All types of artificial nail enhancement products and tip adhesives undergo exothermic reactions. Some types of products are more noticeable than others. Of course, you cannot feel the heat released from just two monomers. But remember, billions of monomers react to form a single nail enhancement. Can you feel the heat of this many monomers as they interact? Definitely yes! This heat is called an **exotherm.** Under certain circumstances it can be quite noticeable or even painful, especially when using wrap resin systems, UV-light-cured products, and fast-set monomer liquid/powder systems. Unless the heat causes your clients to become uncomfortable, you should not be overly concerned. A slight warming will benefit the enhancement by providing additional energy for the curing process, especially with liquid/powder systems. However, exotherms that burn the client's nail beds can cause damage to the tissue and may weaken the enhancement *FT* . Why do wrap, fast-set monomer liquid/powders, and UV gel systems generate more heat? There are several reasons. Mostly it depends on how quickly the heat is released. Products that release heat very quickly will feel more intensely hot. If the same amount of heat is released more slowly, it would only feel warm or might not even be noticeable. In other words, rapid heat buildup is the problem. Below are four other factors that may cause a noticeable exotherm:

1. *Temperature of the room and/or product.* The warmer the artificial nail product, the faster it will cure. This is much more important for heat-curing products but also true of light-curing products to a lesser degree. If the room is too warm or if you use a halogen table lamp or incandescent bulb higher than 60 watts, the extra heat makes monomers react faster. Sometimes your clients will feel their nail beds become very warm, even hot!

Solution: Use low-wattage or fluorescent bulbs and don't store monomers in warm locations. Also, never put any type of professional nail product in a window, car trunk, or other warm location. Keep them cool but not cold. This will improve the shelf life and protect product quality. Also, control the temperature around your work area. It is best to maintain 68–77°F (20–25°C) to ensure proper set of artificial nail enhancements.

2. *Excessive initiator or catalyst.* Faster is not always better. It takes time to do things right. To meet the demands of busy nail professionals, some manufacturers increase the level of initiator or catalysts to make faster-curing products. Faster set means more heat is released in a shorter time. This can lead to uncomfortably warm exotherms. Excessive initiator or catalyst also may cause enhancements to lose flexibility, lower toughness, and badly discolor. Wrap catalysts must be used exactly as recommended in order to prevent painful exotherms. Some specially formulated brush-on wrap products don't require the application of a catalyst. But these products harden and cure more slowly.

UV-light-curing products can also produce high amounts of heat, especially if the initiator levels are too high or if the product is cured with a mismatched UV lamp. In other words, UV gel products are designed for curing with a specific UV lamp. The product and lamp are designed to work together for best performance, just as monomer liquids must be used with the correct powder. It is obvious that the best results will be achieved when there is a proper balance between the UV lamp, the UV bulb, and the UV gel product. These three UV partners should work together in unison to ensure the balance is maintained. One great way is by ensuring to use the correct UV replacement bulbs in your UV lamp.

Different UV lightbulbs generate different amounts of UV light energy. Don't just go by the wattage of the UV light. Wattage can be very misleading! Some 27-watt UV lamp units create more UV light energy than other 36-watt lamp units. The wattage of the light is *not* the amount of UV light energy released by the bulb. **Wattage** is the amount of electrical power that the bulb will consume while producing light ⒻⓉ. Wattage tells you how expensive the bulb is to run, not how much UV light they produce. Don't choose a UV lamp based on its wattage. Instead, only purchase the UV lamp that was designed for the UV gel system you choose. Remember, it is very important to use the correct UV light with the proper UV gel.

Solution: If clients complain of heat, do not use fast-set products on their nails. Make sure you're using the correct UV light and properly applying the UV gel. The more thickly the product is applied, the more heat it will release. The same is true for liquid/powder enhancement products.

3. *Unhealthy or damaged nail beds.* Damage to the nail bed is one of the leading reasons for clients' complaints of burning sensations. Damaged nail beds are like a sore tooth. Tapping with your finger on a healthy tooth doesn't hurt, but don't try it on an aching tooth! Normally nail beds are not very sensitive to heat. But a damaged nail bed is highly sensitive and can feel exotherms much more easily. Common causes for damaged nail beds are overfiling and overpriming with acid-based primers. Heavy abrasives or aggressive filing techniques can friction-burn nail beds, leaving them sore and tender. Abrasive grits between 60 and 120 and electric files used directly on nail plates can friction-burn the beds, making them more sensitive to normal product exotherms.

Excessive amounts of methacrylic acid primers, especially on thinned nail plates, can seep through to the sensitive nail bed tissues and cause damage (*FT*). If your clients experience painful exotherms on all fingers, it could be that their nails have been abused by either overfiling or excessive use of acid-based primers. But if they complain of heating on only one or two fingers or the thumbs, overfiling is the more likely reason. Either way, when it comes to filing and primers, remember: less is more.

Solution: Use light abrasives and a light touch on the natural nail. Only remove the shine. Filing should only remove oils, not rough up the nail. Oils are what makes the nail plate shiny and causes product to lift. Don't use the heavy-handed approach when filing. No more than 5 percent of the nail plate should be removed. Also, avoid using excessive amounts of acid-based primer (containing methacrylic acid). With acid-based primers, all that is needed is just enough to barely wet the nail plate.

4. *Metal sculpting forms.* Metal can act as a catalyst. Sculpting on metal or metallized forms may cause mild exotherms. Healthy nail beds will experience minimal warming only. As mentioned before, this warming can actually be beneficial to the curing of the enhancement.

Solution: Usually no special action is required since the exotherm is quite mild and beneficial to the curing process. But if the warmth causes clients to complain, try switching to a plastic or paper form.

Yellowing, Brittleness, and Other Signs of Aging

Yellowing and premature aging of nail enhancements can be caused by many things. There are many reasons why nail enhancements become dingy or develop an off color. Some technicians just accept yellowing or brittleness, thinking this cannot be avoided. When enhancements become brittle or develop an off color, something is wrong! If you take the time to find the problem, it can usually be solved. Don't be satisfied with your work until you can create color-stable, durable nail enhancements. Below, you will find a list of reasons for these problems. Use this information to avoid these common pitfalls.

1. Simple polymers (i.e., wrap resins) can absorb color between the chains, causing stains. Nail polish, household cleaning products, and some types of sunscreen-containing lotions and bronzers may all be absorbed into the surface to cause artificial nail discoloration. These types of stains can usually be filed away. If this is so, you have an important clue. If the stain is only on the surface, something has come in contact with the surface of the enhancement to cause a discoloration. This clue makes identifying the cause much easier. In this case, try using a base coat or wearing gloves to prevent discoloration.

2. If a nail enhancement discolors immediately upon application, this may be a sign of product contamination. Brush contamination is a likely cause. Some nail technicians store their brushes upside down with the hairs pointed upward. Monomer may run into the base of the brush, collect there, and become

discolored. Eventually the discolored product will run back into the hairs of the brush, causing yellowing of new product. If your brush has a wooden handle, monomer contact with the handle inside the metal ferrule can leave discolored monomer in the brush. If you use more than one type of enhancement product, always use a separate brush for each different product. Cross-contamination between products can occur and lead to discoloration of normally color-stable products. Always lay brushes flat when not in use. Store them in a clean, dry, covered container. The brush's hairs should never touch anything except the enhancement product and a clean wiping towel.

3. Improperly cleaning brushes can also contaminate them. Residues from detergents and oils may cause discoloration and lifting. Liquid monomer users should clean the brush with the same monomer. A good rule of thumb is that nail technicians should always use a different brush for each product. Why? No one will take the proper amount of time nor will they want to use enough monomer to properly clean the brush. It would take several changes of the new monomer in the dappen dish (and extra time) to ensure that all the old monomer had been rinsed from the brush. That's just not time-saving or cost-effective! Using the same brush for two different monomer liquids is a bad idea no matter how you look at it. Brush contamination is a leading cause of enhancement discoloration and lifting. Dedicated brushes help ensure that clients will be satisfied with their services. They also make the nail tech's job easier, since you'll be doing fewer repairs. That's cost-effective and time-saving, too!

Never use soap or detergent on your nail brushes. Avoid using solvent-based cleaners, since they can dry out the hairs over time. Solvents can also soak into wooden handles and allow contaminates to leach back into the belly of brush. Value and properly maintain your tools. Clean brushes correctly and never use soaps, detergents, or oils to clean or condition them.

4. Dappen dishes and pumps can also be a source of contamination. Dappen dishes should be cleaned between clients. Never leave product in them overnight. Never add fresh monomer to a dirty dappen dish or pump. Monomer residues can build up inside pump containers, so clean them regularly. Finally, always fill dappen dishes and pumps from a 4-ounce container. Avoid filling from larger containers (FT). Repeatedly opening and closing the liquid monomer container allows for excessive evaporation. This affects the quality and composition of the product. After many repeated openings, discoloration and service breakdown may begin to occur. If you purchase a large (8- to 32-ounce) container of monomer:

- Use this to refill your 4-ounce container.
- Be sure to use all of the product before it expires. Out-of-date product can be a cause of discoloration.
- Pour out only the amount of monomer needed for the service. Never pour unused monomer back into the container. This can dramatically affect the quality of the product and cause yellowing and other types of service breakdown.

5. Monomers must be mixed with the correct amount of polymer powder. Using the proper ratio of liquid to powder is critical. Too much liquid or powder can have disastrous consequences. Yellowing and brittleness are some of the effects of improper consistency. Use a medium bead consistency; avoid a mixture that is too wet or too dry. More information on this extremely important topic will be given in the next chapter.

6. Many problems, including yellowing and brittleness, can be traced back to incorrect use. Nail technicians often fail to realize the importance of exactly following manufacturer's instructions. For example, monomer liquids are designed for use with a specific polymer powder. Never use polymer powder and monomer liquid from two different manufacturers ⒡. Use only the powder designed for the monomer liquid. It is risky to create custom products, unless directed to do so by the manufacturer of each of the involved products. For example, some manufacturers teach nail technicians how to custom-blend colored "nail art" powders to achieve a wide range of colorations. This is fine, as long as the manufacturer's recommendations are followed. Creating custom blends by mixing powders (or liquids) made by different manufacturers is risky and irresponsible. Such practices can cause allergic reactions. If the client develops a serious problem, you are legally responsible for your actions. It will be difficult to explain why you did not follow directions. Never mix systems or break apart systems that were specifically designed to work together. Also, never alter manufacturer's products by mixing or adding other ingredients.

7. Topcoats are very useful products, but they contain ingredients that can yellow. If you apply them directly over nail enhancements, they can discolor over time. In most cases, once the topcoat is removed the discoloration disappears. Use care when applying topcoat over unpolished nail enhancements. A discolored topcoat can leave a yellow stain on the top surface of the enhancements. A good base coat can help prevent this from happening.

8. If enhancements become yellow or brittle after several days or weeks, sunlight and the environment are most likely the causes. UV light from the sun or tanning bed can discolor enhancements. **Ozone** (a component of smog) can also create brittleness. UV light and ozone are responsible for cracks in car dashboards. Sunlight contains so much UV light that it can badly yellow a newspaper in one afternoon. Proper application, as well as the product's formulation, often determine a nail enhancement's resistance to these environmental factors.

9. Improperly formulated products are more prone to yellowing. Properly formulated products are highly resistant to yellowing and premature aging. You will learn later that some products use special absorbers to filter out damaging UV light. Fast-setting monomer liquid/powder systems often yellow and become brittle because of excessive catalyst or initiator levels. Also, products are not all the same. They usually contain different combinations of ingredients or special "secret" additives to enhance performance. In general, a poor choice of ingredients leads to poorly formulated products that discolor and become brittle. As the old saying goes, you get what you pay for. If the least expensive products are used,

don't expect them to perform like more expensive products. It's a simple rule of economics—if a manufacturer can charge more for a product, it can put higher-quality ingredients into the formulation. Manufacturers of low-cost products must keep ingredient costs as low as possible. That's no surprise! If discoloration occurs, contact the manufacturer's customer support to find out how to prevent it from occurring. Give the manufacturer a chance to solve your problem. If nothing they suggest seems to work, review your technique and make sure it is correct from beginning to end. Then, if all else fails, try another product. But remember, if your techniques are the problem, then changing products won't help. The best way to know is to test the products. For example, it's easy to evaluate products for color stability. Try the following:

- Adhere several of your favorite tips to wooden pusher sticks.

- Overlay or sculpture a nail enhancement on to the tips, following your normal technique. If testing UV gels, be sure to test the clear gels. The same is true for polymer powders. Be sure to test monomer liquids using a clear or translucent powder. Pink, natural, or white powders can cover up product discoloration. Of course, you can use this same test to determine the color stability of other products. Apply your current product to one set of tips and do the same with the test product. The product that you currently use will be the baseline or standard for comparison.

- Properly label each tip so they can be identified later, then place the test tips in direct sunlight for a few days.

- Check them each day and compare the test product to your current product's performance to see which yellows first. A properly formulated product will not yellow, even after days of exposure.

- Repeat the test if you are still unsure. Test as many products as you need to convince yourself that the results are correct.

- You can use this same method to test polishes, topcoats, and treatments as well.

Porosity and Permeability

Some people will tell you that artificial nail enhancements that are more porous are better. They can even give you some convincing-sounding reasons why they believe this is true. But some will argue that less porous enhancements are better, and their arguments sound just as convincing. Which is correct? Neither! Confusion arises because this term is used incorrectly. **Porosity** is a measure of how many voids or spaces there are in a solid substance. It is the ratio of the volume of voids to the total volume of the substance. The more voids, the greater the porosity. It's as simple as that. Soil, paper, and sponges are examples of substances that have lots of empty spaces, making them highly porous.

Actually, porosity is not as important as some believe when it comes to artificial nails. When properly applied, there shouldn't be any significant voids in the artificial nail. Of course no solid material is flawless. Even the most solid substance, including diamonds and steel, are slightly porous and contain microscopic voids and flaws. To some degree these exist in all types of solids and all types of artificial nail enhancements. Generally, these microscopic voids are unimportant and go unnoticed by the nail technician or client. It is incorrect (and unimportant) to claim that one type of artificial nail enhancement is more or less porous than another, since they all have about the same degree of porosity—very low! Excessive shrinkage, as described above, may be the one exception. Excessive shrinkage can increase the level of porosity by making small bubbles and voids grow larger. This is why shrinkage is important to avoid. It can cause internal flaws to grow and weaken the enhancement.

Permeability is the ease with which a liquid moves through a porous substance. This property is much more important to artificial nails than porosity. The more permeable a coating, the easier it will be for a liquid to penetrate its surface. For instance, enhancements with too much permeability will allow stains to be absorbed into the upper layers and cause discoloration. Discoloration may come from dyes in nail polish or clothing, food, cigarette smoke, tanning lotion, household cleaners, and so on. Of course, permeability is only a problem when it is excessive. Some amount of permeability can be a good thing as long as it's properly controlled. For instance, artificial nail enhancements would not soak off in solvent if the solvent couldn't penetrate its surface. Fiberglass and silk wraps are highly permeable to solvents used in product removers, such as acetone. Therefore, they are quickly and easily removed when soaked in these removers. Liquid/powder enhancements are less permeable to product removers, so they take two to three times as long to remove. UV gel enhancements tend to be the least permeable to solvents and therefore are the least affected by soaking in product removers, which explains why they are the most difficult to remove with solvents.

TO ABSORB OR NOT TO ABSORB . . . THAT IS THE QUESTION

Natural oils and moisture travel from the nail bed through the nail plate to maintain the proper oil and moisture balance needed for flexibility and durability. Water and certain oils can also be absorbed into the top surface of the nail due to the plate's permeability. Wraps, liquid/powder enhancements, and nail polish may also absorb certain oils, increasing their durability as well. UV gels are less permeable and therefore absorb much less of these oils, so the benefits aren't as dramatic. But this is only half the story.

Some oils are made of large and bulky molecules that cannot easily penetrate nail plates or enhancements. In general, oils that don't easily penetrate the skin (for example, massage oils) won't absorb very well into a nail coating. So both surface permeability and the oil's ability to be absorbed are important factors to consider when choosing conditioning oils for natural nails or artificial enhancements.

EVAPORATION COATINGS: UP, UP, AND AWAY

Nail polishes, topcoats, and base coats will form another type of coating on the nail plate. These products are entirely different from artificial nail products. The main difference is they do not polymerize Ⓕ . These products contain no monomers, oligomers, catalysts, or initiators. They work strictly by evaporation of solvents. Approximately 70 percent of the ingredients are volatile (quickly evaporating) solvents. Special polymers are dissolved in the solvents. These polymers are simple polymers with no cross-links, so they dissolve easily. As the product evaporates on the nail plate, a smooth polymer film is left behind. Artist paints and hair sprays work in the same fashion. Of course, the strength and durability of simple polymers are much lower than for cross-linked enhancement polymers, which explains why nail polish is so easily removed with solvents.

Nail Polish Chemistry, from the Roaring Twenties to Now

Modern nail polish has been in use since the late 1920s. Much has changed since then, but the basic chemistry of the products remains the same. Nail polish is also called enamel, lacquer, or varnish. These are different names for the same type of product. At first glance, polishes may seem to be nothing more than a paintlike coating for the nail plate, but their chemistry is actually much more complex. The simplest way to look at them is as a strong film created by evaporation of a volatile solvent. But these coatings must withstand severe abuse without losing color, gloss, or adhesion. Luckily, clever formulators have a wide range of ingredients from which to choose. With careful selection, the properties of the polish can be greatly enhanced.

A typical formulation for nail polish consists of several major types of ingredients. Table 8–1 shows examples of these ingredients and why they are used.

Tosylamide/formaldehyde resin or **TAF resin** is a copolymer resin produced by polymerizing together monomers. It is not the same as formaldehyde. TAF

Table 8-1 *Typical polish formulation*

Type of Ingredient	Chemical Name	Use Levels
Simple polymer	Nitrocellulose	10%
Copolymer	TAF resin	10%
Plasticizer	Citrate esters	5%
Solvent	Ethyl alcohol	5%
Solvent	Ethyl acetate	20%
Solvent	Butyl acetate	15%
Solvent	Toluene	25–30%
Suspension agents	Clay	1–2%
Pigments/dyes	Various colorants	0.5–1%
Stabilizers	Benzophenone-1	0.2–0.4%

resin is a copolymer used to improve adhesion and toughen the polish coating. TAF resin sticks strongly to the nail plate, but it is too soft and has a dull appearance. TAF resin is currently the best nail polish resin on the market. Another alternative to TAF resin is an ingredient called toluene sulfonamide/epoxy resin. But this copolymer suffers from poor stability. To date, nothing compares to TAF resin for strength and durability.

Nitrocellulose (NYE-troh-SELL-you-lohse) produces very hard shiny surfaces but does not stick to the nail plate and is too brittle. TAF resin and nitrocellulose make a great pair. TAF resin increases flexibility and toughens the nitrocellulose while improving adhesion. On the other hand, nitrocellulose improves the TAF resin by making a hard and shiny surface. Nitrocellulose is called the **film former** because it is responsible for creating the continuous coating on the nail plate. It is a naturally occurring simple polymer (cellulose comes from plants) and the first polymer to be successfully modified by chemists and commercially produced (1860). Its main drawback is its tendency to yellow when exposed to sunlight or UV light. This has driven inventors to constantly look for replacements. Recently, a new type of cellulose, cellulose acetate butyrate or CAB, was developed that is much more resistant to yellowing. CAB is currently used in non-yellowing topcoat formulations.

Suspension agents are added to make the product easier to use. They are usually finely ground clays, such as stearalkonium hectorite and montmorillonite. They give nail polishes a unique feature, making them **thixotropic.** In other words, they are thick in the bottle but become thinner while being brushed on the nail! Ketchup is another common example of a thixotropic liquid. Hitting the bottom of the bottle or shaking it causes the ketchup to temporarily become thinner and pour more easily. The same is true for nail polish. Rolling a bottle of nail polish between your hands will cause it to become temporarily thinner and easier to apply. Suspension agents also keep the pigments from settling.

Pigments are the heart of the polish. They provide the color and covering power. A white pigment called titanium dioxide (TiO_2) is frequently combined with colored pigments to increase coverage or produce pastel colors. Other pigments, such as bismuth oxychloride and the mineral mica, are coated with a thin layer of titanium dioxide or other colorants to create many beautiful iridescent shades. Dyes are also occasionally used to modify the color. What's the difference between pigments and dyes? Pigments do not dissolve in the nail polish formulation. They are finely ground solid particles of color. But even when ground into tiny particles, pigments are still far too large to penetrate the nail plate and cause staining. Dyes are soluble and dissolve in the formulation. Food colorings used to color Easter eggs are examples of soluble dyes. Notice how easily the dye soaks into the surface of the egg to stain it?

Plasticizers increase flexibility and wear of the product (FT). As the name suggests, plasticizers make the polymer coating more like plastic. Plasticizers increase flexibility of the coating, allowing it to give or bend when stressed. Nail polish polymers by themselves are too brittle and quickly crack or chip. The proper blend of plasticizers, polymers, and copolymers helps to produce a tougher film.

Solvents are used to improve application and flow. Solvents keep the polymer and additives dissolved, as well as helping adjust the product's thickness. They are an important key to proper application. After the polish is applied, the solvent evaporates, leaving behind the remaining ingredients to coat and color the nail plate.

Color stability is very important for nail polish, both on the nail and in the bottle. Special stabilizers are added to prevent the colors from changing or fading. Nitrocellulose is usually the culprit, since it is discolored by UV light. A solution of nitrocellulose will change from clear to yellowish brown after only a few hours of exposure to UV light or sunlight. Pigments and dyes may also discolor after longer periods of exposure. The lighter shades have less color stability than the darker shades. Also, polish colors closer to the blue side of the visible spectrum shift and change more easily than those that are closer to the red side. To help slow discoloration, nail polish formulations use **UV light absorbers.** These special ingredients absorb UV light and convert it into harmless blue light and heat (infrared energy). They act as "sunscreens" for the product.

With this background, it is easier to understand why some polishes perform differently than others. Performance has nothing to do what the product is called; varnish, polish, lacquer, or enamel. The formulation determines performance, not the name. For example, formulations with too little plasticizer or too much nitrocellulose will be brittle. Add too much TAF resin and the polish will be soft and scratch easily. Poor coverage usually means the formulation contains too much solvent or doesn't contain enough titanium dioxide or pigment. Polish that bubbles easily or has an uneven surface after drying usually contains solvents that evaporate too quickly. Usually bubbling issues are magnified during periods of high temperatures and humidity. If the polish seems to quickly thicken in the bottle before it is half used, then the formula contains too little solvent. Some manufacturers do this intentionally to give the polish a thicker, richer feel upon application. But such formulations quickly become too thick and unusable before half the bottle is finished, so product waste is much higher. **Polish thinners** are solvents that are sold to combat this problem. Unfortunately, they cannot return the polish to its original composition and consistency. Polish that has

WHAT'S A RESIN?

Technically speaking, any solid or semisolid polymer (natural or synthetic) that melts over a broad temperature range is a **resin.** So cyanoacrylates—also called fiberglass wraps or silk wraps—are not resins at all. They are not polymers, they're monomers. But, TAF is a true resin that meets these criteria.

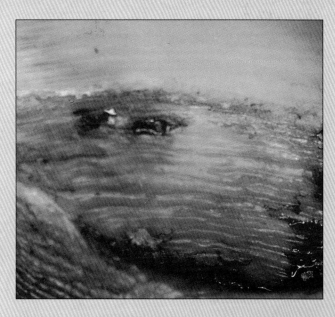

Color Plate 1
Cuticle

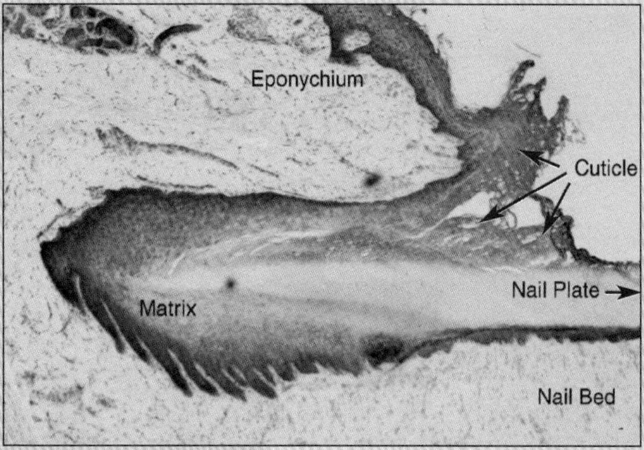

Eponychium

Cuticle

Nail Plate →

Matrix

Nail Bed

Color Plate 2
Grooves in the dermis of the nail bed

Color Plate 3
Solehorn tissue adhering to the underside of the nail plate's free edge

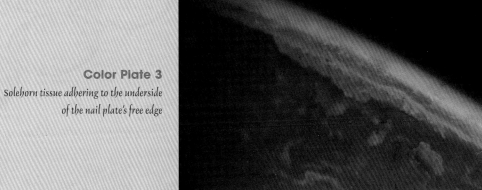

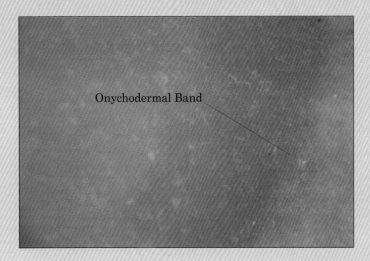

Onychodermal Band

Color Plate 4

The onychodermal band

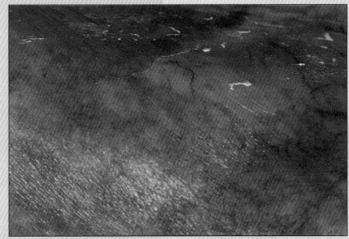

Color Plate 5

Capillaries in the nail fold

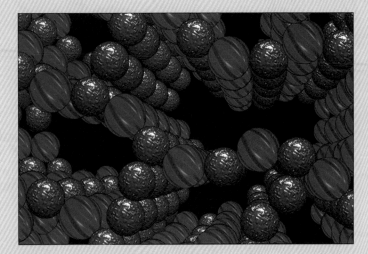

Color Plate 6

A three-dimensional representation of the structure of the nail plate

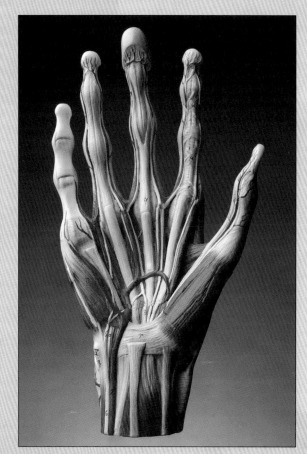

Color Plate 7
The structure of the hand and wrist

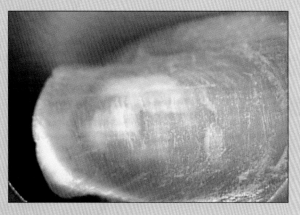

Color Plate 8
Damage created by pinching artificial nails into dramatic
curvatures before fully hardened

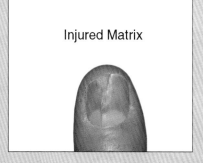

Injured Matrix

Color Plate 9
Permanent split caused by damage in
the matrix area

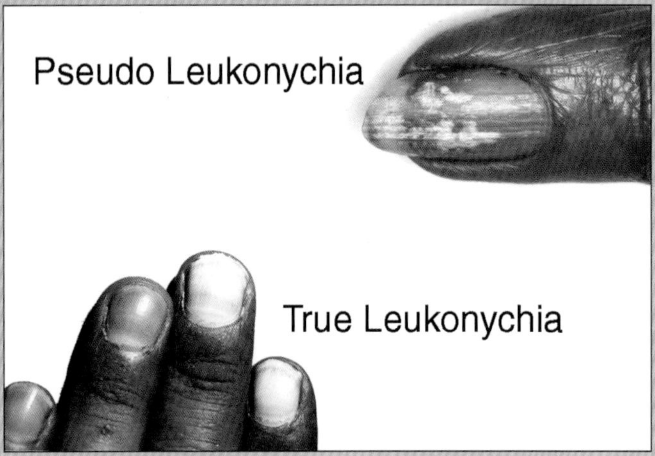

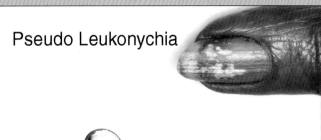

Pseudo Leukonychia

True Leukonychia

Color Plate 10

True leukonychia and pseudoleukonychia

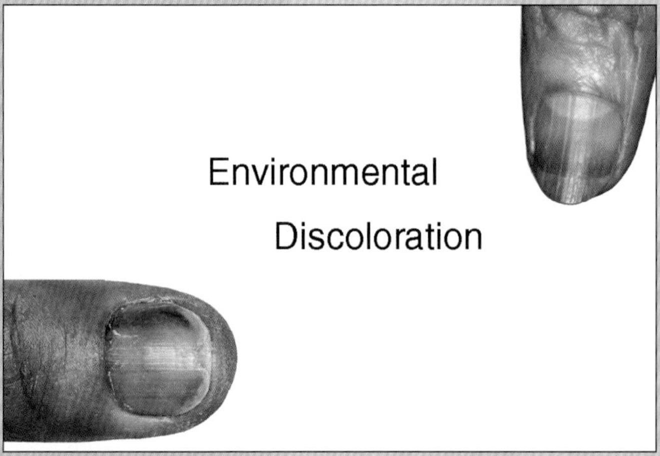

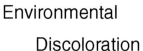

Environmental

Discoloration

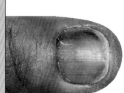

Color Plate 11

Natural nail discoloration

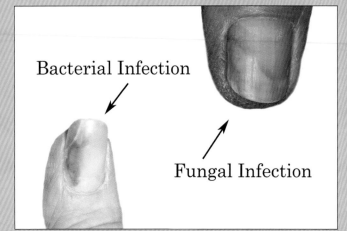

Bacterial Infection

Fungal Infection

Color Plate 12

Examples of bacterial and fungal nail infections

Color Plate 13

Most athlete's foot infections come from floors and carpets, especially in hotels, health clubs and gyms, swimming pools, and other places where many people walk barefoot

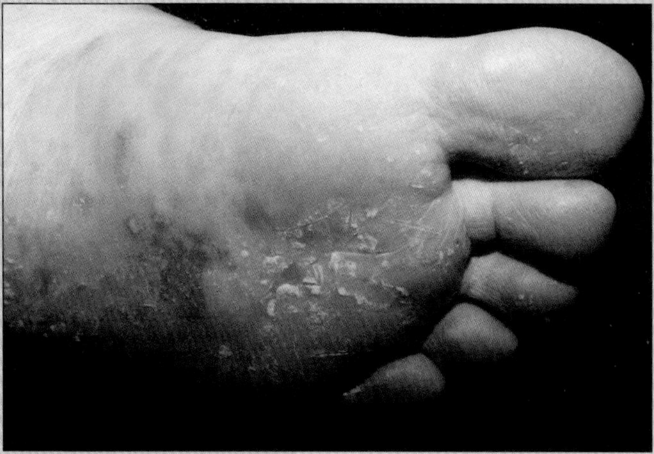

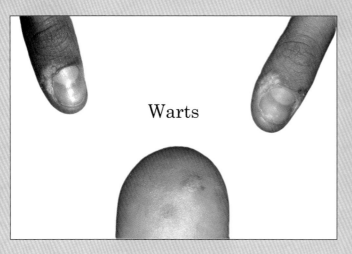

Warts

Color Plate 14

Warts around the nail plate and on the fingertip

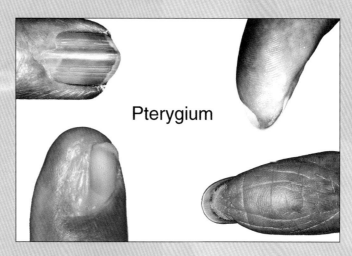

Pterygium

Color Plate 15

Pterygium is an abnormal winglike growth of skin; the term pterygium should never be used to describe the cuticle or any other normal growth of skin

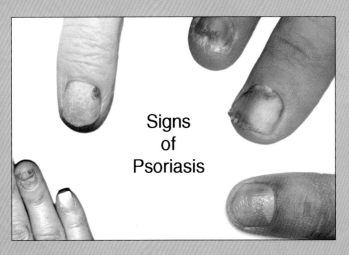

Color Plate 16
Cysts and paronychia

Mucoid Cyst

Paronychia

Color Plate 17
Signs of psoriasis

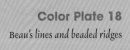

Signs
of
Psoriasis

Color Plate 18
Beau's lines and beaded ridges

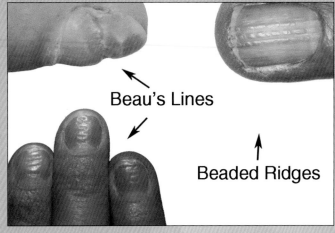

Beau's Lines

Beaded Ridges

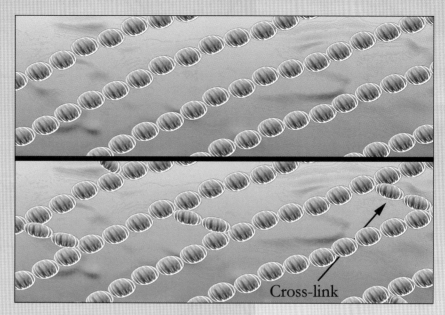

Cross-link

Color Plate 19

Simple versus cross-linked polymers: the simple polymer chains appear in the upper half of the image, the cross-linked chains in the lower half

Color Plate 20

UV nail bulbs emit both visible light, mostly from the blue and violet part of the spectrum, and light in the UV-A region, shown in Color Plate TK as the darkest blue zone to the left of the violet and indigo on the color spectrum

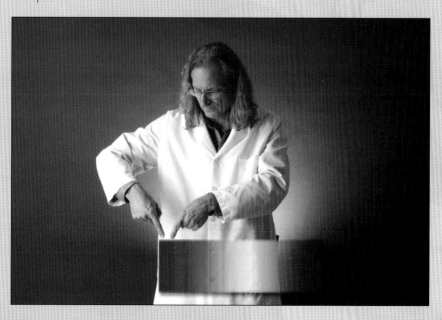

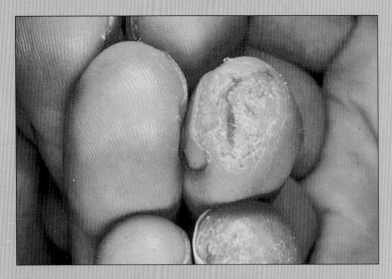

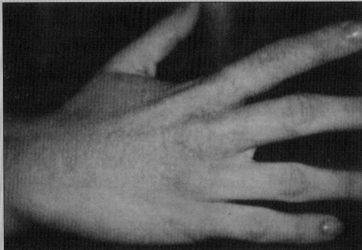

**Color Plate 21 and
Color Plate 22**

*Irritant contact dermatitis on cosmetologists
whose hands were always wet*

Color Plate 23

*Artificial nail–related skin allergy caused by
overexposure — note the redness and skin peeling,
both potential signs of allergy*

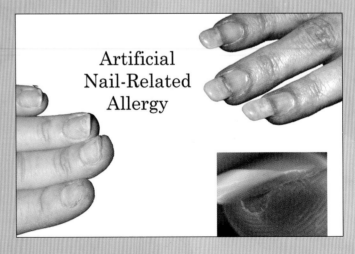

Artificial
Nail-Related
Allergy

been treated with a thinner will perform poorly when compared to the original product. So it's best to avoid using thinners if possible. One way to avoid using them is by ensuring that polish caps are cleaned and tightly sealed after use.

Finally, a variety of highly specialized additives are available to the skilled polish formulator. Even very tiny amounts of these special additives can give dramatic differences in performance. Some examples are ingredients used to improve wetting and adhesion or to stabilize colorants. Of course, there are also examples of additives that serve absolutely no function other than to increase consumer appeal (for example, proteins, calcium, vitamins, minerals, fibers). These ingredients do nothing for the nail plate or the polish but sound great on the label!

Contains No Formaldehyde

This claim is seen on some nail polishes. Should formaldehyde be a concern for nail polish users? In most cases, no! The negligible amount found in polish is extremely safe. In the United States, nail hardeners may legally contain up to 5 percent **formaldehyde** as **formalin** (a stabilized form of formaldehyde that is used in nail hardeners). Nail-hardening products are quite different from nail polishes. Using a product with a formaldehyde level greater than 1 percent dramatically increases the risk of allergic reactions and may cause the natural nail to rapidly become brittle *F1*. For these reasons, formaldehyde is rarely used at such high concentrations. Nail-hardening products usually contain between 0.3 and 1 percent formaldehyde. Clients usually are confused when the nail plate loses flexibility. They think their nails are getting stronger. Clients assume that harder and stiffer nails must be stronger, but they are wrong! Although the plate will bend less, it has actually lost strength and durability. Prolonged or overuse of formaldehyde hardeners can cause the nails to become split, dry, and brittle. This does not happen with nail polish, since it contains less than 0.002 percent formaldehyde. This extremely tiny amount comes from using TAF resin as an ingredient. Formaldehyde is used to make TAF resin, so it contains tiny residual amounts. These traces of formaldehyde are far too low to cause concern unless the client is already allergic to formaldehyde, perhaps from previous repeated overexposures to formaldehyde nail hardeners.

The only way to eliminate this tiny residual of formaldehyde from nail polish is to use an inferior copolymer. Hypoallergenic polishes usually replace TAF resin with a polyester resin. This makes the polish about 10–20 percent less durable. Put another way, superior nail polish formulations containing TAF copolymer have almost no detectable amounts of formaldehyde. The only reason for using the inferior resin is so that marketers can make the "no formaldehyde" claim. Because they are less durable, these products offer little benefit for the user. The only exception is the occasional client who is allergic to formaldehyde. Allergic clients have no choice but to use the inferior formaldehyde-free nail polish.

Toluene-Free: Why All the Fuss?

Toluene has been safely used in nail polish since the late 1930s. In 1993 toluene became a very controversial ingredient. Paranoid politicians passed a state law in California that basically says that safe is not safe enough. The California law requires exposure to be thousands of times below the federally recognized safe exposure level. Because of a lawsuit involving nail polish, the state of California asked for a study to determine the level of toluene in the average salon. The results were very interesting! This study proved that the toluene levels in salon air are exceedingly low; the very highest levels of toluene found were more than 200 times lower than the federal standards for safety! In other words, the air would still be safe to breathe even if the toluene vapors from 200 salons were put into just one salon. That's pretty safe!

Toluene is used to dissolve other ingredients in nail polishes and treatments. Nail products with toluene will go on more smoothly and produce more brilliant colors that resist peeling. No other solvent does as good a job as toluene. Toluene-containing nail polishes are clearly superior. Strangely, before the results of the California salon air quality studies were completed, manufacturers of retail nail polish settled out of court. They made the mistake of promising to never use toluene again. Now it's too late for them to change their mind. This lucky turn of events is a tremendous break for professional nail salons. Now, only professional nail polishes are allowed to use toluene. This means that clients who want superior nail polish will have to buy it from a salon. Otherwise, they can only purchase inferior, toluene-free retail products from the drugstore or supermarket. In short, there is no reason for nail technicians to worry that toluene levels in salon air might be unsafe. That question has been answered.

Finally, a 1988 study claimed that toluene causes the natural nail to peel and split. This effect was seen when nail clippings were soaked for three days in toluene and then examined under a high-power microscope. Obviously, no one would soak the nail in toluene for this long. Therefore, toluene should still be considered safe for use on healthy nails. Of course, if your client already has nails that easily peel or split, it might be wise to avoid toluene-containing products or perhaps nail polish in general. Such nails could be adversely affected by solvents used in nail polish removers.

Base Coats and Topcoats

Base coats and topcoats are formulated with many of the same ingredients as polish. Most base coats contain a high percentage of TAF resin to improve nail plate adhesion. Topcoats generally have high amounts of nitrocellulose (or CAB) with extra plasticizer and no pigments. All of this should make more sense now, based on what you have learned about nail polish. Both topcoats and base coats are important and will improve nail polish performance. Base coats improve adhesion and block staining. Topcoats improve wear by coating the polish with a protective shield while increasing gloss.

Waiting for a polish to dry is tiresome. But the more slowly the coating dries, the better! Slower-evaporating solvents produce brighter colors. If a polish is forced to dry quickly by heat or chemical dryers, it may result in more shrinkage and cracking. Some brush or spray-on polish dryers incorporate natural oils into the formulation to help plasticize the coating and minimize this problem. A less successful approach is to use high amounts of rapidly evaporating solvents to shorten dry times, as in fast-dry polish. These products have a tendency to bubble and pit or produce uneven, dull surfaces. Blowing on polish will not speed dry times, but it can lower the gloss and cause clouding. The best results will be obtained with a base coat, two coats of a professional polish, and a topcoat applied to a properly prepared nail plate. Take your time and pause (as long as is reasonable) between each coat you apply. Slowing down the drying process by even a few minutes will produce a smoother, more brilliant surface. Applying the second coat of polish too quickly or too thickly is a major reason for the "orange peel" or rough, textured appearance of the surface. This effect is especially pronounced during times of high temperatures and humidity.

What's Up?

Until recently, most nail polish research was focused on faster drying times and improved durability and adhesion. The new focus is on improving the nail plate's health. This is presently one of the hottest topics of interest for consumers. So the search is on for ingredients that provide benefits for nail plates. A nail polish that improves the toughness of the nail or provides solutions for yellow, dry, brittle, and splitting nails would be hugely popular and beneficial. The first step toward this goal is the development of water-based nail varnishes (containing 50 percent or more water as a solvent). It will take a while, but once water-based products equal the current solvent-based technology, they will become the preferred formulations. With a successful water-based technology, it would be possible to use a wider variety of important additives. This could then lead to the Holy Grail of nail polishes—one that truly prevents or helps treat common nail problems and disorders.

FAST TRACK Ⓕ

- Ⓕ Billions of molecules must react to make just one sculptured nail.
- Ⓕ Chemical reactions that create polymers are called polymerizations.
- Ⓕ A monomer is a molecule that makes polymers.
- Ⓕ Homopolymers are polymers made from one type of monomer.
- Ⓕ Copolymers are polymers that are made from two types of monomers.
- Ⓕ An initiator molecule starts polymerizations.

(FT) Oligomers are short chains of monomers.

(FT) Solvents unravel simple polymer chains, causing them to dissolve.

(FT) Cross-links create netlike structures of great strength and flexibility.

(FT) Sunlight is made of many colors, called the visible spectrum.

(FT) Each color we see is a different level of energy.

(FT) Red is the lowest energy of visible light, and violet is the highest.

(FT) The next energy level above violet is called ultraviolet or UV light.

(FT) Light energy just below the color red is called infrared light, or heat.

(FT) Catalysts make initiators more effective.

(FT) Chemical reactions that release heat are called exothermic reactions.

(FT) Excessive exotherms damage the tissue and weaken the enhancement.

(FT) Wattage measures power consumption, not UV light output.

(FT) Excessive amounts of acid-based nail primer can damage the nail bed.

(FT) Nail polishes and treatments form coatings but do not polymerize.

(FT) Don't fill dappen dishes from a large container of monomer liquid.

(FT) Never mix liquid and powder from different manufacturers.

(FT) Evaporation coatings, such as nail polishes, topcoats, and base coats, do not polymerize.

(FT) Plasticizers increase the flexibility and wear of nail products.

(FT) Prolonged use of formaldehyde can make nail plates dry, brittle, and split.

Review Questions

1. What are coatings? Name the two main types.
2. Every type of product used to create nail enhancements does so by a chemical reaction called _____.
3. Polymers created by using two different monomers are called _____.
4. What are monomers and polymers? Define each and explain the differences.
5. What is the difference between a simple polymer and a cross-linked polymer?
6. After the monomers react and a hard polymer is created, have all the chemical reactions finished? Explain your answer.
7. What are the main two sources of energy for initiator molecules?
8. Why do polymers shrink when they are created?
9. What is an exotherm? How can you tell when it is happening?

10. Do nail polishes and topcoats polymerize on the nail? Explain.
11. At what salon temperatures do artificial nail products work best?
12. How can you tell if a product truly cures with UV light?
13. Name three products that can cause high amounts of exotherm.
14. How should nail enhancement product brushes be stored?
15. What is the largest container that should be used to refill your monomer dish?

Chapter 9

Liquid and Powder Product Chemistry

Objective

In this chapter you will learn how to apply your knowledge of enhancement product chemistry to better understand its inner workings. You'll learn about the basic technology behind liquid/powder enhancement products. You'll learn how they work, what they're made from, and how to avoid common pitfalls.

FAMILY TIES

Nail technicians use many types of products to create artificial nail enhancements. UV gels, liquid/powder combinations, wraps, and no-light gels all seem totally different and unrelated, but nothing could be further from the truth. The main ingredients used to make each of these are very closely related. In fact, they all come from the same chemical family, the **acrylics** (FT).

The first artificial nail enhancement products were called acrylic nails. As you might imagine, they weren't very good by today's standards. But neither were the first cars, computers, or airplanes. All new products need time to reach their full potential. Unfortunately, many people still associate the word *acrylic* with those outdated products. They don't realize that all artificial nail enhancements are based on ingredients from the acrylic family. Of course, just because these products are based on the acrylic family doesn't mean they're all the same. That's like saying all Americans or all Australians are the same. Liquid/powder systems are based on one branch of the acrylic family called the **methacrylates** (FT). Wraps, no-light gels, and tip adhesives are based on another directly related branch, the **cyanoacrylates** (FT). UV gel products until recently were based strictly on ingredients from a third branch, called the **acrylates,** but newer, more advanced products based on methacrylates have become available (FT). Each category has advantages and disadvantages. There are no perfect product types. None is ideal in every way or in every situation. In the next two chapters we will explore how they differ. We will also look at the advantages and disadvantages of each.

LIQUID/POWDER SYSTEMS

The original nail enhancement products were liquid/powder systems. These are still the most widely used type of artificial nail enhancement in the world. Many years of experience and scientific research have brought these products far beyond those used by the first generation of nail technicians (see Table 9–1). The liquid is a complex mixture of monomers, stabilizers, catalysts, and other additives. The powder is a polymer that contains the initiator, colorants, and other additives.

These liquid/powder products are the most sophisticated, high-tech products used in the entire beauty industry! In fact, this is true of artificial nail

Table 9–1 *Major categories of artificial nail enhancement products*

Cyanoacrylates	Methacrylates	Acrylates
Wraps	Monomer and polymer (odorless and non-odorless)	UV light gels
No-light gels	UV light gels	
Tip adhesives		

products as a whole. Methacrylates, acrylates, and cyanoacrylates are used in life-saving medical devices, computers, commercial jets, and even the space shuttle. You learned in the last chapter that monomers join to create polymers. So it might seem strange to mix liquid monomers and powdered polymers to create another polymer, but this is exactly what happens during the creation of artificial nails. Let's look at the powdered polymer first and understand its role in nail enhancement chemistry.

POLYMER POWDER

Polymer powder particles (beads) act as carriers for other ingredients (FT). Several of the ingredients needed to make nail enhancements are embedded inside each powder bead as well as coating the outside. A mineral called titanium dioxide (TiO_2) is used to alter the color and opacity of the artificial nail. TiO_2 is a white pigment that does not dissolve when mixed with monomer liquid. This is the same pigment used to whiten artist paints, paper, and artificial teeth. This useful pigment is used in sunscreen lotions, cosmetics, and hundreds of thousands of other applications. In artificial nail products, this pigment is the whitening agent in white tip powders used to simulate the free edge of a nail. In lesser amounts it is used to create a translucent, natural-appearing enhancement. Figure 9–1 shows a highly magnified bead of polymer powder coated with TiO_2. This pigment is also sometimes incorporated both outside and inside the bead to create higher

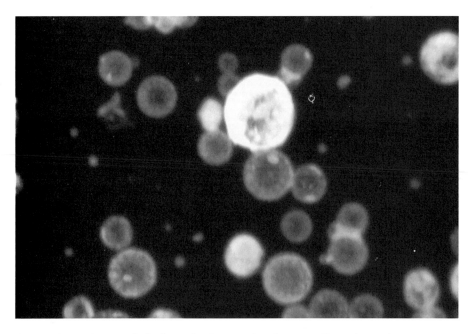

Figure 9–1 *Polymer powder beads coated with* TiO_2 *and small amounts of benzoyl peroxide, an initiator*

opacity. White tip powders are used to create extensions beyond the free edge and to give a "French manicure" look. An extra-white tip polymer contains additional titanium dioxide, and clear polymer powders contain no titanium dioxide. This mineral is used because of its fantastic ability to whiten. Nothing does a better job. Strangely, as a fine powder it is extremely white, but a large crystal of titanium dioxide is absolutely crystal clear and more brilliant than a diamond. Unfortunately, it is too soft and easily broken to be used as a gemstone.

Other color pigments are often blended with the polymer powder to make colored powders used to create nail art. Dyes are sometimes added to give the polymer a pinkish or blush color. These colors give a very pleasing appearance to the nail bed. Pink dyes will cover up product discoloration and natural nail defects. Blue colorants play a special role by acting as an **optical brightener.** An optical brightener makes colors look brighter. Whites look whiter when a small amount of blue is added.

The polymer also carries a heat-sensitive initiator. In the last chapter, you discovered that an initiator was needed to energize the monomers and cause polymerization to occur. Monomer and polymer systems are heat-curing, because the initiator used in these systems is sensitive to heat. The initiator is **benzoyl peroxide,** the same ingredient used in acne creams (FT). The heat of the room or finger provides enough energy to break a molecule of benzoyl peroxide in half. This occurs rapidly when the benzoyl peroxide is mixed with the proper catalyst, found in the monomer liquid. Each half is capable of exciting or energizing a monomer. When an initiator molecule breaks in half, it creates a **free radical.**

A RADICAL REACTION

Free radicals are very excited molecules that cause many kinds of chemical reactions. They can be found almost everywhere. For instance, free radicals cause newspaper to discolor and help hydrogen peroxide lift and deposit hair color. Our bodies use free radicals to perform thousands of vital functions each day. Free radicals also play a role in the wrinkling and aging of skin. Many skin care products contain chemicals that eliminate free radicals. So you see, some free radicals are useful, while others are not. The free radicals found on skin are very different from those used in nail enhancement products.

Free radicals are very important to nail enhancements. But don't worry that they will injure nail plates. The benzoyl peroxide has no damaging effects on the nail plate. Once it passes a jolt of energy to a monomer, the free radical is completely eliminated. Let's review what was learned in Chapter 8 to get a better picture of how these products work.

1. Monomer is mixed with a polymer containing benzoyl peroxide (initiator).

2. The catalyst found in the monomer uses heat energy to break the initiator in half, creating two free radicals.

CAN'T STOP ME NOW

The monomers and oligomers used to make artificial nail products are so tiny they can only be seen with the most sophisticated scientific instruments available. Cracks created as a result of aggressive filing techniques (such as improper use of heavy abrasives or electric files) are thousands of times larger than any monomer or oligomer. It is a myth that these cracks can block the polymerization process. They can't possibly be blamed for this. Once polymerization starts, cracks can't stop the enhancement from curing. But once formed, these tiny cracks can later lead to larger cracks and service breakdown, so aggressive filing techniques should be avoided.

3. Each free radical will combine with a monomer and energize it.

4. The energized monomer attaches to another monomer's tail (covalent bonding).

5. After attaching and bonding, the newly energized monomer gives up the extra energy to its new partner.

6. The second monomer doesn't want the energy either, so it attaches to the tail of another monomer and passes the energy again . . . and thus the chain begins.

This cycle repeats itself billions of times, reaching very long polymer chain lengths. Notice that the polymer powder isn't mentioned in the reaction. That's because it is the carrier and does not chemically react. The powder carries the initiator to the monomer and monomer is needed to make new polymer. The polymer powder is important in other ways. The powder plays an important role in toughening the enhancement, as explained below. But it does not become part of the new polymer chain. As these growing chains lengthen, they wrap around and completely encase each tiny bead, even penetrating their surfaces. This fuses the polymer bead into the artificial nail.

SECRET SAUCE

The polymer powder contains other additives as well. Sometimes color stabilizers are added to prevent yellowing. Sunlight is one major cause of yellowing. It contains very high amounts of UV light and can discolor nail enhancements, leading to brittleness. **UV absorbers** are additives to prevent this type of damage. They absorb damaging UV light and change it into blue light or heat (FT). In a sense, UV absorbers are like sunscreens for enhancements. They work on the same principle.

Calcium is sometimes added to polymers, but its benefits are highly questionable. Calcium certainly does not strengthen the nail plate. Neither can it stimulate nail growth. In fact, calcium provides no benefit at all for the nail plate. Some believe that a small amount gives the product a slightly creamier consistency. But in high concentrations, calcium can weaken enhancements and cause premature service breakdown.

MAKING A POLYMER POWDER

All polymer powders start out as monomers. Monomer is placed in a large mixer, which may hold over 1,000 gallons (3,785 liters). Water is then used to dilute the monomer. Then initiator and catalyst are added while mixing rapidly. After several hours, the monomer polymerizes into tiny beads. The water is drained away, the beads are dried, additives are blended in, and the mixture is then packaged up for sale. The bead sizes vary greatly depending on manufacturing conditions. The size of very small items such as polymer powder beads are measured in **microns.** A thick human hair is about 100 microns in diameter. Therefore, a 1-micron particle is 1/100th the diameter of a human hair, and a 50-micron particle is half as thick as a hair. Most polymer powder beads are around 50–80 microns. But they can be as large as 125 microns or as small as 10 microns (1/10th of a hair's thickness). The polymer powder beads shown in Figure 9–1 are highly magnified. You can see that they are not all the same size.

A common misconception is that these powders are made by grinding and sifting. Grinding and sifting would be very expensive and unnecessary. It would also produce an inferior polymer powder. Manufacturers can easily control the bead size when the polymers are made. In other words, when the polymer is dried, it is already the correct size. Another misconception is that the polymer powders are sifted many times. This is untrue. The polymer is passed through a screen to remove large chunks, making additional sifting unnecessary. The extra sifting would be costly, and it would not make the product any better—just more expensive.

SISTER, SISTER

As shown in Table 9–1, liquid/powder formulas are based on a family of monomers called methacrylates. There are many kinds of methacrylates, but only a few are useful for artificial nail polymers. These different types are so similar, they may be thought of as sister chemicals. Still, even sisters are different in many ways, and the same is true for methacrylate monomers. Powders are usually made from two sister monomers called **methyl methacrylate (MMA)** and **ethyl methacrylate (EMA).** Methyl methacrylate was used for many years to make artificial nails, but is no longer sold by reputable manufacturers, since nail enhancement products made with this monomer causes excessive nail damage and significant numbers of allergic reactions. But a polymer made from methyl methacrylate is both safe for the natural nail and unlikely to cause allergic reactions. In fact, most manufacturers use MMA polymer in nail polymer powders blended with EMA polymers. When used in the correct combination, their properties complement each other. Ethyl methacrylate is the most widely used monomer in the nail industry and the ingredient of choice for liquid/powder systems.

HOMOPOLYMER VERSUS COPOLYMER

A polymer made of only EMA or only MMA is called a homopolymer. *Homo-* means "same." In other words, the polymer was made entirely from one type of monomer, such as EMA homopolymer. Homopolymers are usually simply referred to as polymers. The homopolymer made from EMA is usually called PEMA or polyEMA. *Poly-* in this case indicates that the monomer has been polymerized into a long chain. A homopolymer can be made from methyl methacrylate monomer as well; this is called **methyl methacrylate polymer (PMMA)** or polyMMA. Usually, both EMA and PMA are blended together to create polymer chains with unique properties. In other words, the polymer chains contain both sister monomers, instead of just one. Polymers made from two different types of monomers are called copolymers. In this case, *co* means "two working together."

Homopolymers made from EMA are slightly softer and more flexible than homopolymers made from MMA. But homopolymers made from MMA are harder, stronger, and more rigid. Which is better, homopolymers or copolymers? In general, copolymers offer a wider range of properties and are more versatile than homopolymers Ⓕ. For example, what would be the result of blending EMA and MMA into a copolymer? Recall from Chapter 2 that toughness is a combination of strength and flexibility. By properly blending both EMA and MMA into a copolymer, a tougher material is created. By using two monomers with different properties, manufacturers can create "designer blends" of polymers customized to perform specific functions. A polymer is made harder by using more MMA or made more flexible by adding additional EMA monomers to the chain. Clearly, copolymers offer many advantages over homopolymers.

MONOMER MAKES IT HAPPEN

The monomer liquid is the most important part of the nail enhancement. Non-odorless nail enhancement products contain mostly ethyl methacrylate monomer, but other monomers and additives are used as well. Ethyl methacrylate makes only straight polymer chains and cannot form cross-links. Recall from the last chapter that monomers normally join together in a head-to-tail fashion, unless special cross-linking monomers are added to obtain a tough, three-dimensional, netlike structure.

Besides cross-linkers, many other additives are used to create monomer liquids. For instance, UV absorbers are also included to prevent discoloration from the sun or tanning beds. Some monomer blends can be simple mixtures containing only a few ingredients. But others are complex blends containing several types of monomers, cross-linkers, and many special additives. A common myth is that all products are alike. This is completely false! Manufacturers of less expensive products promote their products as the same as the more expensive brands, but it just isn't so. A good rule to remember is that you get what you pay for. As you would imagine, economy products use basic formulas with a minimal amount of special or expensive ingredients. Special additives increase performance but can also dramatically increase costs. Flow modifiers, catalysts, and wetting agents are a few examples of specialty ingredients. A **flow modifier** is an ingredient that reduces brushstrokes on the surface, causing them to melt away or "self-level." Flow modifiers also improve bead pickup and workability. Wetting agents improve adhesion to the natural nail plate, as discussed in detail in Chapter 7.

BUT NOT WITHOUT A CATALYST

Choosing the proper catalyst is extremely important. By itself, the initiator molecule is much too slow. A catalyst is needed to speed things up. Without the catalyst, it would take days for the enhancement to harden. Remember, the initiator is the starting gun, but the catalyst is the trigger. Catalysts are usually only about 1 to 2 percent of the total monomer blend, but they make all the difference. If the improper catalyst is selected or too much is added, the artificial nail enhancement may become weak or brittle and may also badly discolor. The excess catalyst can make the reaction happen too fast and cause too many polymer chains to start growing. The result is an enhancement with excessive amounts of short polymer chains and very few long chains. This gives the surface a softer set or makes the enhancement too flexible. When enhancements are too flexible, they bend and break more easily. So you can see, more flexibility isn't necessarily better. Some flexibility is important, but too much will lower toughness and durability. Flexibility and strength must remain in balance for tough nail enhancements.

INHIBITORS IMPROVE SHELF LIFE

Inhibitors are ingredients that prevent monomers from joining into chains before they are mixed with the polymer powder. Inhibitors are used to prevent premature polymerization and are added to the monomer blend to improve shelf life. They prevent the monomer from turning into a thick, jellylike substance and then hardening into a glassy lump inside the container. Not surprisingly, this premature reaction is called **gelling.** It's a natural process for monomer liquids to slowly turn into polymers while sitting on the shelf, unless an inhibitor is added to prevent it from occurring. Without inhibitors, all artificial nail enhancement products would harden in their containers within a few months. Inhibitors prevent nail enhancement products from gelling for up to 18 months from the date of manufacture, assuming the product is properly stored. Improper storage deactivates the inhibitor and causes artificial nail enhancement products to harden in

THE INHIBITORS

The three most commonly used inhibitors are hydroquinone (HQ), hydroquinone monomethyl ether (MEHQ), and butylated hydroxytoluene (BHT). The inhibitor is added by the manufacturer of the basic ingredients used to make monomer liquids. Inhibitors are used with all the main ingredients found in artificial nail enhancements, such as methacrylate or acrylate monomers and oligomers.

Inhibitors are necessary to ensure the shelf life and stability of the artificial nail enhancement products. Each of these inhibitors are added in extremely low amounts, typically less than 0.002 percent. At these exceedingly low levels, they are recognized as safe, effective, and necessary additives.

the container. Excessive heat is the most common reason for liquid/powder products to harden in the container; it will also affect wrap resins, UV gels, and tip adhesives. These types of products should never be stored in a warm location and must be kept away from windows. Store these products in cool, dry locations. Keep all products away from sources of heat, open flames, or sparks. Never put any of your professional nail products in the trunk of your car, especially during the summer. Even if there is no obvious gelling, your enhancements may be weaker and more prone to lifting. Nail enhancement monomers will often begin gelling at the bottom of the container, while the top portion remains a liquid. Once this process begins, it affects the quality of the product. Partially solidified monomer liquids should not be used and should be immediately discarded.

Another common reason for product gelling is contamination. Once the monomer is poured out, never pour it back into the original container. This will destroy the inhibitors and cause product gelling to occur. Unused monomer can be stored in a separate, properly marked container and used to clean your brushes. Once poured from the original container, monomer liquid should be either used or disposed of properly. For information on proper disposal, see Chapter 11. Finally, preserve the shelf life of your liquid monomer by filling dappen dishes from a 4-ounce container. Each time you open a bottle of monomer liquid, small amounts of vapor will escape from the bottle. If you open a large container many times a day, the evaporation will slowly change the chemical composition of your monomer liquid. These changes will affect the quality of the product and can lead to service breakdown. Also, if the room's humidity is very high, moisture from the air may get inside the container and contaminate the product. Purchase large containers of liquid monomer to refill your 4-ounce container. It is unwise to work directly from a large container of any type of product. In general, bulk products should be used only to refill smaller containers used to perform your services.

OXYGEN INHIBITS TOO!

Many types of nail enhancement products are affected by oxygen. Some types of artificial nail enhancements cannot properly polymerize if too much oxygen is around. Oxygen will stunt the growth of the polymer chains and dramatically affect the surface of the nail enhancement. When this occurs, the short chains of monomers result in a sticky, gooey layer that rolls off when filed (FT). This layer is called the **inhibition layer** (it is sometimes incorrectly called the dispersion layer). You'll learn in later chapters that oxygen-related problems most commonly occur in UV gel products or odorless liquid/powder systems. Why does this happen? An oxygen molecule can act as a "cap" at the end of growing polymer chains. Once oxygen reacts with the end of the chain, the chain can no longer add new monomers or cross-links. Therefore, oxygen disrupts chain growth on the surface of the enhancement and causes the surface inhibition layer. The molecules that lie under the surface are shielded from oxygen, so they are free to create long polymer chains and cross-links. *Caution:* In Chapter 12 you'll learn that the inhibition layer contains many unreacted ingredients that can cause skin irritation and/or allergy. You must avoid prolonged or repeated skin contact with the inhibition layer.

PERFORMANCE THROUGH CONSISTENCY CONTROL

Consistency is determined by the amount of polymer powder blended with the monomer liquid (FT). Consistency is also called the **mix ratio.** It is not possible to create a monomer liquid that can be used at any mix ratio. If the proper consistency is used (see below), the nail enhancement will contain the correct amount of polymer powder. For non-odorless products (those based on EMA), the enhancement will contain between 30 and 40 percent polymer powder, depending on the mix ratio used. The polymer powder has other dramatic effects on the artificial nail enhancement's performance. The powder actually gives the enhancement much of its durability (FT). Figure 9–2 shows a magnified view of monomer and polymer at both correct and incorrect ratios. When the monomer polymerizes, it completely surrounds each tiny bead. The polymer beads act like tiny crack arrestors, blocking cracks from spreading. The importance of the powder shouldn't be underestimated. Polymer powders greatly reinforce the entire enhancement. In a nutshell: too little polymer powder will mean that the enhancement contains too few crack arrestors and therefore will have less reinforcement and lower toughness. Cracks will grow and spread more easily if the enhancement contains too little powder.

Nail technicians sometimes add extra monomer liquid to smooth the enhancement surface, not realizing that this alters the mix ratio, reducing durability and color stability and possibly leading to excessive breakage. The greatest enhancement durability is obtained when using the correct ratio of monomer liquid to polymer powder. Table 9–2 shows actual laboratory data that demonstrate

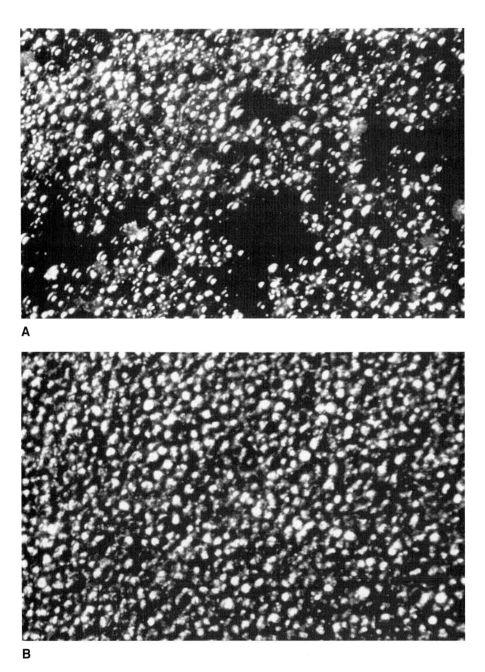

Figure 9-2 Incorrect ratios of monomer to polymer create voids where no polymer can be found. The monomer-rich areas show up as black spaces in this highly magnified view. Part A shows a bead with too wet of a consistency; the bead in part B has the correct consistency.

Table 9-2 *Toughness of artificial nail enhancements at varying mix ratios*

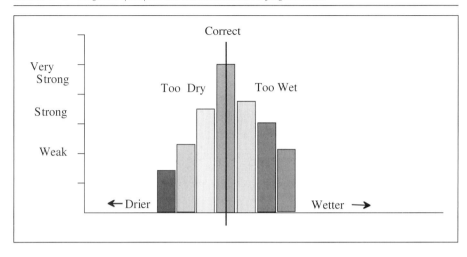

the toughness of enhancements at different mix ratios. As you can see, too much monomer liquid or too much polymer powder can lower the enhancement's toughness. Achieving the correct ratio takes a little practice, but the rewards are great! Clients will be happier and need fewer repairs. Techniques for achieving proper mix ratios will be discussed in the next section.

BE A CONTROL FREAK

Controlling product consistency is an extremely important part of being a nail professional. Product or bead consistency is determined by the ratio of monomer liquid to polymer powder. Extra amounts of monomer will create a wetter bead consistency. A drier bead consistency is made by increasing the amount of polymer powder in the mixture. (See Table 9–3.) Improper consistency is the number one reason nail technicians fail when using these products. The correct ratio of monomer liquid to polymer powder must be used. Too dry a consistency causes breakage and lifting, but too wet a consistency is worse. If you use too much monomer liquid, the enhancements may seem strong and flexible and will adhere well to the nail plate, but don't be fooled—all is not well! Too wet a consistency is one of the leading causes of allergic reaction in clients and nail technicians. Also, using the improper consistency causes enhancements to lose their durability.

Table 9-3 *Bead consistencies are altered by changing the ratio of monomer liquid to polymer powder*

Wet consistency	2 parts monomer to 1 part polymer
Medium consistency	1½ parts monomer to 1 part polymer
Dry consistency	1 part monomer to 1 part polymer

BRRR . . . IT'S COLD IN HERE

Fast-setting liquid/powder enhancement products aren't just for veteran nail technicians with a need for speed. They are actually more suitable for cold, drafty salons. Fast-setting liquid and powders contain more initiator and/or catalyst, so they'll set up twice as fast as products with standard set times. The shorter set times will occur no matter what the salon temperature—cold, medium, or warm. These faster-setting products will set up at just the right speed in colder salons, but in warm salons they can be blazingly fast—oftentimes too fast for novice nail technicians.

Using a wetter bead will slow down the set time, but this will make the consistency too wet and can lead to allergic reactions and/or service breakdown. Nail technicians who complain that a fast-setting product isn't all that fast are probably working with much too wet a mix ratio. *Caution:* Don't be tempted to use a wetter mix ratio to slow down fast-setting products. Instead, switch back to a standard-setting product. Fast-setting products aren't for everyone or all salons, but those who use them must use them correctly.

Wet consistencies may improve adhesion, but they lower the enhancement's overall durability. This is because the artificial nail contains less polymer powder. Recall that the polymer powder improves toughness and prevents cracks from spreading through the enhancement. So using the right amount of powder is important. Using too wet a consistency can mean big trouble in other ways as well. You'll learn in Chapter 12 that an overly wet mix ratio can cause allergic reactions. Wet consistencies can also lead to cracking and lifting. Table 9–2 shows that dry consistencies have equal amounts of monomer liquid and polymer powder. The extra powder offers improved durability but lowers adhesion, because adhesion comes from the monomer liquid. Medium consistencies give the best of both worlds. Medium-consistency enhancements are tough, durable, and flexible and also have good adhesion to the natural nail plate. How can you know if the mix ratio is correct? Here's an easy way to determine the proper consistency for liquid/powder enhancement products:

1. Use a clean brush to make a normal bead.

2. Carefully lay the bead on top of a clean, unfiled artificial nail tip, placing it directly over the center or apex of the tip. Do not pat or push down on the bead.

3. Watch the bead for 10 seconds and carefully note what you see. Determine which of the following best matches your observations:

    • Does the bead begin to settle and flow out almost immediately?

    • Does the height of the bead drop halfway or more within 10 seconds?

- Does the bead seem to lose most of its original shape?
- Can you see a ring of excess liquid around the base of the bead?
- Would this bead be difficult to control, or would it flow into the skin surrounding the nail plate?

If you answered yes to any of the questions above, your bead is probably a wet consistency. If you answered yes to all of these questions, your ratio is probably 3 parts liquid to 1 part powder (or more). If this is the case, you are using the product incorrectly. Nail enhancements made with excessively wet mix ratios are prone to develop tiny stress fractures, cracks, and lifting near the cuticle area or sidewalls. Also, discoloration becomes more likely, and there will be an increased chance of developing an allergic reaction to the product.

- Does the bead melt out fairly slowly and have a "frosted glass" appearance?
- After 10 seconds, does the bead hold a smooth, domelike shape?
- Does the overall height of the dome drop only 1/4 of the original height?
- Does all of the liquid stay in the bead without a ring of excess liquid around the base?
- Is the bead easy to control, and does it retain its shape once it's placed?

If you answered yes to all of the questions, you are probably using a medium mixture, so good for you! Make sure you always stick to this procedure. You will be much less likely to have problems.

- Does the bead hold its original shape and/or melt out very little?
- Does the bead height and shape remain unchanged after 10 seconds?
- Does the bead look lumpy or have a crusty appearance?
- Is the bead difficult to control and shape into place?

If you answered yes to any of these questions, you are probably using too dry a bead consistency. Only odorless products require technicians to use dry mix ratios for durability, as well as to lower the risk of developing allergic skin reactions. But a dry mix ratio can cause nonodorless products to undergo massive lifting as well as brittleness and discoloration.

Nail technicians are often fooled into using a wet consistency. They mistakenly believe that there are advantages to this practice. For instance, using wetter consistencies is a quick way to make the surface smooth. But it causes far more problems than it solves. A high-quality nail enhancement product performs best at medium ratios.

ALL THAT GLITTERS

Excessive amounts of colored pigments, glitter, and other types of decorative art can cause enhancements to crack or break more easily. Too much can actually seed the formation of cracks. How much is too much? That depends on what you're using. But one thing's for certain—any foreign object added to the polymer powder can cause the resulting artificial nail to be weaker. A good rule of thumb is that the more that's added, the weaker the nail enhancement. For example, if you add just a little pigment, the nail enhancement will be just a little weaker . . . a lot of pigment, a lot weaker. The same holds true for glitter, crystals, feathers, whatever! Any foreign body in the artificial nail can cause weakness and may create service breakdown. So, if you use these decorative additives and are having more service breakdown, they should be the first thing you suspect when you start troubleshooting your problem.

Remember:

- Never go back and smooth the surface with more monomer.
- Never use pure monomer to clean around the edges or under the nail or sidewalls.
- Never touch any monomer to the skin (including gels and wraps).
- Avoid using overly large brushes for product application.

Using an overly large brush can throw off the mix ratio. How? Large brushes hold a considerable amount of liquid monomer. If this excess liquid is pressed from the belly of the brush into the enhancement, the mix ratio could become too wet. Very large brushes do not save time. And they increase the risk of allergy in two ways, both by creating overly wet beads, with too much monomer, and by increasing the risk of skin contact with monomer liquid. It is very difficult to keep the edges of an overly large brush from touching living skin. Using smaller brushes will improve the quality of the enhancement as well as help protect sensitive clients from developing skin allergies. As you will see in the following chapters, many problems can be related to using monomer liquids improperly. Don't fall into these traps. These bad habits are ghosts from the early years of the nail industry, when there was no proper education. Don't be a victim of past mistakes and myths.

PLASTICIZING ENHANCEMENTS

Plasticizers are another important example of special additives in artificial nail enhancement products. Plasticizers improve flexibility and toughness (FT). How? If you could shrink down to the size of a molecule, the enhancement would look like a jungle of interwoven polymer vines. Between the vines would be many small spaces. Empty pockets exist between the millions of tangled polymer chains and cross-links. These pockets are far too small to see, even with a microscope. The spaces may be small, but they are important. Just as motor oil lubricates a car engine, the plasticizer lubricates the polymer chains. Plasticizers allow chains to slide and shift when they are bent, flexed, hit, or stressed. This extra movement allows the polymer chains to absorb shocks and impacts without breaking. Plasticizers prevent cracking, increase flexibility and make nail enhancements much tougher. In Chapter 2, the importance of plasticizers to improve natural nail durability was discussed. The same arguments hold true for the artificial nail. Recall from Chapter 8 that plasticizers increase the durability of nail polish.

Certain natural oils are small enough to penetrate through these pockets and soak deep into the artificial nail, just as they do in the natural nail. Through the daily use of penetrating natural oils, nail enhancements can be kept flexible and tough. Plasticizing oils are a valuable and important way to help ensure that clients' artificial nails will be trouble-free and long-lasting.

SAFE AND PROPER REMOVAL

The natural nail may be damaged if artificial nails are improperly removed. Artificial nail products should never be removed by prying them from the plate. Sometimes impatient nail technicians will use nippers to force the product off the nail plate, but nipping can lead to lifting. The more you nip, the more the product will lift. The nipping action creates weaker adhesion under the remaining artificial nail. Impatient clients may use their teeth to remove the enhancements. This can cause extreme damage and injury! Warn clients against removing their own artificial nails. The damage created while improperly removing nail enhancements can lead to nail infections. Caution must be used while removing nail enhancements to avoid harming the nail plate, bed, or surrounding tissues.

To speed removal, enhancements can be filed down with an abrasive before immersing in a solvent. If you remove the majority of the product, the remaining thin layer is more easily dissolved by solvents, since there is less product to remove. Also, solvents will absorb more easily into rough surfaces than smooth ones. The rough surfaces have much more exposed surface area for solvents to be absorbed into. Whatever you do, avoid overly aggressive filing techniques to prevent friction burns to the delicate nail bed.

Cross-linking makes liquid/powder enhancements more resistant to solvents (FT). Unfortunately, this makes product removal more difficult. Un-cross-linked polymers (i.e., wraps and nail polish} easily dissolve in solvents, but cross-links prevent other types of enhancements from dissolving. Then how should these products be removed? Solvent-based removers will swell the polymer network until it breaks into pieces. The same effect can be seen when a roll of paper towels is put into a bucket of water. The water doesn't dissolve the paper, but the roll will eventually break into shreds. The roll will break up even faster if you poke it with a stick. The same is true of enhancements, which also may be removed more quickly by using a wooden stick or other implement to gently scrape away pieces of softened polymer. The enhancement will swell and break apart more quickly if the solvent is slightly warmer then body temperature. Slightly warming product removers/solvents can significantly reduce product removal time, but this is a professional technique that requires proper training and understanding to be performed safely. In Chapter 6, you learned that warming nail enhancement product removers will considerably shorten the time required to safely remove artificial nail enhancements. Of course, warming any solvent should be done with great care and caution. Many solvents are highly flammable. Never warm solvents in a microwave oven, on a hot plate, or over an open flame. Be very careful when warming flammable solvents. Please refer to Chapter 6 as well as the manufacturer's instructions before warming enhancement product removers. Other very useful techniques can speed removal of enhancements (see the "Nice and Easy" sidebar in Chapter 6).

The most commonly used solvent for removal of nail products is acetone (FT). Acetone is used for two reasons: it is extremely fast and very efficient. When properly used, it is one of the safest solvents available to nail technicians. Non-acetone removers can't compare for speed and safety. More will be said about acetone and non-acetone products in later chapters.

NO PORCELAIN NAILS

The term *porcelain* is incorrectly used to describe liquid/powder systems. There have never been porcelain nails and never will be. Porcelain is made from a blend of special ceramic powders that are mixed with water, then heated slowly to over 1,500°F (815°C). Sound like any nail enhancement application process you've ever seen? Of course not! This is one of many old-fashioned ideas passed down from the days when our industry had no real education or proper information. Sadly, some still use this word to describe or market their products.

METHYL METHACRYLATE

In the early 1970s nail technicians used monomer liquid and polymer powder obtained from local dentists or medical supply stores. Some became highly allergic to these dental products, mainly because they didn't avoid skin contact. The culprit was the monomer methyl methacrylate. Once it was determined that methyl methacrylate was the cause, the FDA confiscated certain MMA-containing nail products and warned against future use of this monomer.

In recent years, MMA usage has increased, and it has become one of the most controversial topics in the professional beauty industry. Unfortunately, there are many myths and misunderstandings surrounding the use of this ingredient. Most nail technicians have heard that they shouldn't use products containing this ingredient, but very few know why! Many believe that MMA is too toxic to use safely. This is untrue. Relatively speaking, MMA is not as toxic as some believe. In fact, for many years MMA has been safely implanted in the body as a bone repair cement. MMA is not a human cancer-causing agent, it is not absorbed through the nail plate, it is not dangerous to inhale in the salon environment, and it does not cause brain tumors. All these are silly, irresponsible myths spread by people who don't understand the issues. Here's the truth! MMA is a safe monomer when used in the proper applications. Artificial nail products should not be based on MMA monomer as an ingredient. There are four main reasons that MMA monomer makes a poor ingredient for artificial nail products:

- MMA nail products do not adhere well to the nail plate. To make these products adhere, nail technicians must shred the surface of the nail plate. This thins the nail plate and makes it weaker.

- MMA creates the hardest and most rigid nail enhancements, which makes them very difficult to break. When a nail enhancement gets jammed or caught, the overly filed and thinned natural nail plate will often break instead of the MMA enhancement, leading to serious nail damage.

- MMA is extremely difficult to remove. Since it will not dissolve in product removers, it is usually pried from the nail plate, creating still more damage. Since MMA products tend to discolor and become brittle, they must be removed more often than EMA-based products, and the difficult removal process often causes a lot of nail damage.

- The FDA and most state boards of cosmetology say not to use it. This clearly is the most important reason. The FDA bases its prohibition on the large number of consumer complaints resulting from the use of MMA nail enhancements in the late 1970s, and it continues to maintain this position today (FT).

For these reasons, several countries, many states, and most professional nail associations have taken a stance against the use of MMA liquid monomer as an ingredient in artificial nail liquids—not because MMA monomer is overly toxic, but because it is an unsuitable ingredient. MMA monomer is used around the world and has a long history of safe use in medical and dental products. MMA monomer is fine for making bulletproof windows and shatterproof eyeglasses, but not artificial nails. That's the real problem with MMA monomer.

How can you tell if MMA-monomer-containing products are being used in the salon? Some have tried to devise test kits that could be used to spot MMA monomer usage in salons. Unfortunately, these tests are not accurate. The only way to determine if MMA monomer is being used is to perform an expensive laboratory analysis, called GCMS testing. Only the monomer liquid can be tested, not the artificial nail enhancement or polymer powder. MMA is only a problem in monomer form. In places where MMA usage has been prohibited, these regulations only apply to MMA monomer in its liquid form. MMA monomer is fine when used to create nail polymer powders or PMMA. Even so, it is not possible to prove that MMA monomer is being used without spending hundreds of dollars for a laboratory test. However, one clue is that MMA-containing products have a different smell. The monomer smells slightly sweeter and stronger than traditional products.

Nail technicians who knowingly use MMA are endangering their clients' nails, their professional licenses, and the salon's reputation, as well as the reputation of the entire professional nail industry. If you know of a nail technician who buys MMA-containing products, you'd be doing yourself and the industry a favor if you reported your suspicions to your state board of cosmetology.

AVOIDING ALLERGIC REACTIONS

Allergic reactions occur in every facet of the professional salon industry. Nail, skin, and hair services can all cause problems for sensitive clients. Fortunately, the vast majority of fingernail-related problems can be easily avoided if you understand how! Allergic reactions are caused by prolonged or repeated contact *(FT)*. Therefore, skin problems do not occur overnight. Artificial nail products are good examples of this. In general, it takes from four to six months (or longer) of repeated exposure before sensitive clients develop skin allergies *(FT)*. Nail technicians are also at risk. Simply touching monomers doesn't cause skin sensitivities; usually months of improper handling must occur before sensitivities develop. For example, nail technicians sometimes develop sensitivities between the thumb and pointer finger. Why? From constantly smoothing monomer-soaked brushes with their fingers. Eventually the pads of the fingers become sore and inflamed. Touching the client's skin with any monomer liquid has the same effect. With each service during which skin contact occurs, the risk of allergy increases with sensitive clients. The problem is, you never know who they are until it's too late. For this reason, it is extremely important that you always leave a 1/8-inch (3-mm) margin between the product and the skin for every client. *Never intentionally touch any nail enhancement product to the skin* *(FT)*. For more information on avoiding allergic reactions with nail enhancement products, see Chapter 12.

MIXING POWDERS

Can liquids and powders from different manufacturers be used interchangeably? Monomer liquids work best when used with the correct polymer powder. Besides having different chemical compositions for different powders, manufacturers use different levels of initiator in their powder. Using a powder with the wrong level of initiator is like using the wrong mix ratio! If there is too little initiator, the enhancement may be weak and the risks of developing an allergic reaction are greatly increased. Also, if there is too much initiator, then discoloration and brittleness become more likely. In short, you should always use the polymer powder that was designed for the monomer liquid of your choice and at the correct mix ratio. It is not very wise to work with a mismatched liquid and powder. The polymer powder must contain the right amount of initiator to ensure proper cure. Upset the delicate balance with too much initiator or too much catalyst and the client's enhancements may suffer. For example, unreacted monomer can remain trapped inside the enhancement and may soak through the nail plate and nail bed to cause a nail bed allergic reaction. The truth is, there is no such thing as a liquid monomer that works with any powder or vice versa Ⓕⓣ.

DAMAGE CONTROL

It's a common misconception that artificial nail products "damage" or "eat" the nail plate. Of course this is absolutely false! Verify this for yourself by taking a small clipping of natural nail plate and placing it in a tightly capped bottle filled with monomer. You can keep this bottle at your station and show it to anyone who believes that monomers damage the nail plate. The same can be done with any of the products you use. None will damage the natural nail, including primers.

Nail products do not damage nails—nail technicians damage nails! Improper application and improper product removal cause most of the nail damage seen in salons. These problems can usually be traced back to a lack of knowledge, understanding, and awareness. Injury and nail damage are easy to avoid, but not by blaming the products. If a client's nail plates or surrounding soft tissue are in bad shape, the nail technician may be to blame. It's your job as a professional nail technician to keep the entire nail unit as healthy as possible. Accept that responsibility and you will be a success. Turn your head the other way or place the blame elsewhere and you will be a bad nail technician who will probably fail. In fact, clients, manufacturers, and good nail technicians will be hoping you fail quickly. Face the facts: the industry has no need for nail technicians who have little regard for their own or the client's health. The information presented in this book will make you better-educated than the best nail technicians of the past. Use this knowledge and strive to be the best you can be. You'll find it is much easier in the long run and far more rewarding.

EXCESSIVE SHRINKAGE CAUSES LIFTING AND BUBBLES

Pocket lifting under liquid/powder enhancements usually occurs on or near the center or **apex** of the nail plate. As the nail enhancement product shrinks, internal stresses build up inside the enhancement. This is especially true if the nail technician uses a wet mix ratio (see "Shrinkage" in Chapter 8). Just as a magnifying glass focuses sunlight into a small, intense spot of light, the curvature of the natural nail plate focuses the stress forces of shrinkage toward the apex. It is at the apex where these forces will meet and collide. When these stress forces become excessive, the product can lose adhesion and separate from the natural nail. The result is a small, bubblelike void or pocket between the enhancement and natural nail, centered directly over the apex of the natural nail. The deeper the

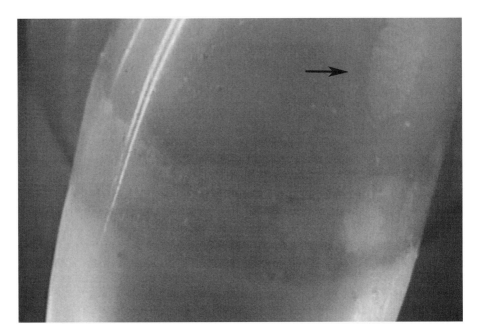

Figure 9-3 *In this example, the arrow points to a void, or lifted pocket, under the artificial nail, that was caused by undercuring of a UV enhancement, but similar-looking round voids can appear at the apex of the nail with liquid/powder systems*

curvature of the nail, the more likely that a center pocket lift will occur. But there is another, more important reason center pocket lifting happens. Using too wet a mix ratio will greatly increase shrinkage. Changing from a wet ratio to a medium consistency will usually solve this type of problem. (See Figure 9–3.)

Bubbles and voids can also be caused by excessive shrinkage, especially if the bubbles appear after the product has hardened. **Voids** are large, irregularly shaped bubbles that appear almost anywhere on the nail plate. They look very much like center pocket lifting except for their irregular shapes. Voids usually form under UV gel enhancements that are not exposed to enough UV light and have undercured. Of course, excessive curing can also be a problem.

Very tiny, nearly invisible bubbles always occur inside the artificial nail. In most cases, these bubbles remain unnoticed unless viewed under a microscope. But when shrinkage becomes excessive, these bubbles can expand and become visible. When tiny bubbles appear only after the product has hardened, this is a sign that the mix ratio is too wet. In general, the wetter the mix ratio, the greater the shrinkage *FT*. Figure 9–4 shows a highly magnified portion of the artificial nail before cure. Figure 9–5 shows the same portion of the artificial nail after the product has set up and turned hard. As seen in this figure, bubbles can grow to very large sizes when the mix ratio is too wet. The best way to prevent problems like this is to avoid using overly wet ratios of liquid monomer to polymer powder, no matter which artificial nail enhancement product you're using.

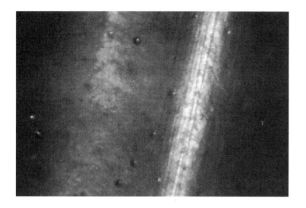 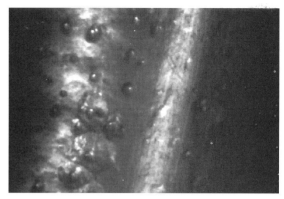

Figure 9-4 and Figure 9-5 *Very tiny, nearly invisible bubbles can grow in size after curing when the improper ratio of liquid and powder is used*

FAST TRACK Ⓕ

- Ⓕ All enhancements are based on the same chemical family, the acrylics.
- Ⓕ Liquid/powder systems are based on methacrylates.
- Ⓕ Wraps, no-light gels, and nail tip adhesives are based on cyanoacrylates.
- Ⓕ UV-curing gel products use both methacrylate and acrylate monomers.
- Ⓕ The polymer powder is the carrier for several key ingredients.
- Ⓕ The polymer carries an initiator called benzoyl peroxide, which is heat-sensitive.
- Ⓕ UV absorbers prevent discoloration and brittleness by absorbing damaging UV light.
- Ⓕ Copolymers give better toughness than homopolymers and offer a wider range of properties.
- Ⓕ Oxygen inhibition results in a sticky, gooey surface layer that rolls off when filed.
- Ⓕ Consistency is determined by the mix ratio of monomer liquid to polymer powder.
- Ⓕ The polymer powder gives the enhancement much of its durability.
- Ⓕ Plasticizers improve nail enhancement or nail plate flexibility and toughness.
- Ⓕ Cross-linking makes nail enhancements more resistant to solvents.
- Ⓕ Acetone is a commonly used solvent because it is safe and extremely efficient.

(FT) Liquids based on methyl methacrylate monomer should never be used in salons.

(FT) Allergic reactions are caused by prolonged or repeated contact.

(FT) In general, allergies can develop after four to six months of repeated skin exposure.

(FT) Never intentionally touch any artificial nail enhancement product to the skin.

(FT) It is impossible to make monomer liquids that work with all polymer powders.

(FT) The wetter the mix ratio, the greater the shrinkage.

Review Questions

1. What is the chemical family name for all nail enhancement coatings and tip adhesives?
2. What is a UV absorber and how does it work?
3. In microns, how large are most polymer powder particles?
4. What effects do excessive amounts of monomer liquid have on nail enhancement durability?
5. Why are inhibitors used in nail enhancement products?
6. Too _____ a consistency, using brushes that are too _____, and using the _____ polymer powder with the monomer liquid are some of the leading causes of allergic skin reactions to nail enhancement products.
7. When performing the bead test described in this chapter to test a bead mix ratio, describe what a medium bead should look like.
8. Why shouldn't products based on methyl methacrylate monomer be used in the salon?
9. What should you do if you suspect that someone is selling methyl methacrylate liquid monomer?
10. A medium-consistency mix ratio contains _____ parts liquid to _____ part powder.
11. A _____ _____ is an ingredient that reduces brushstrokes and improves workability.
12. How is MMA physically and chemically different from PMMA?
13. Bubbles in the artificial nail product that appeared after the product hardened are probably caused by _____ _____ .
14. The curvature of the natural nail plate focuses the _____ _____ of shrinkage toward the apex.
15. The _____ the mix ratio, the _____ the shrinkage.

Chapter 10

UV Gel and Wrap Chemistry

Objective

This chapter will build upon the information you learned in Chapters 7, 8, and 9. Many of the terms and concepts introduced in those chapters will be important to understanding this information. This chapter delves into UV gel chemistry and how to use these products safely. We'll also be exploring the details behind wrap resins and their catalysts.

SAME YET DIFFERENT

In the last chapter you learned that UV gels are based on acrylic monomers and oligomers and are similar in many ways to liquid/powder products (FT). These similarities apply to wrap resin products as well. Each of these product types relies on similar chemistries and ingredients. For example, each uses initiators and catalysts to polymerize monomers and/or oligomers into long chains of polymers. Each type of system polymerizes by using energy to create free radicals. These free radicals in turn activate the monomers and/or oligomers. Each type can be used safely, and none is more "natural" or chemically "organic" than another. But each type of artificial nail enhancement product is different. If you understand these differences, you will be more successful when using these products. Each has advantages and disadvantages. The more you understand these, the better off you and your clients will be.

EFFICIENCY MATTERS

What's the main difference between the chemistry of liquid/powder wraps and UV gels? For many reasons, UV gels are more difficult to properly cure. In other words, they are not as efficient at curing as the other types of artificial nail enhancements. This causes many of the problems associated with this technology. Why? Both undercuring and overcuring are possible with UV gels. Either situation may cause problems if not avoided.

Both heat (room and body) and UV light are forms of energy used to cure artificial nail products. From a chemical point of view, there are several reasons why using UV light is a less efficient way to cure artificial nail products. UV light cannot penetrate very deeply into most substances, including UV gels. UV light is usually absorbed by the upper surface layers of UV gel or may even be reflected away (FT). When thick layers of UV gel are applied to the nail plate, most of the UV light is absorbed by the upper layers. In other words, the upper layers act like an umbrella to shield the lower layers from UV light. So it is much more difficult for UV light to penetrate thick layers of UV gel. This is why UV gels cure more thoroughly when applied in thinner layers (FT). White-colored UV gels, used to create the appearance of a white free edge, contain high amounts of a mineral called titanium dioxide (see Chapter 9), which easily absorbs and reflects UV light. Other colored pigments can also create an umbrella-like effect by absorbing and reflecting UV light. This is why white or colored UV gels are more difficult to cure (FT).

Curing is often inefficient even at the upper layer of the UV gel. Here's why. You learned in the last chapter that oxygen in the air prevents UV gels from curing on the surface, creating an oxygen inhibition layer. Thicker than normal oxygen inhibition layers are often seen when the artificial nail is undercured (FT). UV light's inefficiency as an energy source for curing artificial nails contributes to the formation of these layers. Of course, more powerful UV lights could be used, but these could have an adverse effect on clients' skin. These lamps must be safe for the client's skin and nails. That is why more-powerful lamps are not used in the professional nail industry.

EFFICIENCY OF UV LAMPS

The UV nail lamps contain special bulbs designed to create light from a unique part of the spectrum (Figure 10–1). These bulbs create both visible and invisible light. The visible light is from the blue and violet part of the spectrum. The invisible light is from the ultraviolet or UV range, as shown in Color Plate 20.

UV bulbs emit both visible and invisible light. The visible bluish glow that comes from the bulb is from the blue and violet part of the spectrum. The amount of UV-A light emitted by the bulbs used in the nail industry range from roughly equal to the UV found in summer sunlight up to almost three times more UV. Since these lamps are covered and the client's hands are in them for a relatively short period, UV nail lamps are safe and when properly used do not pose any significant risk to clients or nail technicians. Of course you should read, understand, and follow all manufacturer's instructions and warnings to ensure that you are safely and correctly operating the unit. One of these warnings is to avoid looking into the opening of the light.

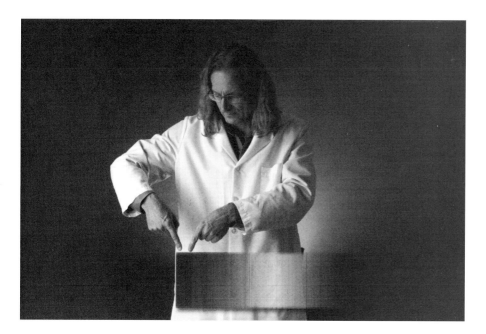

Figure 10-1 UV nail bulbs emit both visible light, mostly from the blue and violet part of the spectrum, and light in the UV-A region, shown in Color Plate 20 as the darkest blue zone to the left of the violet and indigo on the color spectrum

UV bulbs need to be changed regularly. Recall from earlier chapters that UV light intensity is different from wattage. The wattage will always stay the same, but the UV intensity of the bulb will slowly degrade with usage. Remember, the UV gel product and lamp are designed to work together for best performance, just as monomer liquids are designed for use with the correct powders. Different lamps and bulbs generate different amounts of UV light energy (Figure 10–2). Don't go just by the wattage of the UV lightbulb. Some 27-watt UV lamps deliver more UV light to the nail than many 36-watt units. Wattage measures how much electricity the bulb will consume when it's on. Also be careful when selecting table lighting. Many types of table lamps produce UV light. True-color bulbs and those designed to mimic natural sunlight usually produce significant amounts of UV light *FT*. In fact, they produce enough UV to affect products sitting directly underneath them, especially if the lamp is within a few feet of the product container. This type of exposure can cause UV gel products to partially cure and form small, soft lumps in their containers. Partially cured product can lead to many types of service breakdown issues, including lifting, rubbery or overly flexible nails, and discoloration.

Halogen and fluorescent bulbs will produce much smaller amounts of UV light. As long as these are kept three or more feet from the UV gel product, exposure will be minimal and probably will not contribute to premature curing. UV gel products can be slightly sensitive to visible light, especially blue light. Care

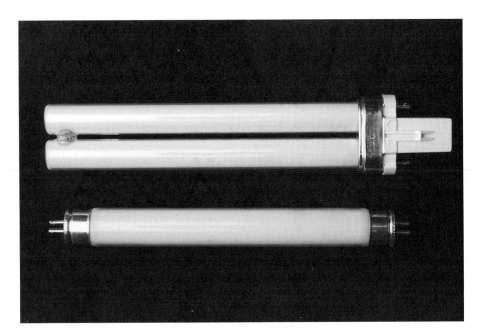

Figure 10-2 *A UV nail lamp may have between 4 and 45 watts, depending on the number of bulbs that are used; the double or U-shaped tube is a 9-watt bulb, while straight bulbs may emit either 4 or 6 watts*

should be taken to cover containers when not in use. It is important to minimize exposure to all sources of light, not just UV. Of course, sunlight, true-color lights, and UV lights are far more likely to cause premature thickening in the container. Remember, especially if you work near a window, be sure to take precautions to shield your product containers from all light exposure—use blinds, curtains, and UV-absorbing window films or coatings. You don't have to work in the dark, but you do have to protect your product from intense visible light or direct UV light exposure.

TIME FOR A CHANGE

A fresh set of UV bulbs will quickly begin to emit less and less UV light, even though they will continue to emit blue and violet visible light. Depending on how often you use the lamp, the bulbs may not be producing enough UV light to properly cure the product. In general, after about two to four months of regular use, the entire set of bulbs must be changed (FT). Eventually these bulbs will produce too little UV light. When this occurs, undercuring of the artificial nail is likely. Undercuring makes artificial nails more prone to staining, lifting, and breakage and creates a higher potential for allergic skin reactions (FT). When UV bulbs become weakened, less UV light reaches the lower layers of product. The result is that there's not enough energy to convert all of the oligomers and monomers into polymers. This creates an undercured zone of the product near the nail plate. Small sections may lose adhesion and lift away from the natural nail, creating small pockets or voids. These small pockets look like air bubbles but are actually spaces caused by the product's separation from the keratin surface of the natural nail. Also, coatings that lose clarity and become cloudy in appearance may also be a sign of undercuring. If any of these symptoms occur and it has been more than two months since you changed your UV bulbs, it would be wise to put

FINE FROM AFAR

Here's a very interesting fact about UV light: intensity is drastically diminished by distance (FT). As a rule, every time you double the distance between you and a light source, the intensity drops by a whopping 75 percent! This is true for all types of light. That's why flashbulbs on cameras don't help if the subject is more than a few feet away. An artificial nail held one inch from a UV lightbulb receives three times more UV light energy than one held two inches away. This demonstrates how easy it is to avoid overexposing eyes to UV light. Unless the client makes a habit of looking directly into an exposed UV bulb from a few inches away, there's very little risk of eye injury. Casually or occasionally looking at a UV nail light from several feet away for brief periods poses virtually no risk.

in new bulbs. Other indicators of improper cure are thicker than normal oxygen inhibition layers, soft or dull surfaces, weak enhancements, or bare spots where the coating has been easily wiped or filed away.

LESS IS MORE

As discussed in Chapter 8, initiators cause polymerization to occur in all types of artificial nail systems. In liquid/powder and wrap systems, these initiators use heat (from the body or room) as the energy source. UV gel systems use initiators that rely on UV light as the energy source. Light-sensitive initiators are called **photoinitiators.** Photoinitiators absorb UV light and convert it into the energy needed to drive the polymerization process (FT). So photoinitiators control the process and play an important role in the resulting artificial nail. In general, the more photoinitiator there is in the formula, the faster the cure. But more isn't always better. Too much photoinitiator can cause problems.

For example, UV gel products can quickly heat up, even to the point that clients will pull their fingers from the lamp. This can happen with formulations that contain excessive amounts of photoinitiator. It's also more of a problem in clients whose nail beds have been friction-burned by aggressive filing techniques. Excessive exotherms are also more likely when overly thick layers of UV gel are applied to the nail plate. Extreme exotherms that cause clients to pull their fingers from the lamp may prevent products from being properly cured (FT). What's the result of an improper cure? Improper curing of UV gel enhancements can lead to skin allergies. When undercured, unreacted ingredients are left inside enhancements. Normally, these ingredients would react and become a permanent part of the artificial nail. But unreacted chemicals can be fairly mobile. In other words, they can slowly migrate through both the artificial and natural nail until reaching the soft, living tissue of the nail bed. When these types of skin irritations or allergies occur, clients often complain of "itchy" or "warm" nail beds. They also make allergy-related onycholysis more likely (see Chapter 4). To ensure proper curing, it is important to use both the correct lamp and bulbs. Always use the UV lamp and bulbs designed for use with the UV gel system of your choice. In Chapter 12, you will learn more about allergic skin reactions and how to avoid them.

Choosing the proper photoinitiator for a UV gel and using the correct amount are two of the most difficult tasks facing scientists who formulate these types of products. Three of the most important factors in UV curing are:

1. A proper balance between the photoinitiator and UV lamp
2. The intensity of available UV light
3. The duration of the UV exposure

Photoinitiators are key to the success of a UV gel system. Many photoinitiators can cause yellowing and/or brittleness, especially when excessive amounts are used. Photoinitiator remaining in the enhancement after curing can still

CLEAR AS NIGHT AND DAY

Photoinitiators are like photographic film—they come in different speeds. Films designed for use in darkness are very sensitive to very low levels of light, while films used for bright days are much less sensitive to light. You wouldn't use the less sensitive film in a dark room or vice versa. Your pictures would be under- or overexposed. Photographic film must be matched to the available light. The same is true for UV gels. Different UV gels have very different sensitivities to UV light. That's why it's important to use the UV lamp designed for the UV product of your choice. There's no such thing as a UV lamp that works with any UV gel product.

react with UV light from the sun, tanning beds, and so on. It is a myth that all curing stops as soon as the hand is removed from the UV lamp. Curing can continue for days, but at a much slower rate (FT). This helps explain why continued UV light exposure can lead to age-related brittleness. Some UV gel formulations undergo severe age-related service breakdown, forcing nail technicians to remove the enhancements every three to four months, creating problems for both nail technicians and clients. A properly formulated UV gel enhancement should remain flexible and trouble-free throughout its lifetime on the fingernail. Nail technicians should never have to remove the product from their clients' hands because of age-related service breakdown. Why is this important? UV gel products are the most difficult to remove. If not removed carefully and correctly, nail damage is more likely to occur (FT). (See the "Nice and Easy" sidebar in Chapter 6 for removal tips.) For this reason, it is better to use a UV gel nail product that does not require periodic removal.

HONEY, I SHRANK THE NAIL!

In Chapter 8 you learned that all polymers shrink when they are created. Wrap resin products shrink between 4 and 7 percent, liquid/powder systems shrink between 7 and 11 percent, and UV gel enhancement products shrink between 12 and 18 percent. UV gel products containing acrylates shrink much more than those made from methacrylate monomers and/or oligomers. A little shrinkage is normal, but greater than 12 percent causes many problems. Lifting, tip cracking, and other types of service breakdown are often caused by excessive shrinkage.

Why does shrinking occur? Recall that monomers and oligomers wander aimlessly around the container, always avoiding each other and never touching. But when they join to form polymers, each embraces the other tightly. As you can imagine, when billions of monomers and oligomers suddenly move closer together, a great deal of shrinkage can happen. Excessive shrinkage can cause small pockets to form under the enhancement. Product shrinkage can also cause cracking, lifting, even pain. Clients can sometimes feel the effects of excessive shrinkage and may comment that the enhancement feels like it is tightening or throbbing. The symptoms usually occur after a few hours, depending on how much the product shrinks. Excessive shrinkage not only is uncomfortable but can cause damage or trauma to the nail bed. For example, the nail plate may separate from the bed. The first sign may be a small white area at the free edge or hyponychium. Over time, excessive shrinkage may squeeze the nail plate, causing it to "jump off track" and separate from the bed (see Figure 1–6). Once separation begins, it travels further under the nail plate. In Chapter 1 you learned that the hyponychium forms a watertight seal that prevents bacteria, fungi, and viruses from attacking the nail bed. Spaces under the nail plate create the perfect environment for infections to take hold. Remember, trauma to the nail plate can lead to infection.

SKIN SENSITIVITY

As discussed in previous chapters, using the wrong polymer powder with a monomer liquid or using an incorrect (usually too wet) bead consistency can lead to improper cure. Just as monomer product residues may cause allergic reactions, the same can occur with UV gel systems. Some unreacted ingredients can increase the potential for allergic skin reactions, so it is important to ensure a proper and thorough cure. Several factors determine the degree or percentage of cure. The more important ones are listed below:

- Thickness of applied UV gel layer
- Color and opacity of the uncured UV gel
- Position of hand and fingers under the UV gel lamp
- Time that the UV gel spends under the lamp
- UV bulb quality, age, and condition
- Whether the UV lamp has been designed for the gel system

The thickness of the UV gel coating has a great effect on the degree of cure. As a rule, the thicker the coating, the less efficient the cure. It is much better to use three or four thin coats rather than one or two thick coats. This may take a little longer, but thinner coats allow more UV light to penetrate and deliver energy into the deepest layers to ensure a proper cure. This is especially important for white-tipping UV gels and colored nail art UV gel products, since these can absorb and reflect large amounts of UV light.

The amount of time the enhancement spends under the UV lightbulbs is extremely important. The same is true for the positioning of the hand and fingers. The longer the enhancements remain properly placed under the UV light, the more likely it is that they will properly cure. Curing the enhancement with the correct amount of UV light means less unreacted ingredients and a more durable artificial nail. Remember, just because the enhancement has hardened does not mean that it is properly cured. Always use a timer to ensure that the correct cure times are observed. Some UV lamps come with built-in timers to help ensure proper curing. Make sure to never shorten the recommended time, and teach clients the importance of correctly placing their hands and fingers.

UV bulb quality and condition are vital to the success of UV gel enhancements. Not all UV bulbs are alike. Some quickly lose their ability to create UV light, while others are weaker and produce lower amounts of UV light. UV bulbs can look identical, even if they are from different manufacturers. Different manufacturers' bulbs emit significantly different amounts of UV light and lose strength at different rates. In general, higher-quality UV bulbs (which usually cost more) have a higher UV output and will maintain these levels for much longer. So buyer beware! Saving a few dollars when purchasing UV bulbs may not be in your best interest.

Regardless of which UV bulbs you use, they must be regularly changed. Heavy users should change all of the UV bulbs in their lamp at least every three months. If the nail enhancements seem to be setting more slowly than normal or are showing signs of undercuring, change the UV bulbs immediately! It is a good idea to keep a spare set of bulbs around. Dirty bulbs will also lower UV strength. Clean the dust and other debris from bulbs whenever needed. At least once per week is recommended. If the bulbs have UV gel product adhered to the bottom of the bulb, flip it over in the socket so the product is on the top of the bulb and not blocking UV light from reaching the product on the nail If both sides have product adhered to them, discard the bulbs and replace them. Skimping on UV bulbs will cost far more in repairs and problems. Make sure you always unplug your lamp before changing bulbs. Be sure to refer to the manufacturer's instructions for information on how to safely clean your UV lamp and bulbs. Finally, be sure to use the proper UV lamp with the UV system of your choice. It is impossible to make a UV lamp that works with every UV gel system.

"BETTER FOR THE NAIL" CLAIMS

Some claim that UV gel enhancement products are "better" or "safer" for the natural nail than liquid/powder systems or wrap resin systems. This is absolutely false! In fact, it could be argued that UV gels are more damaging to the natural nail since they are more difficult to remove. Also, some UV gel formulations utilize glutaraldehyde or acrylic acid as adhesion promoters, and all contain photoinitiators. Each of these substances may cause allergic skin reactions if prolonged and/or repeated overexposure occurs. Glutaraldehyde and acrylic acid should never be used in artificial nail products since they have such a tremendous potential to cause allergic skin reactions. Luckily, recent advances in the development of new photoinitiators and adhesion promoters have made it easier for scientists to formulate UV gel products with a lower tendency to cause allergic skin reactions. But remember, no type of artificial nail enhancement product is better for the natural nail or safer to use than others when properly applied by a trained professional Ⓕ. Nor is it true that some enhancement products are more "natural" or chemically "organic." These are bogus marketing claims design to scare nail technicians away from competitive products. What is truly "better for the nail"? That is easy to answer. The best thing for the natural nail is a highly skilled, educated, and conscientious nail professional who understands how to properly apply and maintain clients' artificial nails. This kind of nail technician is the natural nail's best friend. Good nail technicians protect and nurture the nail plate. Don't be fooled by fear-based marketing claims! Professional nail enhancement products don't damage the natural nail when used properly. Nail technicians must take responsibility for much of their clients' nail damage. Any product can be applied and removed safely. It is up to nail professionals to use their knowledge and skills to do this while protecting their client's natural nails.

WRAP RESINS AND CATALYSTS

The chemistry of wrap resins is discussed in detail in Chapters 7 and 8. To recap, wrap resins are monomers from the acrylic family called cyanoacrylates (FT). This book uses the terms *resin* and *cyanoacrylate monomers* interchangeably. It is also important to note that cyanoacrylate monomers are used as adhesives for artificial nail tips as well. Cyanoacrylates can polymerize very rapidly, especially when moisture is present. Try this experiment. Put a small amount of water on an artificial nail tip that has been freshly coated with cyanoacrylate monomer. The product will cure so quickly that it will turn an opaque, chalky white. This is because the rapid curing process shatters the coating, forming millions of microscopic cracks that cloud the coating.

Catalysts are used with all wrap resin systems. Catalysts trigger polymerization, but they are not needed for the process to occur. In fact, tip adhesives cure quite nicely without them. All the cyanoacrylate monomers need is a tiny amount of initiator and they will rapidly polymerize. What is the initiator for cyanoacrylate monomers? You saw in the experiment that cyanoacrylates are moisture-sensitive. In other words, moisture is the initiator for all systems that are based on cyanoacrylate monomers. Moisture in the air, skin, nail plates, and even the wrap fabric react with cyanoacrylate monomers to cause polymerization. Once contact occurs, polymerization is almost immediate. Very long chains of single-link polymers are created within a tiny fraction of a second. Since wrap resin products contain no cross-linkers, the polymers formed are like long, spaghettilike strands. This creates both advantages and disadvantages. The disadvantages may be why this technology has limited usefulness. A discussion of these advantages and disadvantages will provide a better understanding of this useful technology.

ADVANTAGES OF CYANOACRYLATES

Recall from Chapter 8 that simple polymers harden when the chains become intertwined into a tangled mass that resembles a very dense undergrowth of vines in the rain forest. But if this tangled mass is soaked in the right solvent—such as acetone—it will unravel and fall apart into smaller chunks. This makes removal of cyanoacrylate enhancements a quick and easy task. Another important advantage is that cyanoacrylate-containing enhancement products are unlikely to cause skin allergic reactions. Why? Before a skin allergy can develop, allergy-causing ingredients must be absorbed into the upper layers of the skin. Since the skin is filled with moisture, it is unlikely that cyanoacrylate monomers will get very far past the topmost surface layers. The skin's natural moisture will initiate its hardening (curing) on the skin's surface. It is interesting to note that because cyanoacrylate resins break down in the presence of moisture over time and rarely cause allergic skin reactions, they are often use by doctors to close wounds.

In relatively rare instances clients may become allergic to the stabilizers used to prevent premature polymerization in the container and improve shelf life, such as HQ and MEHQ. This type of allergic reaction is rare, since these stabilizers are usually less than 1/200th of 1 percent of the formulation.

Cyanoacrylates are fast-setting and create very clear coatings with tremendous adhesion to the natural nail, which is why they make great artificial nail tip adhesives (FT).

DISADVANTAGES OF CYANOACRYLATES

Most of the disadvantages associated with wrap resins and catalysts can be avoided or controlled if you understand how. For example, quick solvent removal is an advantage for cyanoacrylate polymers, but it is also a disadvantage. Other solvents besides acetone also dissolve cyanoacrylate polymers. Even soaking in water will cause these simple polymers to break down. It's clear that nail polish removers can weaken wrap resins and artificial nail tip adhesives unless precautions are taken. This type of solvent can seep into tiny nooks and crannies on the surface and become absorbed. As more and more solvent is absorbed, the nail enhancement begins to swell as the individual chains break apart, causing the artificial nail to crumble. Luckily, this is easy to avoid. The working strength of nail polish removers can be adjusted by adding small amounts of water. For use with wrap resins, dilute the acetone with one part water for every ten parts acetone. This blend will quickly remove the nail polish color without damaging the artificial nail. Also, add a drop or two of penetrating nail moisturizing oil to the diluted acetone to help replenish the lost skin and plate oils.

Artificial nails made with cyanoacrylate monomers are more likely to be discolored by surface stains. Stains from food, tobacco smoke, nail polish, household cleaners, and so on are more common with wrap enhancements. Again, this is because they are not cross-linked. Just as solvents are more likely to penetrate wrap enhancements, so are stains. Usually these can be easily removed by lightly buffing the nail plate's surface. Most of the stain is usually deposited in the upper two or three layers of the plate. Because of this, it is wise to use a good base coat over wrap enhancements to help prevent staining by nail polishes.

Rapid curing also has advantages and disadvantages. Cyanoacrylate resins are usually applied over fiberglass, linen, or paper to reinforce and strengthen the coating. Without one of these fabriclike materials, the coating is weak and frag-ile. Since these materials can contain moisture, the wrap monomer may poly-merize before being thoroughly absorbed into the fabric mesh. Without proper penetration and a complete "wetting out" of the fabric mesh, air bubbles will be trapped against the fabric, creating an unsightly appearance, as seen in Figure 10–3. Air bubbles can also be trapped between the product and the natural nail, which leads to poor adhesion. Oils can block penetration of the wrap monomer into the fabric. It is wise to avoid touching fabrics with bare fingers.

Another disadvantage comes from the rapid curing of these products. Po-tentially damaging exotherms can result when these products are cured improp-erly. Each time a monomer or oligomer reacts to form a polymer, a small amount of heat is released. Heat is released with each new linkage that is formed as a polymer chain grows in length. The heat created from the joining of billions of monomers or oligomers is what creates these exotherms. Clients don't feel the heat when it is released over a few minutes, unless their nail beds are irritated or damaged. But if the same amount of heat is released over a few seconds, it can create a painful heat spike. Wrap catalysts are designed to shorten the cure time to seconds. If these are sprayed from too close a distance and/or a thick coating of cyanoacrylate resin is applied, excessive exotherms may occur. The potentially

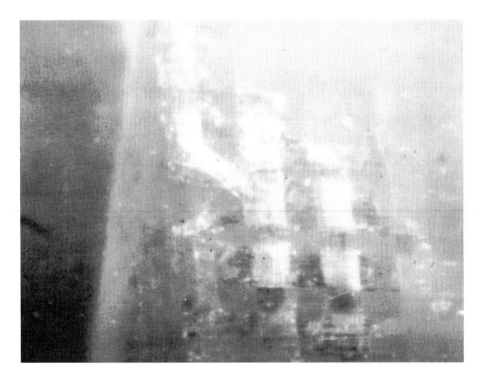

Figure 10-3 *Highly magnified section showing how cyanoacrylate resins can improperly wet fiberglass fabrics*

damaging spike of heat may reach 120°F (49°C) and could lead to onycholysis. These problems can be avoided by following manufacturer's directions. Always spray wrap catalysts in a controlled fashion and at the appropriate distance from the nail. It is important to use proper ventilation to avoid long-term overexposure to the vapors and mists created by wrap catalysts. Overexposure to vapors and mist becomes more likely when spraying a substance into the air. Wrap catalysts contain low amounts of ingredients, such as n,n-dimethyl-para-toluidine (DMPT), that may cause injury if large amounts are absorbed through the skin. Fortunately, this is an unlikely occurrence if these products are used safely and correctly. Because these ingredients are in low concentrations, usually less than 1 percent of the formulation, skin overexposure can be easily avoided with good housekeeping and common sense. Avoid spraying wrap catalysts directly on your own skin. The client is exposed to an occasional misting, which is unlikely to cause skin overexposure. Nail technicians should wear disposable nitrile gloves to lower the potential for skin overexposure. A mist-rated mask should be used when spraying products into the air *FYI* . These masks are thicker and are designed to prevent overexposure and inhalation of fine mists. You will learn more about dust and mist masks in Chapters 14 and 15.

As with all professional nail enhancement products, wrap resins and catalysts must be used with appropriate ventilation. This is especially important when spraying wrap catalysts. Proper ventilation is necessary to avoid inhaling excessive amounts of the vapors or mist generated by spraying wrap catalysts. With proper ventilation and safe handling, these products can be used safely. Proper ventilation is one of the most important steps you can take to improve safety in the salon and to ensure that your health is protected. You'll also learn about the precautions you can take to protect yourself from long-term overexposure to mists and sprays of all types. One of the most important steps is good housekeeping. Be sure to clean tabletops and surfaces regularly. Always avoid resting your arm or hand on any surface that is not clean and free from dust or nail product residue.

You have learned that cyanoacrylates have tremendous adhesion to keratin and rapidly polymerize in the presence of moisture. This is also both an advantage and disadvantage, especially if skin or eye contact occurs. A large droplet can release enough heat to damage the skin. Should this happen, don't panic! Cool the area as quickly as possible with cold tap water. Skin is instantly bonded together by cyanoacrylates. If the fingers become bonded, soak them in acetone until the bond dissolves on its own. Never attempt to pry the skin apart *FYI* . This will tear the skin, only increasing the potential for damage. The same is true of clothing or other items. If another object becomes bonded to skin, soak the bonded area in acetone until they dissolve apart. Never open or use wrap resins or tip adhesives over your lap or near your face. Wearing gloves while using cyanoacrylate products will greatly reduce the chance of accidents.

Many accidents with wrap and tip adhesive monomers involve the eyes. Usually, these occur while removing stuck caps or pulling out pin closures. Always point the tip of the container away from yourself and your client when opening these products. Also, always wear safety eye protection when using any product containing cyanoacrylate monomers (FT). *Warning:* Accidents become more likely if you carry these products in your purse. Some types of containers might be mistaken for eyedrops or nasal spray and their contents accidentally poured into the eyes or squirted into the nose. Also, children may be injured if these products are left in their reach. Remember, serious damage can occur if cyanoacrylate monomers get in the eyes. If this ever happens, quickly cool the eye with lots of cold running water to prevent burns. Do not rub or touch the eye area, and see a doctor immediately. Rubbing may seriously scratch the eye. A qualified medical doctor can separate the eyelids without damaging the eye or eyesight.

NO-LIGHT GELS AND POWDER DIPS

The term *no-light gel* is misleading. The name suggests that these products are similar to UV gels but don't need UV light. Not true! These products are cyanoacrylate monomers that have been thickened to have a gel-like appearance. They should be used and handled like other wrap-type products. They have most of the advantages and disadvantages of other wrap products. Many feel that the gel wrap product is easier to use. But thicker monomers will not wet out the fabric very easily and can affect the artificial nail's appearance.

Cyanoacrylate resins have great adhesion, but they are low in strength and durability. As described above, the wrap fabric is used to reinforce and add durability to the cyanoacrylate coating. Another way to reinforce the coating is to borrow an idea from liquid/powder technology. Methacrylate polymer powders will also strengthen cyanoacrylate resin coatings. These polymer powders are the same except that they do not contain the initiator that is added for liquid/powder systems. In fact, powders designed for use with methacrylate monomer liquids should not be used since they do contain initiator. Benzoyl peroxide is the initiator, and it may cause discoloration and brittleness in cyanoacrylate coatings. The purpose of the polymer powder is to become a part of the coating and toughen it. The powder offers some improvement over the fabric, but these systems still can't stand up to daily abuse and wear like liquid/powder or UV gel systems. Wrap resin systems are best used as protective overlays for the natural nail, not to extend the free edge or for sculpting. As a protective overlay, it is a very useful service. However, it is best to sprinkle or shake the powder over the coating; if the dipping technique is used, dispose of the powder between clients to avoid unsanitary conditions.

FAST TRACK (FT)

(FT) Like liquid/powder products, UV gels are based on acrylic monomers and oligomers.

(FT) Many substances absorb UV light at the surface or reflect it away.

FT Light must completely penetrate the UV gel for proper curing, so thinner coatings of UV gel cure more thoroughly.

FT White or colored pigments can block UV light penetration and prevent proper curing.

FT Oxygen blocks surface curing, causing an oxygen inhibition layer to develop, and thicker-than-normal inhibition layers indicate undercuring.

FT True-color and natural-sunlight bulbs create significant amounts of UV light.

FT UV lightbulbs should be changed after two to four months of regular use.

FT Undercuring can cause staining, lifting, and breakage and creates a higher likelihood of allergic reactions.

FT UV light intensity is drastically diminished by distance.

FT Photoinitiators absorb UV light and start the polymerization process.

FT Extreme exotherms may cause clients to react by pulling their hands away from the light, resulting in improper curing.

FT UV gel enhancements can continue to slowly cure for days.

FT Improper removal of UV gels can damage the natural nail plate.

FT No enhancement product is safer or better for the natural nail than another when used properly.

FT The monomers used to create wraps are called cyanoacrylates.

FT Certain types of cyanoacrylates are used as tip adhesives.

FT Wear a mist-rated mask to avoid excessive inhalation of sprays.

FT Never attempt to pry bonded skin apart.

FT Safety eye protection can protect eyes while using wraps or tip adhesives.

Review Questions

1. Gel products are based on which family of monomers and oligomers?
2. An _____ is a short chain of monomers that is not long enough to be a polymer.
3. List the five factors that determine the degree or percentage of cure in UV gel systems.
4. Which types of UV gels are the most difficult to properly cure?
5. As a rule, every time you double the distance between you and a light source, the intensity drops by what percentage?

6. _____ absorb UV light and convert it into the energy needed for polymerization.

7. Which are more likely to cause skin allergies, UV gels, wrap resins, or tip adhesives?

8. Which is the least likely to cause skin allergies, UV gels, wrap resins, or tip adhesives?

9. Which type of nail enhancement product is best or safest for the natural nail?

10. What is the chemical name of the wrap resin monomer?

11. The initiator for wrap resins is _____.

12. Which type artificial nail enhancement product shrinks more: wrap resins or UV gels?

13. Which is more susceptible to staining, wraps or UV gel nail enhancements?

14. What should be done if skin becomes bonded together with wrap resins or nail adhesives?

15. Name three important pieces of safety equipment required for working with wrap resins.

Chapter

11

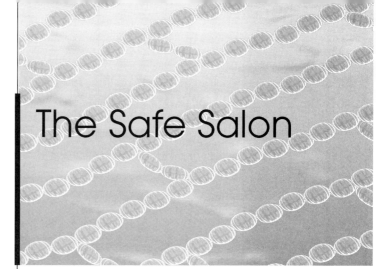

The Safe Salon

Objective

In this chapter you will learn the basics of working safely. You will find that every product in the professional nail industry can be used safely if you know how (FT). You'll discover that safety is under your control if you have the understanding needed. You'll also see how easy it is to use your products cautiously, correctly, and wisely.

CHEMOPHOBIA

What is a chemical? Most people believe chemicals are dangerous or toxic substances. If you asked them to name some chemicals, most would think of pesticides, toxic waste, or pollution. That's because people associate the word *chemical* with something that is dangerous. Nothing could be further from the truth! Actually, everything you can see or touch is a chemical, except for light and electricity. Air is a combination of many chemicals, including oxygen, hydrogen, and nitrogen. Clean, pure mountain stream water is a chemical. Newborn baby skin is 100 percent chemicals, as is every molecule in your body. We can't escape chemicals because we *are* chemicals.

If this is so, then why do people only think of chemicals in a negative way? It is because of the overdramatized and exaggerated images created by the media. These images are misleading, inaccurate, and designed to frighten you. The truth is, over 99 percent of the chemicals you will come in contact with in your life are completely safe and beneficial (FT). Unfortunately, most reporters have journalism degrees and no understanding of chemistry. They almost always use the word *chemical* in a scary, negative way. The media has created a negative information plague called **chemophobia**—the fear of chemicals. Like most phobias, the fear isn't based on facts. What is the cure for chemophobia? Knowledge and understanding! We are not afraid of the things we understand, only what we don't understand. Getting to know and understand your chemical tools will put you in complete control. That's the good news! Working safely is very easy to do if you know how.

Water is the most common salon chemical and one of the most deadly! In fact, water is such a dangerous chemical that a small amount can kill you in minutes. Don't believe it? Try sticking your head in a bucket of water for five minutes. Of course no one would do such a foolish thing. But why wouldn't we do this? Because since you were a very young child your parents have taught you about the dangers of water. Your parents taught you that it is dangerous to swim after a big meal and never to use a blow dryer in the bathtub. We learned not to drive too fast on wet pavement and then slam on the brakes. We learned all the rules for using this potentially deadly chemical, so we can use it with relative safety. The same is true for salon chemicals. There are rules that must be obeyed when working with any and all chemicals. Disobey these rules and you may suffer the consequences. But remember, these consequences are easily avoided. Every chemical can be safe, and every chemical can also be dangerous. It is up to you and how you use it!

If you are serious about being a professional nail technician, you must take the time to learn the rules of working safely. Why risk the consequences? Instead, learn to use products correctly and safely. Start by reading and understanding the manufacturer's educational literature and warning labels. Always use products in strict accordance with the manufacturer's instructions. Remember; safety and health come first!

TWELVE RULES FOR WORKING SAFELY

Is it possible to work safely with potentially dangerous chemicals? Of course it is, but safety doesn't just happen. Still, it's pretty easy to do. All you must do is learn the facts and then apply your knowledge. The best way to ensure you're working safely is to follow the 12 safety rules described below:

Fact #1: No Chemical Can Be Harmful Unless You Overexpose Yourself

One of the most important things to learn about chemicals is the **overexposure principle.** This principle says that every chemical has a safe and unsafe level of exposure. You won't be harmed unless you repeatedly exceed the safe levels ⒻⓉ. When used correctly, professional products are safe. They're designed to be that way. Problems only occur if you repeatedly exceed safe exposure levels for long periods of time. The length of the exposure is very important. Brief or short-term exposures are much less risky. Short-term exposures cause symptoms such as dry or irritated skin, mild headaches, or itchy and watery eyes. It is fairly rare for illness or injury to be caused by professional salon products. This is especially obvious when you consider the many millions of products that have been used over the last 20 years. But occasionally problems can occur, especially if care is not taken to prevent long-term overexposure. Of course, some chemicals are dangerous even in tiny amounts, but these are not used in nail salons. Professional products are formulated to be as safe as possible. Still, no beauty or cosmetic product is free from all risks. It would be impossible. We live in a world full of risks! Even normally safe products can become dangerous if used incorrectly. No matter if you're a gardener, chef, or artist, everyone who works with any chemical must work safely or risk injury.

Rule #1: Always Look for Ways to Reduce Your Exposure to Safe Levels

If you follow this one rule, you will be much safer in the salon. Everything you will learn in this chapter will teach you how to reduce your exposure. You can also find important information in the **Material Safety Data Sheets (MSDS)** for the product. These product sheets are an important source of many types of safety information ⒻⓉ.

MATERIAL SAFETY DATA SHEETS (MSDS)

MSDSs provide information to all chemical workers, including nail technicians. MSDSs help firemen clean up large spills. They help doctors treat accidental poisonings or allergies and cosmetic product formulators to make safer products.

MSDSs provide important information about each professional product that you use. Any professional product that contains a potentially hazardous substance has an MSDS. What is a hazardous substance? Lots of different things qualify as hazardous, ranging from slippery gels or oils that could cause a fall to products that are poisonous if swallowed by children, flammable solvents, and eye irritants.

Here is a brief list of the many important things you can learn from an MSDS:

- All potentially hazardous ingredients found in a product
- Information that will help you to avoid potential hazards
- The best way to handle and properly store products
- How to prevent fires, falls, burns, and other accidents
- Ways to keep hazardous substances out of your body
- Early warning signs of product overexposure
- The short- and long-term health effects of overexposure
- Emergency first-aid advice and emergency phone numbers

Federal regulations require that salons keep MSDSs for all products on the premises and available for anyone to see during normal business hours. Federal regulations also require manufacturers and distributors of professional products to provide MSDSs to all product users. You can contact your local OSHA office for more information about the "Employee Right to Know" regulation and how MSDS sheets can help you work more safely. Contact information for your local office can be found at their Web site, www.osha.gov.

HOW'D THAT GET IN HERE?

There are only three ways that a chemical substance can enter your body. These three ways are called the **routes of entry** Ⓕ. Blocking these routes will automatically reduce your exposure. These routes are:

1. **Inhalation** by breathing vapors, mists, or dusts
2. **Absorption** through the skin or broken tissue
3. Unintentional or accidental **ingestion** (swallowing)

The MSDS will warn you about each route of entry. For instance, it may warn users to avoid inhaling sprays or mists. Or you may be warned to wash hands to prevent skin overexposure. Lowering your exposure is easier if you know when you need special ventilation, masks, eyewear, aprons or gloves, and so on (see Figure 11–1).

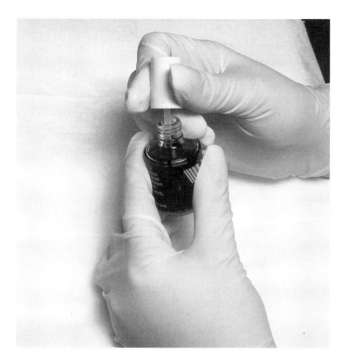

Figure 11-1 *Wear gloves to prevent skin overexposure*

HEALTH EFFECTS EXPLAINED

The MSDS explains both the short- and long-term effects of overexposure. Short-term or **acute effects** occur within approximately six months. Short-term effects are early warning signs of overexposure (FI). These signs and symptoms usually disappear when overexposure stops. Some examples are headaches, nausea, scratchy throat, coughing, or rashes. Long-term or **chronic effects** may also occur with extended overexposure or misuse. Chronic effects usually occur after six months, and in some cases it may take several years of overexposure before they show up. But remember, when the MSDS describes the acute and chronic effects, these are not necessarily what will happen. Quite the contrary! These are potential dangers that *could* happen if you misuse the product or work unsafely, especially over a long period. The longer the overexposure continues, the more likely it is that problems may occur. No problems may ever develop. But long-term exposure increases the risks. That's why ignoring potential overexposure is risky! Products used in nail salons are professional tools, not toys. Treat them with respect and you can easily avoid injury or other problems.

WHAT IF IT DOESN'T GO AWAY?

Do you think you have acute symptoms of product overexposure? Once you discontinue exposure, your symptoms should go away. If they do not begin to disappear, they may not have been related to the exposure.

Not all skin rashes, headaches, or watery eyes are caused by overexposure. If you have hay fever or other similar allergies, you'll also suffer with the same symptoms. Even so, if any symptoms continue for too long, don't ignore them. Consult with a medical doctor or at least ask your pharmacist for advice.

SIGNS AND SYMPTOMS OF OVEREXPOSURE

The human body is very rugged and sophisticated. Our bodies usually give us early warning signs that we are overexposing ourselves. Problems occur if we ignore these early warning signs. What are the signs? Overexposure to certain inhaled solvents can make you feel very tired or keep you from sleeping. This type of overexposure can cause headaches, nausea, irritability, nosebleeds, coughs, dizziness, tingling fingers and toes, dry or scratchy nose and throat, puffy or red and irritated skin, itching, and many other symptoms. It is very important that you be on the lookout for such symptoms and understand their meaning. This will help ensure that you avoid more serious problems. Listen to your body. Symptoms are your body's one way of talking to you. Your body is asking you to reduce your exposure. Remember, if you lower your exposure, acute symptoms will go away. Why suffer with these problems when they are easy to avoid?

EMERGENCY AND FIRST-AID TREATMENT

If a serious accident happened in your salon, what would you do? Should you induce vomiting or give the victim something to drink? Use a hot compress or cold? Elevate the feet or the head? Wash with warm or cold running water? Use soap? Sometimes we discover that we are unprepared for accidents after it is too late!

Fact #2: Accidents Usually Occur When They Are Least Expected

The MSDS will answer your questions during a time of crisis. It provides specific instructions for accidental spills, splashes, or ingestion. Keep MSDSs handy—they will prove to be very useful when you need safety information. The next rule is a familiar one, or should be.

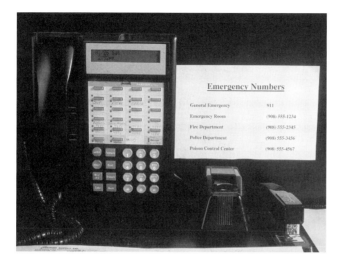

Figure 11–2 *Post a list of emergency numbers by the phone so that you don't need to fumble around for the information after a serious accident or injury*

Rule #2: Be Prepared! Plan Ahead for Accidents

What would you do if a small child grabbed your acid-based primer from the table and drank it? Or a client has a heart attack in the salon? Yikes! Similar incidents happen many times each year. By the time you find the phone number for the hospital or poison control center, it could be too late. Plan ahead! Keep the poison control center and hospital emergency room phone number posted in plain view, along with a list of all other important emergency phone numbers (see Figure 11–2). Obtain the MSDSs for all products in the salon and read them before you need them. Keep the MSDSs in alphabetical order by product name and highlight critical information such as first-aid and cleanup procedures. Meet with others in the salon at least twice a year and go over the salon's emergency response plan. You should discuss fire and accident prevention ideas and have a plan for what to do and whom to call in case of emergency.

SAFE HANDLING TECHNIQUES AND TIPS

Every profession uses different tools and techniques. Understanding how to handle your professional tools properly is critical. A seamstress wouldn't use a knitting needle to hem a skirt. A chef wouldn't boil an egg in a frying pan. The same is true for professional salon chemical products. Each product requires different handling. For example, all nail enhancement products (liquids, resins, and gels) require appropriate ventilation to ensure safe use. Safety glasses should be used to prevent disinfectants from splashing in the eyes, and gloves should be used to prevent skin contact. Flammable solvent must be kept tightly capped and stored in a cool, dry location to prevent fires. Products such as acid-based primers should be kept out of the reach of children.

Manufacturer's instructions and the MSDSs are important sources of information that can help guide you. The technology of nail products is changing faster than any other part of the professional beauty industry. To keep up with these changes, you must stay informed. What you learn in beauty school is just the tip of the iceberg. Your education doesn't end when you leave school. It is just the beginning!

BLOCKING THE ROUTES OF ENTRY

Working safely is surprisingly easy! Still, each year some unfortunate nail technicians suffer from needless harm or avoidable injury. The rules of safety are designed to protect you and prevent problems. It's up to you to understand and follow these guidelines. Guarding the routes of entry is one important way to lower exposure. In the following sections you will learn more about blocking these exposure routes.

Fact #3: All Liquids Evaporate and Create Vapors

Just because you don't smell anything doesn't mean there are no vapors in the air. Not all vapors have odors. Volatile solvents, such as ethyl acetate (non-acetone polish remover), evaporate quickly. Some liquids evaporate slowly, but they all create vapors *(FT)*. Certain monomer liquids are very volatile, while others are not. So what's the best, easiest, and least expensive way to block entry and avoid excessive inhalation of vapors?

Rule #3: Keep Products Capped or Covered When Not in Use and Empty Waste Containers Often

If you prevent the vapors from escaping into the air, you prevent inhalation and lower exposure. Keeping product containers closed will drastically reduce the amount of vapor in the air *(FT)*. For instance, a large marble makes a great cap for monomer dappen dishes. It is especially important to keep artificial nail monomers tightly closed. This prolongs the product's shelf life and keeps it fresh and effective. The more volatile ingredients there are in a nail enhancement product, the more quickly it will evaporate. Rapid evaporation can change the product's composition and cause poor workability, yellowing, lifting, and excessive breakage.

Fact #4: Mists Are Difficult to Control and Potentially Hazardous to Breathe

Pressurized aerosol containers produce very fine and lingering **mists.** A large cloud of spray mist can contain millions of tiny liquid droplets. These mists are

METAL MAKES IT!

Quickly wipe up all spills with absorbent paper towels and toss them into a metal waste can with a self-closing lid. These cans help keep vapors out of the air while reducing the risks of fire. That's why metal is better—it will help suppress fires. They are the only waste receptacles that should be used in nail salons.

Also, don't forget to regularly empty all waste receptacles throughout the day *(FT)* . The longer this waste is in the salon, the more vapors that can escape into your breathing air.

largely made up of volatile solvents, which rapidly evaporate. Mists can also leave a thin residue on a surface after the solvent evaporates. Prolonged or repeated contact with these residues can lead to skin irritation or allergy. Fine mists are more easily inhaled than heavy sprays. In general, spraying any chemical into the air increases the risk of skin, eye, and inhalation overexposure. Pressurized aerosol mists can spread out over large areas, far from the intended target. The finer the mists, the greater the risk. Non-pressurized, pump-type sprayers create larger droplets that don't travel very far. In general, it's best to avoid spraying excessive amounts of product into the air and to use pump sprayers whenever possible.

Rule #4: Control Mists and Vapors by Avoiding Pressurized Spray Cans and Using Metal Waste Receptacles with Self-Closing Lids

Looking for ways to control vapors? Don't think about dust masks. Masks designed to block dust are completely ineffective against vapors! They cannot prevent inhalation of vapors *(FT)* . Dust masks should only be used to keep dust particles out of your mouth, nose, and lungs! Vapor molecules are so small that they pass easily through a dust mask. These masks provide zero protection against vapors. They don't even help a little! Use them only as protection against dust particles. You should remove your mask when not filing. It serves no purpose to leave it on after you are finished using abrasives.

Fact #5: Vapor Molecules Are Hundreds of Times Smaller than the Smallest Dust Particle

Certain types of masks are specially designed for mists and sprays. Not surprisingly, they are called **dust/mist masks** *(FT)* . These masks provide protection from both dusts and mists. These masks are thicker and better-fitting on the face, which is very important. If the mask does not fit well, your protection will be lowered. If used properly, these masks will provide excellent protection against sprays and mists, but they will not block vapors and are not a replacement for proper ventilation.

> ## GET CERTIFIED!
>
> Look for masks that are **N95-certified.** These masks have been tested and shown to block 95 percent of the tiniest dust particles. They are effective against invisible dusts that are 300 times smaller than the diameter of a human hair. Since the smallest particles can be inhaled deeper into the lung, using a mask with this rating is a good idea. You can even find masks with a small valve that allows you to exhale more easily. The valve is a one-way opening that does not allow air to come into the mask but will allow air to leave the mask. This prevents moisture from building up inside the mask (or fogging eyewear) and increases wearing comfort.

Rule #5: Select the Right Tool—Use a Dust Mask to Protect Yourself from Dusts and a Mist Mask When Spraying Anything into the Air

It is always best if nail technicians use masks to prevent inhalation of excessive amounts of dusts while filing. Proper local exhaust ventilation can also help minimize inhalation. These types of devices and their importance are discussed in Chapters 12 and 13.

DUSTS AND FILINGS

It isn't surprising that prolonged, excessive inhalation of nail filings may be harmful. It's not that nail filings are a particularly dangerous type of dust. Breathing large amounts of any dust for long periods may be harmful, even house dust! In the old Western movies, what does every good cowboy do when a dust storm appears on the horizon? He ties a bandanna over his mouth to block out dust.

Fact #6: Over Long Periods of Time, Any Type of Dust May Cause Overexposure

Lungs can handle many types of dust, and lots of it. Our lungs have defenses against dusts, but excessive amounts can overwhelm these defenses. Your risk of overexposure increases if you inhale large amounts of dusts. Wearing a dust mask can prevent inhalation overexposure by blocking this route of entry. These masks are great for protecting nail technicians from breathing excessive amounts of dusts. These masks are most effective if worn while filing artificial nails. You should always wear a dust mask when filing, especially if you use an electric file *FT*. Hand filing with an abrasive creates larger, heavier particles. Electric files create much smaller, lighter particles. Smaller particles stay afloat longer in the salon, travel farther, and can lodge deeper in the lungs. Larger, heavier particles fall on the table or floor and cover your lap. The larger size of these particles makes them less hazardous. The opposite is also true: the finest dusts pose the greatest risks. Since smaller particles are more easily inhaled, they are potentially more hazardous. Just about any particle you can easily see is considered large. Large particles are visible and easier to spot and control. Small particles are nearly invisible and may float around for 40 minutes or longer before coming to rest, only to be launched into the air again by the slightest breeze. Nothing you can buy will protect you from dusts better than a simple dust mask. These masks filter the air as it enters your mouth, removing even the smallest dusts from your breathing air. These masks are inexpensive and can filter out particles that are 300 times thinner than a human hair. But these masks won't last for very long. Throw them away after a week of use. They're designed to be disposable and become ineffective if used too long.

Rule #6: Always Wear a Dust Mask When Filing, Especially with an Electric File

What if your client asks to wear a dust mask, too? That's fine if it makes the client feel better. But can your client be overexposed to nail dust? No way! Remember the overexposure principle? Inhaling dusts found in the salon isn't harmful unless overexposure occurs. Even then, problems occur only when safe exposure levels are exceeded for prolonged periods (months or years). Your clients run no risk of being overexposed to dusts or vapors in the salon Ⓕ . They aren't there long enough or often enough. As a nail professional, the level of exposure to salon chemicals you receive every four days is equal to most clients' exposure for an entire year! But while you're handing dust masks to your clients, take a moment to explain the overexposure principle. Tell them they are not at risk. Explain to them that you're taking steps to protect yourself from the risk of long-term overexposure. Do this and your clients will gain more confidence in your abilities and will be more at ease with their services.

DANGEROUS MISCONCEPTION

What is the most dangerous misconception about chemicals in the salon industry? Many believe that they can tell a dangerous chemical simply by its odor. Wrong! A chemical's smell has absolutely nothing to do with its safety Ⓕ . Some of the most dangerous substances have very sweet, pleasant fragrances. Many terrible-smelling substances are safe to inhale. In short, it is impossible to determine safety simply by smelling. Ingredients called fragrances are perfect examples. These ingredients are added to make products smell wonderful and appealing. Yet fragrances are the most likely ingredient to cause skin irritation and allergy. People who find themselves sensitive to a product are more likely to be allergic to the fragrance than any other ingredient.

Fact #7: Odors Themselves Are Not Dangerous—They Help You Work More Safely

Products or devices designed to cover up or remove odors from the salon will not protect your health. Getting rid of odors will not make the air safer to breathe. Air cleaners designed for the home are not appropriate for salons. These devices can give you a false sense of security and do little to protect your health. Odors are the nail technician's friend. Odors can warn against a potential risk of overexposure (*FT*). An odor is nothing more than vapors touching the sensitive detectors in the nose. After the vapors leave the nose and enter the lungs, odor is no longer important. Your lungs, liver, or kidneys don't care about odor. You'll be fooled if you use odor to judge product safety.

Rule #7: Never Judge the Safety of a Product by Its Odor

Don't listen to fast-talking sales pitches claiming that a particular system "makes the salon air fresh-smelling" or "will remove chemical odors." This doesn't mean the air is cleaner or safer to breathe. Most of these systems are inadequate for salons. In Chapters 14 and 15, you will learn much more about proper ventilation and how to use it to improve the salon environment.

WORK SMART, BE HEALTHY

What do a coffee cup, a piece of chocolate, and a sack lunch have in common? These are all ways that nail technicians eat their products. Who would eat their products? Unfortunately, nail technicians eat far more product than they realize. Coffee and drinking cups can easily collect dusts. Hot liquids can absorb vapors right out of the air. Think about when someone offers you a piece of chocolate or a cookie. How many people wash their hands before touching the food? A common practice in salons is to keep sack lunches in the same refrigerator where products are stored. While you are working, your food is busy absorbing a dose of chemical vapors. Bread is especially good at absorbing vapors. As you can see, this route of overexposure may be more common than you imagine.

Fact #8: Federal Regulations Prohibit Eating in Areas Where Potentially Hazardous Chemicals Are Used

This applies to salons as well! It is very easy to accidentally ingest product in the salon. If you need to eat in a hurry, never do it at your station. Besides being unsanitary, it is an unnecessary risk to take with your health. Accidents usually happen when we take unnecessary risks.

Rule #8: Don't Eat in the Salon, Store Food Safely, and Wash Your Hands

Never eat, drink, or smoke in the salon. Make sure to always store food away from salon chemicals. Don't forget to wash your hands before and after eating, after going to the restroom, and after smoking.

YOU MAY NEED YOUR EYES

Accidents involving the eyes are a serious danger in salons. Solvents such as polish removers that get splashed in the eye can be very painful and may cause damage. Cuticle removers, acid-based primer, wrap resins and tip adhesives, and phenolic disinfectant solutions in the eyes are much worse! Each of these can cause permanent eye injury or blindness. Imagine what it is like to be blind! It could happen if you are not careful to protect your vision.

Fact #9: Eye Injuries Account for Approximately 45 Percent of the Cosmetic-Related Injuries Seen in Hospital Emergency Rooms

Wear eye protection whenever there is the slightest chance that a liquid could splash into your eyes (Figure 11–3). Eye protection can also protect the eye from flying objects, such as dusts and debris created while using an electric file or

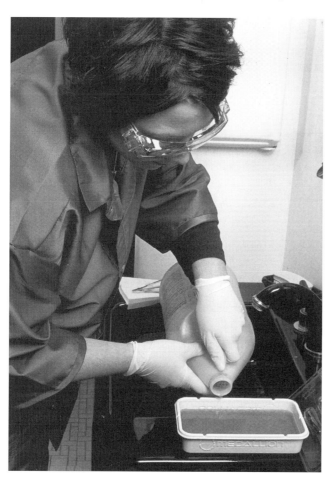

Figure 11–3 *Gloves and eye protection can help prevent accidental overexposure*

nippers. If you wear prescription glasses, you are in luck! Your optometrist can make you a pair of prescription safety glasses. Any safety eyewear you purchase is 100 percent tax deductible and much better than a Seeing Eye dog. Protect your vision! You don't want to damage or lose it.

Rule #9: Wear Safety Glasses When Needed and Give Your Client a Pair as Well

Your client may love you and think you are the greatest nail technician in the world. But if you accidentally splash primer in his or her eyes, you have lost a client (and the income) and gained an expensive lawsuit! Also, clients have sustained damage to their vision or even lost it altogether after being struck in the eye by sharp chunks of artificial nail product sent flying by the nippers of careless nail technicians. As a licensed professional, you are responsible for the client's safety while in your care. If you ignore that responsibility, you may regret it one day.

Fact #10: Soft Contact Lenses Can Absorb Vapors from the Air

Wearing any type of contact lens in the salon is risky. Vapors can collect in soft contact lenses and make them unwearable, even if you're wearing safety glasses. The contaminated lens can injure the eye and may cause permanent damage. If you splash liquid in your eye, it can wick under the lens. This will make proper cleaning of the eye more difficult.

Rule #10: Avoid Wearing Contact Lenses in the Salon and Always Wash Your Hands Before Touching the Eye Area

Many of these rules are just simple common sense. When using salon chemicals, common sense can save you from pain and suffering. Learn these chemical safety rules and follow them!

WHERE TO FIND IT

For technical information about safety equipment call Lab Safety Supply at 1-800-356-2501. Lab Safety Supply sells equipment for every type of business, including salons. Ask for a free copy of their latest general catalog. It contains many useful items ranging from dust/mist masks to gloves and safety glasses. Other great resources include your local or Internet nail supply distributor.

SCARE YOUR CLIENTS?

What if your client sees you putting on safety glasses and a dust mask or following any of the other rules of safety? Some nail technicians may worry that this could scare their clients. It is unlikely that a salon or nail professional will ever lose business because of working safely or showing concern for a customer's well-being. But many have lost their licenses and been ruined because they did not. Can you imagine clients leaving you and going to a salon that doesn't care about safety? Would you if you were in their shoes? If anything, clients will respect and appreciate you even more. Clients want to feel like their salon is a safe haven. Showing your knowledge about the rules of safety will remind them that there's a lot more to doing nails than filing and buffing. You should be more concerned if clients think you're unsafe. In today's world, that can cost you money.

PROPER STORAGE CONDITIONS

Improper storage of your products can create many problems. Improper storage may ruin your product's effectiveness or shorten its shelf life. It may cause a fire or explosion. Freezing temperatures, excessive heat, or sunlight may all adversely affect products. Some products are sensitive to UV light and should be stored in a dark location. Avoid storing product in places where they will be exposed to excessive heat or sunlight *(FT)*. Flammable products must be stored away from heat, sparks, or open flame, including water heaters and windowsills *(FT)*. Don't smoke while using professional products *(FT)*. And never carry any flammable products in a car trunk *(FT)*. Some salon chemicals are more flammable than gasoline. A car's trunk can exceed 150°F (65°C) in the summer. Finally, all professional salon products must be stored out of the reach of children. Hundreds of children have been harmed by improperly stored professional products.

FIT TO FLY?

Airlines regulate flammable substances in personal baggage. You're allowed to fly with flammable substances intended for personal use, such as hairspray, nail polish, remover, and so on. There are limits on the maximum amount you can carry as well as the size of the containers.

Check for the current airline regulations before flying with flammable salon products. Very heavy fines are given to those caught breaking the rules. These regulations are designed to protect you and other passengers, so heed them.

PROPER DISPOSAL—PLEASE CARE!

It's important to consider where your unused products end up. There's a right way and a wrong way to get rid of leftover products and wastes. Of course, specific information for disposing of particular products should come from the product manufacturers. You can get this information in several ways. The first is by requesting a Material Safety Data Sheet from either the manufacturer or the distributor. Many are now available online. Both manufacturer and distributor are required by law to provide you with these important safety sheets for all of your professional products. They are also required to get you this information in a timely fashion or else risk hefty fines from the Occupational Safety and Health Administration. Second, you can call the manufacturer's hotline or information number to ask questions about proper disposal procedures.

Here is some general advice. Products that were not designed to be flushed down the toilet or poured down the sink should always be properly disposed of. Each of us must do what we can to protect our environment. Improperly disposing of professional products is irresponsible and should not be done. Please don't do it! Flammable and corrosive substances should be stored in an appropriate and safe location until they can be properly disposed of. Check with your city or local waste management department for more information on proper disposal policies and procedures. For example, some cities have a special day for hazardous trash pickup day or set up a drop-off point for hazardous or flammable substances.

TOXICITY

What is a toxic substance? Most people believe *toxic* means "extremely dangerous or poisonous, something that must be avoided at all costs." This is false! The news media use the term incorrectly. They use *toxic* mostly to scare people and raise their ratings. Should nail technicians avoid products that are toxic? The answer to this question may surprise you.

Paracelsus, a famous 16th-century physician, was the first to use the word *toxic*. He said, "All substances are poisons; there is none which is not a poison. Only the right dose differentiates a poison and a remedy." Over the last 500 years, we seem to have forgotten what Paracelsus learned. The overexposure principle is the modern-day interpretation of what Paracelsus tried to teach us. This principle also says that overexposure (dosage) can make anything poisonous or toxic. Does that mean you must avoid *everything*, including cuticle oils and skin creams? Of course that's silly. This is not what Paracelsus was trying to tell us. Obviously, something is wrong with the way we think about toxicity. How do scientists define *toxic* and *nontoxic*? They use the following guideline to determine the true risks to humans.

Fact #11: Chemicals Are Considered Relatively Nontoxic if You Can Drink a Quart or More Without Dying

Next time someone tells you a product is "nontoxic," think about this definition. There is no shortage of marketers who use this type of claim deceptively. Even the purest and cleanest salt water is very toxic to drink. Even so, it's safe to swim in the ocean. If ingested, a tablespoon of rubbing alcohol can kill a small child. Bleach and ammonia are also very toxic, but we manage to use these substances safely and easily. Other than foods, very few things are nontoxic. Even so, they can be used safely and without causing any harm. Don't be swayed by fearmongers who use this term to deceive you. Any product can be toxic when used incorrectly. And any product can be safe if used properly!

Rule #11: Treat All Chemicals with Respect and Don't Be Fooled by Marketing Terms Such as "Nontoxic," "Natural," and "Organic"

Do these terms mean what we think they do? When it comes to chemicals, **organic** simply means that the chemical contains the element carbon in its structure[1] (FT). All living things are organic. Other then rocks, sand, metals, water, and air, almost everything else on earth is organic! Cow dung, poison ivy, and road tar are all 100 percent chemically organic and natural, too—but you wouldn't want your shampoo to contain them as ingredients. **Natural** simply means "occurs in nature" (FT). Nature is filled with poisonous and potentially dangerous substances. "Natural" doesn't mean a product is safe, wholesome, or better. Actually, it could mean the opposite. Natural ingredients in products require higher levels of preservatives because they're more susceptible to bacteria and spoiling. Also, the quality and effectiveness of natural ingredients can vary dramatically from season to season and year to year. Finally, most allergic reactions are caused by natural substances, such as pollen, poison ivy, cat dander, and so on. Don't be fooled into thinking that "natural" ingredients are automatically better and safer. They are not! Fortunately, federal regulations are beginning to change the way the word "organic" is used in cosmetics. In the future, this should affect the way consumers view this word. As a result, I suspect that consumers will begin to see how claims have been exaggerated and marketers will be forced to change their tactics. These terms are already losing some of their original luster in the public eye.

---

[1] The Food and Drug Administration has standards for use of the term *organic*, but these apply to food and don't have much meaning or benefit when it comes to cosmetic products.

CARCINOGENICITY

If you believe everything you hear in the news, nearly everything causes cancer, right? Nothing could be further from the truth. The media distort the facts about cancer-causing agents and often misinterpret scientific research. Most reporters have journalism degrees and virtually no knowledge of science, which is why the media do such a poor job of reporting on these subjects. Unfortunately, their ignorance has created a nation that is paranoid about cancer-causing chemicals. In our culture today, it's generally believed that cancer-causing chemicals are everywhere and most of them are man-made pollutants of some sort. Like many common beliefs, this is totally false.

Fact #12: About 20 Million Different Chemicals Have Been Categorized by Scientists, and Only a Few Hundred Are Listed as Suspected Human Cancer-Causing Agents

It is relatively uncommon for a person to get cancer from chemical overexposure. The truth is that cancer-causing chemicals are rare (F). The majority of cancers are caused by smoking and viruses (like the virus that causes hepatitis). Only a small percentage are caused by man-made pollutants or chemicals. It's much more likely that the cancer is caused by hereditary factors. Don't let bogus or exaggerated media reports frighten you. If you work safely, it is extremely unlikely that you'll get cancer from products used in the workplace. The cancer risk from smoking cigarettes is many thousands of times greater than the risk from working with salon products.

Rule #12: Don't Fear What Might Happen—Be Proactive and Prevent Problems

Sometimes people hear what a chemical can do and they become frightened, even if it what they hear about rarely happens or hardly ever occurs! Don't forget, *can* is a whole lot different from *will*. Alcohol can cause liver damage . . . if you drink a quart of hard liquor every day for ten years! You won't get liver damage because you have a glass of wine with dinner every night. Overexposure to some salon chemicals can cause illness or injury, but this is easy to avoid. Professional products can be used safely if used correctly. That's what Paracelsus has been trying to tell us for 500 years.

PREGNANCY AND NAILS

When your clients discover they're pregnant, one of the first questions they will ask you is, "Can I keep wearing my nail enhancements during my pregnancy?" The answer is yes, they can safely wear artificial nails! There is absolutely no reason to believe that it is harmful to wear artificial nail enhancements or polish during pregnancy (F). In Chapter 9 you learned that artificial nail products polymerize and harden within three minutes. This eliminates the chance of any product penetrating beyond the very topmost layers of the nail plate. Besides, exposure during a service is minuscule. It is extremely unlikely that artificial nails are harmful during pregnancy.

But what about pregnant nail technicians? Is it safe for them to work in a salon? Of course they can! But pregnant nail technicians who don't work safely will need to make changes in their work routines. In other words, pay close attention to the rules of safety once you learn about your pregnancy. This will be true regardless of your occupation. When you become pregnant, follow your doctor's advice. A well-informed physician will usually advise mothers-to-be to avoid alcohol and tobacco. Studies have shown that these substances may cause abnormal fetal development. Fortunately, scientific studies indicate there are no such ingredients in artificial nail products. To put things in their proper perspective, smoking is many thousands of times more dangerous to a developing fetus. To be on the safe side, show the MSDSs for all your products to your doctor. And of course, make sure you follow the rules of working safely.

REMEMBER, THERE IS NO NEED TO FEAR CHEMICALS— INSTEAD, BE CAREFUL AND WORK SMART

Ultimately, it is your responsibility to prevent accidents and protect your health! It's all up to you. Learn all you can about working safely and then use your knowledge wisely (FT). You may become the best nail technician in the world, but it won't mean anything if you harm yourself in the process. Don't just talk about working safely—it's only effective if you really do it!

FAST TRACK (FT)

(FT) Every chemical used in the professional salon industry can be used safely.

(FT) Over 99 percent of the chemicals you'll come into contact with in your lifetime are safe and beneficial.

(FT) The overexposure principle says that every chemical has a safe and unsafe level of exposure. You won't be harmed unless you repeatedly exceed the safe levels.

(FT) The Material Safety Data Sheet is an important source of safety information.

(FT) Chemicals can only enter your body via the routes of entry: inhalation, ingestion, and absorption.

(FT) Short-term effects are early warning signs of overexposure.

(FT) All liquids evaporate and form vapors.

(FT) Keep products capped or covered when not in use.

(FT) Regularly empty waste containers.

(FT) Vapors are far too small to be filtered by dust masks.

(FT) Use a mist-rated mask if you spray anything into the air.

(FT) Always wear a dust mask when filing, especially if you use an electric file.

(FT) Clients run no risk of being overexposed to dusts or vapors in the salon.

(FT) A chemical's smell has absolutely nothing to do with its safety.

(FT) A chemical's smell can provide early warning of overexposure.

(FT) Don't keep your products in direct sunlight.

(FT) Flammable products must be stored away from heat, sparks, or open flame.

(FT) Don't smoke while using professional products.

(FT) Never carry any flammable product in a car trunk.

(FT) *Organic* simply means the chemical contains carbon in its structure.

(FT) *Natural* means nothing more than "occurs in nature."

(FT) Cancer-causing chemicals are relatively rare.

(FT) It is safe to wear any type of nail enhancement during pregnancy.

(FT) Learn all you can about working safely and then use your knowledge wisely.

Review Questions

1. What do the overexposure principle and Paracelsus's philosophy have in common?

2. List at least five important pieces of information found on an MSDS.

3. Name the routes of entry.

4. What is the least expensive and easiest way to help keep the vapors out of the salon's air?

5. Why are dust masks ineffective against vapors?

6. Name five potential symptoms of chemical overexposure.

7. To work safely with chemicals you must lower your _____ to _____ levels.

8. What percentage of chemicals in the world are never toxic under any circumstances?

9. Are natural substances safer? Explain.

10. What should you do before flying on an airplane with a large amount of flammable products?

11. Paracelsus said, "All substances are _____; there is none which is not a _____. Only the right dose differentiates a _____ and a remedy."

12. _____ solvents are quickly evaporating.

13. Give three examples of things that are not organic.

14. Products that are sensitive to UV light should be stored in a _____ location.

15. Can clients wear nail enhancements during pregnancy?

Chapter

12

The Healthy Salon

Objective

In this chapter you will learn how to protect your skin and avoid potential problems from product over-exposure. You will learn how to keep your skin healthy and protect your eyes from damage. You'll also learn how to protect your clients and keep them safer while they are in your care.

KEEPING SKIN HEALTHY

Skin disorders of the hands are far too common in nail salons. Nearly half of all nail technicians will suffer from a skin disorder sometime during their careers. These problems are not restricted to nail salons. In fact, they are common in many occupations. Skin disorders are the number one occupation-related disease in America (FT). Skin contact with certain substances can create symptoms ranging from rashes to allergies or serious burns. Salon-related skin problems are usually seen on the fingers, nail beds, hands, elbows, wrists, chins, and cheeks, as well as around the eyes. Skin diseases and allergies force many good nail technicians to give up successful careers. This is especially sad, because it is completely avoidable. No one should suffer from any work-related skin disorder.

Remember the overexposure principle? It says that every chemical has a safe and an unsafe level of exposure. You won't be harmed unless you repeatedly exceed the safe levels. This important principle applies to skin overexposure as well. When nail technicians or clients develop skin disorders, it is tempting to blame the products. Yet the manufacturing workers who make and package them rarely develop skin problems. Manufacturing workers are exposed to both the concentrated raw ingredients and the finished products but manage to avoid skin problems. Why? Because they take care not to be overexposed. Repeated overexposure and improper use are the main reasons nail technicians and clients suffer these problems (FT). Learn to avoid these and you'll avoid the related problems.

DERMATITIS

Inflammation of the skin is called **dermatitis.** Many things can cause dermatitis, including insect bites, heat, cold, sun exposure, plants, animals, cosmetics, perfumes, and foods. For nail technicians, **contact dermatitis** is the most common type. Contact dermatitis is caused by touching certain substances to the skin. There are two main types of contact dermatitis. If the skin becomes irritated by exposure to a substance, it is called **irritant contact dermatitis.** If the skin becomes allergic to an ingredient in a product, it is called **allergic contact dermatitis.** The easiest way to avoid skin problems is to understand the differences between these two types of contact dermatitis.

Irritant Contact Dermatitis

Certain chemicals can damage the upper layers of the skin. Irritants usually affect the skin within a few seconds to a few hours after exposure. The skin's defenses spring into action when damage occurs. First, the damaged tissue is flooded with body fluids. These fluids are mostly water but contain cleansing and healing agents as well. This is the body attempting to dilute the irritating substance and move its defenses into place. This is why swelling often occurs. These fluids also stimulate the cells in your skin, causing them to release chemicals called **histamines.** These chemicals cause the blood vessels around the injured tissue to enlarge. Blood can then rush to the scene more quickly, beginning the healing process. You can see and feel all the extra activity under the skin. The entire area becomes red, warm, and itchy, and it may throb. Histamines cause the itchy feeling that is often felt with contact dermatitis. Afterward, the surrounding skin is left damaged, scaly, cracked, and dry. Special care must be taken to prevent any additional overexposure to the damaged area. Damaged skin is more susceptible to becoming overexposed, especially during the winter months, when skin can become drier. Irritating substances have a greater effect on skin that is already very dry or damaged. So you can see why it's so important to keep your skin healthy. You should use skin moisturizers to protect skin from dryness and irritation in cold climates.

Surprisingly, tap water is a very common salon irritant (FT). Hands that are often wet can become sore, cracked, and chapped. Avoiding the problem is simple. Keep hands dry, and always thoroughly dry them when they become wet. You should use moisturizing hand creams to prevent skin dryness. Take care! You can wash your hands too much. If your hands become cracked and dry because you wash them excessively, that's too much! (FT) Cleansers and detergents can worsen dry skin problems, as shown in Figure 12–1 and Color Plate 21. They worsen the damage by stripping away the protective oily sebum that seals the skin's surface. Prolonged or repeated contact with many solvents can also strip away skin oils, leaving the skin dry or damaged (FT).

As you can see, many things can damage the skin. It will be easier to figure out the cause if you observe the symptoms. The location of the irritation should be your first clue. The symptoms are usually isolated to the contact area. The cause of the irritation will usually be something that has come into contact with that part of the skin.

Corrosives are severe irritants. They can cause rapid, visible, and sometimes irreversible skin damage. Corrosives are at the extreme opposite ends of the pH scale (FT). They are either very acid or very alkaline. They generally have a pH less than 3.0 or greater than 10.0. Strong acid or alkaline solutions affect the skin's normal pH (FT). The pH of normal skin varies between 4.5 and 6.5, and skin has a tremendous ability to neutralize a high or low pH. But products designed to be harshly alkaline or highly acidic can overwhelm the normal balance and cause tissue damage. This is how glycolic acid treatments work on skin. Phenolic disinfectant concentrates have pHs usually in excess of 12.0. Prolonged or repeated contact with these disinfectants can overwhelm the skin's defenses, corrode the tissue, and damage fingernails (see Figure 12–2 and Color Plate 22). High-strength cuticle and callus removers are corrosive, as are methacrylic acid-based nail primers (FT). These are professional tools that can cause serious corrosive injuries if care is not taken. Corrosives can be very fast-acting, causing immediate stinging, redness, and damage. But they can also take more than 15 minutes of exposure to cause damage and hours before more serious symptoms

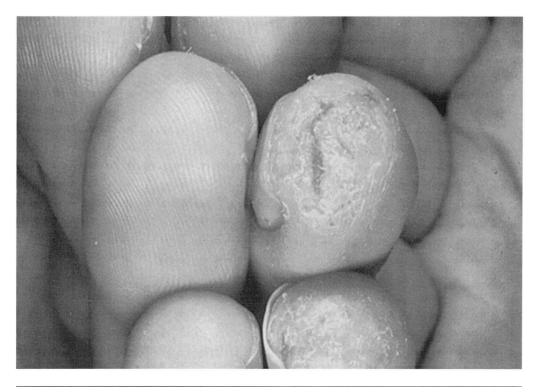

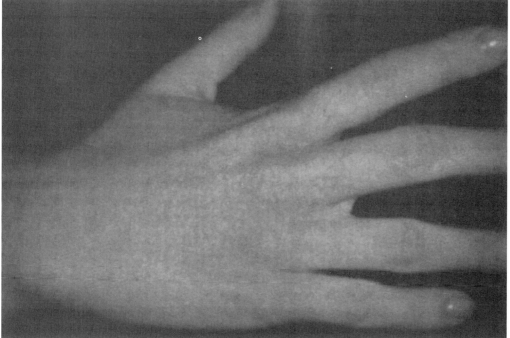

Figure 12-1 and Figure 12-2 *Irritant contact dermatitis on cosmetologists whose hands were always wet*

CARE WITH CORROSIVES

Make sure you know which of your products are corrosive. They require special handling for safe use. Corrosives can be very dangerous for eyes and skin. Keep corrosives out of reach of children and carefully read and follow all product instructions and MSDSs.

Corrosive products can be very useful in the salon if used correctly and safely. They are professional-strength tools that will require your skill and knowledge. Use them with care and caution!

develop. Corrosives may cause painful burns that slowly heal. If proper medical attention is received, the healing process will be accelerated and there is less chance of permanent damage or scarring.

Simply rinsing corrosives off the skin may not be enough. Some are difficult to remove or may have delayed effects on the skin or eyes. It's best to thoroughly wash the area with a liquid soap and plenty of running water. If any injury occurs, see a physician and get treatment. Always use safety eyewear when using corrosive products ⒻⒾ. Corrosives are especially dangerous for eyes. They can cloud or destroy vision permanently! All eye exposure to corrosive substances must be treated immediately by a physician. This is necessary to prevent permanent damage. Corrosives and other irritants can have damaging effects on the fingernail and surrounding tissue. Both can damage the hyponychium, leading to pterygium under the free edge of the natural nail (see Chapter 5, Figure 5–5) as well as onycholysis of the nail plate (see Chapter 4, Figure 4–3).

Methacrylic acid primers are especially corrosive and can cause serious burns if not treated with caution. Should accidental contact occur, immediately wash the area with plenty of cold water and soap. Soap is alkaline and will help neutralize the acid. Cold water will cool the area. If skin redness persists or there is an obvious chemical burn, see a doctor! The damage may worsen over time if not properly treated. If primer is spilled on the clothing, remove the garment immediately. Don't put the clothing back on until it has been thoroughly washed. Be sure to wash contaminated clothing separately from other clothing. If acid-based primer is splashed in the eyes, quick action is required. Flood the eyes with cold water while holding the eyelids open. If your salon has a washbasin with a flexible hose, use it to thoroughly rinse the eyes. Continue to flood them for at least 15 minutes. Don't wait! You should call a doctor immediately, especially if redness, stinging, or pain persists.

Allergic Contact Dermatitis

Studies show that allergic contact dermatitis accounts for approximately 80 percent of all cosmetic-related skin problems. Allergic reactions occur when a person becomes sensitive to a product ingredient. Usually fragrances or preservatives are the culprits. Other ingredients used in cosmetics may also be allergens. These ingredients are beneficial for the vast majority of people, and most never experience any problems. But a small number of people may develop skin allergies when repeatedly exposed. Allergies to cosmetics do not suddenly develop. They may take months or even years to appear. The process of developing an allergy to a particular substance is called **sensitization.** The substance causing the allergy is called either a **sensitizer** or an **allergen** Ⓕ . For example, pollen is a common allergen. The cleansing agents used in shampoos, hand and body washes, and similar products are called surfactants. Previously you learned that excessive hand washing could cause irritation. Many types of surfactants are either irritants or allergens (or both). Allergic contact dermatitis is very similar in appearance to irritant contact dermatitis. But there's a big difference between them! Both share many of the same symptoms—redness, swelling, itching, onycholysis, and pterygium under the free edge of the nail. Irritations and their symptoms go away once exposure stops, but not so with allergies. Once you become allergic, it is for life! Your body remembers that it is allergic to that substance.

The immune system is like a great army that never forgets. This massive fighting force can wage a full-scale war against any foreign aggressor. Your immune system army has privates and generals, spies and assassins, sentries and scouts. When it detects invaders, the immune system springs into action. Certain parts of the immune system act as spies. They roam the body looking for foreign substances. The immune system spies memorize details about the attacking substance and describe it in messages they send back to the generals. They can even bring back prisoners for inspection. The generals then send messengers to alert the immune system army of a possible invasion. They also describe the invading substance so the army can be on the lookout. Once the substance is under control, the immune system strengthens its defenses and patiently waits for the next attack. The immune system is now ready and watching. If skin contact is made again, the immune army will spring into action. When the body reacts in this way, it is called an **immune response.**

Potent allergic sensitizers such as poison ivy can trigger immune responses after just one exposure, but for most substances it usually takes two or more exposures. Fortunately, salon product manufacturers are very careful to avoid using potent sensitizers. Some ingredients (monomers and oligomers) used in nail enhancement products are weak sensitizers Ⓕ . This means they are unlikely to cause allergic reactions under normal conditions of use. But prolonged and/or repeated skin contact with these nail enhancement products can cause sensitive people to become allergic Ⓕ . Prolonged and/or repeated contact is the number one cause for allergic reactions to nail enhancements. Prolonged contact happens when products are allowed to sit on the skin for long periods of time. Repeated contact occurs when the same area of skin is touched many times with the product. Artificial nail enhancement products do not cause clients to become allergic after a single exposure. Skin allergies rarely occur even after several exposures.

Sensitization to nail enhancement products typically takes four to six months (or longer) of prolonged and/or repeated skin contact. So one of the best ways to avoid skin allergies is to avoid prolonged and repeated skin contact. Certain clients' skin may be more sensitive than others. For example, fair skin is usually more sensitive to allergens than darker-pigmented skin. Less sensitive clients may be overexposed for years before becoming allergic, while others develop symptoms much more quickly. Once they become allergic, the symptoms will worsen with each continued exposure.

Through the Looking Glass

Determining the cause of the allergic reaction can be tricky. Unlike irritant contact dermatitis, the symptoms are not restricted to the contact area. Sometimes swelling and other signs may occur far from the point of contact—face, eyelids, armpits, and glands in the throat or groin. But these are less likely and usually happen only in extreme cases. Most people are surprised to learn that allergic reactions usually appear after several months or more of exposure. This can fool nail technicians into believing that the cause was something recent, such as a new polish or lotion. They don't realize it's probably something they've been using (or doing) for months or even years. Luckily, tracking down the source of an allergy is easier if you know what to look for. The first symptoms are a temporary reddening or warming sensation that may go unnoticed. If overexposure continues, the skin may appear dry, tight, flaky, or itchy. In later stages, tiny water blisters or raised bumps are often seen around the eponychium (cuticle area) or fingertip. With continued exposure the symptoms will worsen. The water blisters may develop into open sores. Other advanced symptoms include numbness of the fingertips or an annoying itch underneath the nail plate. Continued product overexposure may result in the permanent loss of the nail plate. All artificial nail enhancement products, including UV gels, wraps, and monomer/polymer systems, can cause allergic reactions, but none of them need cause problems. To prevent this, uncured enhancement products must never come into contact with any living skin, including your own. Each time the product touches the skin you increase the risk of irritation or allergy. Yes, it is easier to slop on product than it is to carefully avoid skin contact. Since allergic reactions occur after many months of repeated overexposures, nail technicians can easily fall into the habit of touching the skin. Since there is no immediate negative effect, they don't realize that they are slowly sensitizing their clientele.

In most cases the symptoms of allergic reactions will be restricted to the area of skin that has been repeatedly overexposed Ⓕ. **Hives** (also called wheals or welts) are the one exception to this rule. Clients can in rare instances develop hives as a symptom of overexposure to artificial nail products. Hives can appear on the wrist, arms, face, or neck. Hives are a smooth, slightly elevated area on the skin. The area is either redder or paler than the surrounding skin and is often accompanied by severe itching. The welts may change size or shape or even disappear within a few hours. Even so, many other things are more likely to cause

BIGGER MEANS BETTER? NOT ALWAYS!

Large, oversize brushes make overly wet beads. The belly of these large brushes can carry enough liquid to make four normal-size beads. Larger-size brushes are more difficult to control, making it nearly impossible to avoid touching the skin. The extra liquid in the belly prevents proper control of the liquid-to-powder ratio.

Brushes that are too large don't save time—they cause allergic reactions and can lead to service breakdown. Yellowing, inconsistent color, lifting, and cracking are just a few of the problems caused by oversize brushes. Overall, medium-size brushes are better tools. In the long run, they'll save you time and create better nails for your clients.

hives, such as foods, medications, plants, or clothing. Artificial nail product overexposure is a much less likely cause.

Overmanicuring the cuticle area can make clients more susceptible as well. Previously irritated, broken, or damaged skin increases the chance of developing an allergy (FT). The skin is a barrier. If that barrier is broken, the risk increases for allergic reactions.

Another main cause of allergic reactions is using too wet a bead consistency. Monomer and polymer products must be used with a medium bead consistency. Wetter ratios may help smooth the artificial nail's surface, but the product is difficult to control and can run into the nail folds. As you learned in Chapter 9, polymer powder must be correctly balanced with the monomer liquid. There must be enough powder to cause all of the monomer to react and polymerize. Using too much liquid throws off this balance and leaves uncured monomer trapped inside the nail enhancement. This monomer can eventually work its way down to the nail bed and may cause overexposure. Some nail technicians believe it is quicker and easier to go wetter, but in the long run both you and your clients will pay the price.

DUTY CALLS

It is your professional duty to avoid skin contact with nail enhancement products. This cannot be overemphasized! Nail enhancement products and chemistry cannot advance until nail technicians accept this responsibility. Many high-tech ingredients cannot be used in products because nail technicians in general are too careless. Don't be one of those who abuse their professional tools.

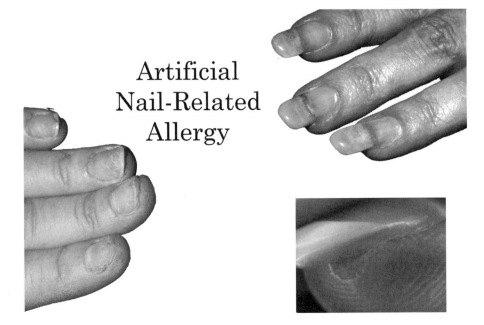

Artificial Nail-Related Allergy

Figure 12-3 *Artificial nail–related skin allergy caused by overexposure — note the redness and skin peeling, both potential signs of allergy*

Another common reason for sensitivity to monomer/polymer systems is mixing product lines. Monomer liquids are designed to efficiently react with a specific polymer powder. Upset this delicate balance and you are asking for problems. When you use the incorrect powder, a high percentage of uncured monomer can remain trapped inside the enhancement. The excess monomer may improve clarity and flexibility, but don't be fooled. This trap catches many nail technicians. Eventually the excess monomer can soak through the nail plate and into the nail bed. This prolonged exposure is one of the leading causes of itchy nail beds and can lead to other symptoms of overexposure. One way to help prevent this is to avoid overfiling the nail plate. The top layers of the plate are composed of very hard, densely packed cells designed to protect and seal the underlying layers. If filed away with an aggressive technique, the nail plate becomes more susceptible to penetration by uncured ingredients. So keep the plate thick and healthy! That's every nail professional's most important job (see Figure 12–3 and Color Plate 23).

WHY TAKE THE RISKS?

Developing a nail enhancement product takes years of scientific education and experience as well as months of testing with high-tech laboratory instruments. It is highly unlikely that a nail technician will accidentally stumble across a better blend or mixture than the one recommended by the product manufacturer. It just doesn't happen that way. If you mix product lines, you may find something that looks whiter or pinker or clearer or seems more flexible. But without extensive testing you can't know if there are any long-term negative effects. If problems develop, what do you do? Where can you go for help?

Imagine what you would do if a client lost all of her natural nails and said it was your fault. If you are a good nail technician and follow instructions, any responsible manufacturer or expert would agree with and defend your actions. Following the instructions and using the best practices is your best defense against these problems. Now imagine the same situation, but pretend it happened after the technician mixed two different polymer powders and two different monomers to create her own "special" blend. What will the experts say about that? What can they say? The nail technician disregarded the manufacturer's instructions. She'll more than likely be found negligent and held liable for her actions. It may seem fun and exciting to "invent" your own special blends. Most nail technicians have a little bit of chemist inside them. But seriously, why bother? If you don't like the product the way it is, change to another. Eventually you will find one that meets your needs and expectations. Don't jeopardize your career or risk harming your clients. Follow instructions and never mix products or make your own blends unless instructed to do so by the manufacturer of the products involved. Highly colored nail art powders are a perfect example. Some manufacturers encourage blending different colored powders together to create new and unique shades. As long as these powders all come from the same manufacturer as the monomer liquid, this would be fine. But even these colored powders should be used with the matching monomer liquid. There are no exceptions to this rule—use the right polymer powder with the right monomer liquid (FT). Don't let anyone tell you differently.

Here are a few other things you should avoid:

- Avoid going back to smooth the nail surface with more monomer (FT).
- Avoid using monomer to clean the edges, the sidewalls, or under the nail.
- Avoid applying product to a client with a skin reaction or infection (FT).
- Avoid touching the hairs of the brush with your fingers (FT).

Once a client becomes allergic, things will only get worse if you continue using the same products and techniques. It is best to discontinue use on that client and figure out what you are doing wrong before more clients develop similar problems. Behind most allergic reactions to nail products is a careless nail technician. Don't let that nail technician be you! If your client becomes allergic to the product, you may have yourself to blame. Medication or illness isn't what makes clients sensitive to nail products. These are just excuses. Only prolonged and/or repeated direct skin contact causes these client allergies.

What if a client with an obvious skin reaction or nail infection insists that you continue giving her services? If you do so, it is at your own risk! You are legally responsible for your client's safety. Even if your client signs a waiver or release form, you can be sued for negligence. Clients cannot sign away their health and safety! Asking your client to sign a waiver is an admission of guilt on your part. You would not ask a client for a waiver unless, in your professional opinion, the services should not be performed. If this is the case, it's your duty to refuse. Refer the client to a physician, dermatologist, or podiatrist for advice. Don't try to fix the problem yourself. Only qualified medical professionals are allowed to treat or cure diseased or infected fingernails or toenails.

CONTROLLING AND AVOIDING OVEREXPOSURE

Below are a few more reasons for enhancement-related skin allergies and some useful tips for avoiding them.

Case #1

UV gels are usually very sticky, adhering tenaciously to brush handles, tabletops, and containers. This can make it more difficult to avoid prolonged and repeated contact. And it's more difficult to remove the gel from hands. Also, UV light is required to harden and polymerize UV gels. Fresh UV bulbs quickly began to emit less and less UV light. After a while, they don't produce enough UV light to properly cure the product. After two to four months (depending on your usage) these bulbs can emit less than half their original levels of UV light. The problem is, the bulbs look as bright and blue as ever. But blue light doesn't cure UV gels. Nail professionals are sometimes fooled because the UV bulb hasn't burned out, so they think it still works. UV light is *invisible*, so you cannot see it fading away. Inexpensive UV bulbs (often with lower quality) may save a little money but may leave UV gel nails partially uncured. Lower-quality bulbs won't last nearly as long as their higher-quality counterparts.

On the other hand, some UV gels heat up, and the sensation can be so painful that the client jerks her fingers from under the light. The longer the client's hands are out, the less thoroughly the enhancement will cure. This creates the same problem that is seen when old UV bulbs are used. Both of these lead to improper curing of the enhancement. What can be the result of improper curing? Ingredients that would normally become a permanent part of the artificial nail are left to migrate slowly into the natural nail. Trace amounts can reach the soft, living tissues of the nail bed, especially if the plates are thin or damaged. When product allergies occur, clients often complain of "itchy" or "warm" nail beds.

Finally, it is very important to avoid soft tissue contact with the gooey surface layer, called the inhibition layer. In earlier chapters you learned that this layer of goo is caused by oxygen, which inhibits or blocks the proper cure of the UV gels. The same thing happens with odorless liquid monomer products. The oxygen in the air over the UV gel prevents or inhibits proper curing at the surface. Weakened UV bulbs will create an even thicker inhibition layer. This layer contains potential allergens, so always avoid skin contact! Alcohol or other solvents used to wipe away this layer can actually carry the allergens through the cotton pad to the fingers, increasing the potential for skin overexposure.

Solutions: Use a plastic-backed pad to remove inhibition layers and prevent allergens from soaking through to the skin. Freshly cured dusts still contain small amounts of uncured ingredients, so avoid them! Use only the highest-quality UV bulbs from a reputable source and replace them three or four times a year, especially if used every day. Clean the bulbs weekly to prevent dusts and/or product buildup. Apply thinner layers of UV gel to prevent excessive heat. That's the beauty of going thinner. The less product you use, the lower exotherm and the more comfortable your clients will feel. It is important to never shorten the recommended curing time under the UV light. Don't forget to make sure your client's hands are positioned correctly under the light to ensure proper cure. Use only the UV light unit designed to work with the UV gels of your choice, just as you should use the correct powder and liquid monomer combination. Different lights may look similar, but these units vary widely in performance, efficiency, and UV light output. Wattage is not the same as UV light output. The wattage is how much power the bulb will consume. Wattage is not an indication of effectiveness or efficiency. In short, choose the UV gel system you like and use the entire system, including the light.

Case #2

Odorless products are more likely to cause client sensitivities than the traditional non-odorless enhancement products. Odorless products must be used with a dry bead consistency (mix ratio), but they are often used too wet. As with all monomer liquid/powder systems, the ratio of monomer liquid to powder must be correct. The powder carries an ingredient needed to cure the enhancement. Using too little powder makes a wet bead that will leave uncured ingredients inside the enhancement. Different companies vary the amount of carrying agents in their powders. They also adjust their monomer formulas to work best with the level of curing agent in their powders. This can dramatically affect the polymerization process and the quality of the enhancement. That is why it's extremely important to use powders specifically designed for that particular monomer liquid. Don't let anyone tell you differently. Uncured ingredients can migrate to the nail bed and cause itching. Allergic skin reactions—for example, water blisters around the nail plate area—can result if brush flags (tips) touch the skin repeatedly. Skin contact can also occur while cleaning up around the sidewalls or under the free edge with the brush. Product overexposure under the free edge can injure the hyponychium and lead to onycholysis or pterygium.

Solutions: Leave a tiny free margin between the product and the eponychium and sidewalls. Regularly check your mix ratio to ensure you're not working too wet. Don't use a brush soaked with monomer to smooth the enhancement surface. Don't work with your face too close to your brush. If you work too closely, monomer and solvent vapors can irritate your eyelids and nasal passages. Wear a dust mask while filing. Wear disposable nitrile gloves while pouring, transferring, or cleaning up monomer liquid or UV gels. Keep your table clean. Throw away monomer-soaked towels by sealing them in plastic bags and dropping them into your trash can often throughout the day. Wash your hands after each client and dry them thoroughly. Also, always use a pump-dispensed skin moisturizer to ensure that hands are properly conditioned.

Case #3

Wrap resins, no-light gels, and adhesives are all made from cyanoacrylate monomer. Although this monomer is highly unlikely to cause allergic skin reactions, people still become allergic. These products contain stabilizers, which prevent them from hardening in their containers while they sit on the shelf. The stabilizers are potential skin allergens, but they are used in such low concentrations that they are not very likely to cause problems. Very few clients will develop sensitivities to them. Why? Cyanoacrylate is a very unique monomer. It reacts almost instantly in the presence of moisture. Once the curing process begins, within a very short time all the monomer has reacted and cannot penetrate the skin to cause allergy.

Solutions: Adhesives are frequently the first product that nail technicians suspect when clients complain of itchy nail beds. Interestingly, they are rarely to blame! Skin allergies can occur with adhesives, wrap resins, and no-light gels, but they are relatively rare. If clients begin to develop sensitivities, it's always best to discontinue use.

WATCH OUT FOR GHOSTS

Take extreme care to keep brush handles, containers, tabletops, and drawers clean and free from product residue (*FT*). Repeatedly handling contaminated items can lead to skin overexposure. Skin allergies and irritation between the thumb and forefinger are often the result of stroking the brush hairs or cleaning the brushes with bare fingers. Uncured enhancement products are not designed for skin contact! If you avoid skin contact, neither you nor your client will ever develop an allergic reaction. Also, avoid touching your face. People touch their faces with contaminated hands way too much. Dusts and product residues can cause blemishes and skin inflammation. The chin and cheeks are especially prone to allergy. Facial skin (especially the eye area) is relatively thin, so wash your hands before touching these areas.

Table towels are another source of skin overexposure. Technicians often wipe their brushes on a table towel. Resting the arm or hand on the contaminated towel will increase the risk of developing an allergy. Fresh dust or filings on tabletops can also cause skin overexposure. Never allow your arm to rest in dusts or filings. Using too wet a bead consistency makes matters worse. Dusts are rich in ingredient residues. The dusts and gooey inhibition layer from UV gel enhancements and odorless enhancement systems are even more likely to cause irritation and allergy. Repeated skin contact with this gooey layer must be avoided.

Some nail technicians have suffered serious problems because they did not avoid skin overexposure. Don't fall into these traps. Some of these bad habits are ghosts from the early years of the nail industry when there was no proper education. Don't be a victim of past mistakes and myths. Irritation and allergic reactions are special challenges for nail technicians and they have forced too many nail technicians to leave the profession. Don't be next! Your best defense is knowledge! Use this valuable knowledge wisely.

THESE GLOVES ARE MADE FOR WEARING

Wearing the right glove is an excellent way to lower skin exposure to professional products that are not designed for prolonged and repeated contact with skin (FT). There are lots of bad excuses for not wearing gloves but no good reasons. "They're too uncomfortable," "It's inconvenient," and "I don't like them" are some common excuses. Sure, wearing gloves may seem uncomfortable and inconvenient. But your shoes would feel uncomfortable and be inconvenient if you had never worn shoes before. Painful rashes, blisters, open sores, and cracked, dry skin are even more uncomfortable. Wearing gloves is far less "inconvenient" than finding a new line of work. Gloves are like seat belts. Once you get in the habit of wearing them, you'll feel uncomfortable without them! Today, hundreds of different types of gloves are available in many types of materials. There are gloves that reach the shoulders, individual finger gloves, and everything in between. You can choose powdered or powder-free, lined or unlined cotton, straight or naturally curved fingers, ultra-sheer to heavy-duty. Some gloves even have a rough texture for improved grip and handling. Table 12–1 lists various materials used to make gloves and their usefulness in the salon environment. Gloves are best worn to prevent prolonged and/or repeated contact with any professional nail product not designed for skin contact. They are especially important to those with existing skin sensitivities.

Overall, disposable nitrile gloves are the best alternative for nail salons. Latex gloves provide very little protection from monomer liquids and many solvents, since these substances can quickly penetrate the glove. Because of this, latex gloves are not recommended. If you must wear them, then it is best to wear two gloves on each hand. The double layering will provide increased protection. Either nitrile or cotton-lined rubber gloves are the best choice in reusable gloves. The cotton lining is important when using rubber gloves to prevent contact dermatitis from the rubber. For those with serious skin allergies, EVOH/PE laminate gloves (Silver Shield/4H glove, North, Inc.) may be the only adequate alternative. These gloves are thin but slightly stiffer and not as comfortable as the reusable nitrile or rubber gloves described above. But they offer the very best in chemical protection. These gloves are more expensive but are washable and worth the expense to those with serious skin sensitivities.

Table 12-1 *An overview of the most useful gloves for salons*

Material	Disposable Gloves
Nitrile	Exceptional chemical resistance and strength. The best disposable gloves available for nail technicians. Highly recommended!
Polyurethane	Excellent chemical resistance and strength—tough and sheer.
Natural latex	Inexpensive, good strength, poor resistance to artificial nail enhancement products.
Polyethylene	Lowest cost, but lower strength and chemical resistance.
	Reusable Gloves
Nitrile	Exceptional chemical resistance and strength. Probably the best overall reusable gloves available for nail technicians.
EVOH/PE	Extreme protection for those who need or want it.
Rubber	Inexpensive, good chemical resistance, tough and flexible.
PVA	Exceptional chemical resistance and strength, lighter than most.
Neoprene	Good chemical resistance and strength, only fair flexibility.

Gloves should be worn to prevent skin contact with products that are not designed to touch the skin, that is, nail enhancement gels and monomers. Disposable gloves should be thrown away after each use. Reusable gloves should be disposed of each month or sooner if needed. Don't use either type of glove for too long. If product contaminates the inside of a glove, it must be disposed of immediately. Remember, no glove is impervious to penetration. Depending on the thickness, eventually products will soak through the glove. Think of gloves as temporary barriers, not permanent shields. Also, try several different types and sizes of gloves. That is a good way to determine which is right for you (see Figure 12–4).

Glove Allergies

It seems strange that a person could become allergic to wearing gloves, but it happens often—usually with powdered latex gloves. Cornstarch is the powder that makes it easier to put on or remove gloves. Cornstarch keeps hands drier as well. Hands that are constantly wet can become irritated. Powdered gloves can help prevent this. But a fair number of people are sensitive to cornstarch. If you are allergic to cornstarch, you must wear powder-free gloves. It might be wise to wear a thin cotton glove underneath as well. The cotton will wick away moisture, keeping the hands drier. It will also prevent your skin from touching the latex. Some people are sensitive to latex as well. Latex comes from rubber sap, an all-natural substance. As you learned in Chapter 11, most allergies are caused by naturally occurring substances. Proteins found in rubber can cause allergic reactions

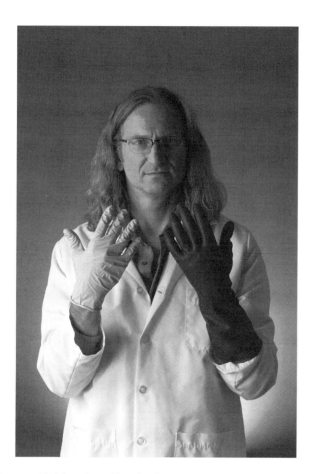

Figure 12–4 *Disposable (left) and reusable (right) gloves, both made from nitrile*

in sensitive people. Also, it is believed that other additives used in manufacturing of rubber gloves can cause problems for some individuals. If you experience any problems wearing gloves, don't give up. If you are allergic to one type of material, then changing to another will probably alleviate your symptoms. You can always wear a light cotton inner liner to protect your skin from the glove. Talk to your distributor or call the manufacturer of the glove. They can suggest alternative materials that will not cause problems. Once you find gloves that are right for you, wear them and keep your skin healthy.

Formaldehyde, Wherefore Art Thou?

Allergies can occur on the skin surrounding the nail plate. Formaldehyde is often the culprit. Nail plate hardeners contain between 0.25 and 1 percent formaldehyde. Products with less than 0.25 percent formaldehyde will not significantly harden nail plates. This is too low a concentration to be effective. Because formaldehyde is a potential skin allergen, products are rarely formulated with more than 1 percent formaldehyde, since this would pose a significant risk of allergic reaction. But even at low concentrations, formaldehyde nail hardeners can cause allergic reactions if used excessively or incorrectly. Typical symptoms are: blue or red nail beds that may throb, onycholysis, peeling skin around the nail plate, or pterygium under the free edge. These problems can be avoided if these products are used correctly.

Unfortunately, once clients become allergic to nail hardeners they usually become allergic to most types of professional nail polish. The very best resin used in nail polish is called tosylamide/formaldehyde resin (TAF resin). Most professional nail polishes contain this incredible ingredient. This resin is more flexible, chip-resistant, and color-stable and has much better adhesion to the natural nail. But this resin has one small disadvantage: formaldehyde is initially used in its creation. Yet only a very small residual amount is left in the final resin. After processing and formulating, nail polishes using this resin contain about 0.002 percent formaldehyde, not enough to cause clients to become sensitive to formaldehyde. Clients rarely become allergic to professional nail polishes unless they have been previously overexposed to formaldehyde-containing nail hardeners. Clients who are allergic to this type of hardener are sensitive even to extremely tiny amounts of residual formaldehyde.

Of course, formaldehyde-containing products can be used safely. They must be kept off the skin, carefully applied, and used only when needed. Formaldehyde-containing hardeners should never be applied to fragile, brittle, dry, split, broken, or damaged nails. The extra cross-links that formaldehyde creates will only worsen their condition. Formaldehyde overexposure on the nail bed can lead to separation of the nail plate onycholysis and seriously damaged skin pterygium under the free edge of the natural nail. Besides, these products are not designed for these type of nail plates. Formaldehyde-containing nail hardeners are best used on weak, flimsy, or overly flexible nail plates. Stop using them once the desired nail plate hardness is achieved and then discontinue use until once again the nails begin to grow out weak. Excessive use of formaldehyde nail hardeners can make nails appear dry and become brittle (*FT*). Actually, these can be signs that the product is being incorrectly or excessively used. Excessive use also increases the risk of skin overexposure and potential allergy. Use these products carefully and only as needed. They are not products that should be used continuously or carelessly.

IF IT QUACKS LIKE A DUCK . . .

"Quack (kwak) is anyone who fraudulently misrepresents his or her ability to diagnose and treat diseases." We like to believe that quacks and charlatans only exist in history or old movies. Sadly, many are still around, taking advantage of their unsuspecting victims. There are medical quacks everywhere, so beware! There is no end to the medical scams that exist today, especially on the Internet. Many of the scams use food and skin allergies to cheat consumers. Muscle testing is an excellent example of an allergy scam. The subject is asked to hold a glass vial containing the supposed allergen. Sometimes a subject holds the vial over the affected part of the body. Weakness in the muscle is interpreted as a positive reaction. Bogus! Here's another example: the Electrodermal Promoter (the infamous "Vega machine") has been declared a medical scam by the FDA and the Canadian health authority, Health Canada. Why? It is impossible to touch a probe to the skin and determine existing allergies or "energy balance." Everything from magnets to feathers to crystals have been used to "diagnose" and "cure" allergies. All bogus!

Some quacks say they can look at your blood under a microscope to determine your allergies. Bogus, too! There are lots of fake blood tests for allergies. Of course, all of the scams have one thing in common: the quacks will charge for these foolish tests, but insurance companies won't pay for most. The insurance companies know they're bogus! There are dozens of these ridiculous tests that do nothing but waste your time and money and don't solve your problem. After you get your diagnosis, most quacks will sell you a treatment (usually something "amazing" or "all-natural"). They may give you a long list of things that you're supposedly allergic to and should avoid. Or they'll frighten you into believing there is a buildup of "toxins" in your blood or body. Really bogus! Then they'll happily sell you vitamins, herbs, blood cleansers, magnetic inserts for your shoes and mattress, air cleaners, water filters, and other so-called remedies. They don't want to help or heal you—they just want your money. They may pretend to be caring and supportive. But they are really just con artists (or misguided individuals) who want your money—that's all! How can you tell the "quacks" from the experts?

Of course, there are some valid test methods performed by qualified allergists who are medical doctors specializing in allergy testing. Or you can schedule a visit with a board-certified dermatologist. **Patch testing** is considered the most medically reliable method for identifying skin allergens *(FT)*. A tiny amount of the suspected allergen is diluted, applied to a small spot on the skin, and covered with a bandage. After a fixed period of time (24–48 hours), the exposed site is examined. A large increase in redness, itchiness, blisters, or other signs of adverse skin reaction at the exposed site is considered a positive result and solid evidence of a skin allergy. Skin scratch-and-prick or puncture tests are also performed *(FT)* . As the names suggest, tiny amounts of the suspected allergen are applied to small scratches made in the skin. Alternatively, they may be injected underneath the skin. Scratch and prick tests are medically valid tests, but they do give more false positives and are not as reliable as patch testing. Applying a substance to scratched skin can create an irritation that mimics a positive reaction. In some cases skin testing might not be appropriate. The best alternative to direct skin testing is called RAST testing. This sophisticated blood test works far better for food allergies, but reasonably well for skin allergies. Remember, though, there are many other blood tests that are phony. Only patch, prick, puncture, or RAST tests are worth the effort (FT). All others are ineffective or completely ridiculous, so don't bother. Save your money!

There are no "cures" for skin allergies. You either prevent them by avoiding the allergen or live with them; those are the only choices. If you're offered any vitamin, herbal supplement, or other such remedy to "neutralize" your allergy, be very, very suspicious. Don't be a victim of a medical scam. There are many more phony tests and remedies than there are real ones. How can you sort the bad from the good? Here are two sources of information that can provide facts to help you avoid quackery and medical scams. The first is www.quackwatch.org. This is a very reliable source of information. It will provide links to other recommended sites. Quackwatch will also warn you away from Web sites intended to deceive or confuse consumers. A good source for medical information and advice is www.mdadvice.com. Be wary and be informed. That's the best way to protect yourself from quacks.

FAST TRACK (FT)

(FT) Skin disorders are the number one occupation-related disease in America.

(FT) Repeated/prolonged exposure is a cause of salon-related skin disorders.

(FT) Tap water is a very common salon irritant. Keep hands dry!

(FT) Excessive hand washing can damage the skin and cause irritation.

(FT) Prolonged and/or repeated contact with many solvents can strip away skin oils, leaving skin dry or damaged.

(FT) Corrosives are found at the extreme opposite ends of the pH scale.

(FT) Strong acid or alkaline solutions negatively affect the skin's pH.

(FT) High-strength cuticle and callus removers and methacrylic acid primers are highly corrosive to tissue.

(FT) Always use safety eyewear when using corrosive products.

(FT) A substance that causes allergy is called a sensitizer or allergen.

(FT) Some ingredients used in nail enhancement products are weak sensitizers.

(FT) Nail enhancement allergies usually occur after months of repeated contact.

(FT) Skin allergies usually occur at the site where overexposure occurred.

(FT) Irritated, broken, or damaged skin increases the risk of allergies.

(FT) Only use polymer powders with their matching monomer liquids.

(FT) Never go back and smooth the enhancement surface with more monomer.

FT Never apply product to a client experiencing a skin reaction or infection.

FT Never touch the hairs of the brush with your fingers.

FT Keep brushes, containers, and tabletops clean and free of product residue.

FT Wearing gloves is an excellent way to lower skin exposure.

FT Excessive use of formaldehyde hardeners can make nails dry and brittle.

FT Patch testing is the most effective way to determine skin allergies.

FT Scratch, prick, puncture, and RAST tests are the only other valid tests for skin allergies, and these should be performed by qualified medical doctor.

Review Questions

1. What is the most common occupational disease in America?
2. Which is more dangerous to the skin, irritants or corrosives? Why?
3. Will an ingredient allergy ever go away?
4. Name two common salon irritants.
5. Allergic contact dermatitis accounts for _____ percent of cosmetic-related skin problems.
6. What is the best type of disposable glove for nail salons?
7. Why can overly large brushes create skin overexposure?
8. The substance that causes the allergy is called a _____ or _____.
9. What is the best way to avoid allergic reactions and irritations?
10. What causes the inhibition layer on top of cured UV gels?
11. What two natural ingredients cause most latex glove allergies?
12. How much formaldehyde is found in professional nail enamels containing tosylamide/formaldehyde resin? Can this make clients become sensitive to formaldehyde?
13. What are the risks of using formaldehyde nail hardeners excessively or improperly?
14. What are the only valid tests for skin allergies?
15. What Internet site will give you the latest information on medical scams?

Chapter

13

Sanitation and Disinfection: The New Reality

Objective

In this chapter, you will gain a complete understanding of sanitation and disinfection in the salon. You will learn how to properly use these practices to create a safe and healthy haven for your clientele. Finally, you will gain a deeper understanding of the value and importance of using universal sanitation to give your clients peace of mind and confidence in your services.

CONTROLLING SALON CONTAMINATION

Preventing the spread of infectious disease is an important part of your job. The reality is that you're responsible for your clients. They depend upon you to ensure their safety. That is why protecting against the spread of infectious disease is required by state and federal regulations. For good reason! You will come in contact with many people, and your services provide clients with great benefits, but proper care must be taken to prevent the spread of disease or illness. Luckily, these problems are easy to avoid. You'll learn how in this chapter.

Look around the room for a moment. What do you see? No matter where you look you'll see some sort of surface. The surface of the table, the wall, the floor, even your own hand—almost everything has a surface. No matter how clean you keep the surfaces, they will eventually become contaminated. Your tools, implements, containers, cases, electric files, and so on can be contaminated by visible dust and debris (dark, dirty layers of "crud"). This also applies to sticky residues even if they are not visible. Nail dust filings in the drawer, hair in a comb, or makeup on a towel—these are all common examples of contaminants. Surfaces are also contaminated by bacteria, fungi, or viruses. Since these can be seen only under a microscope, they are called **microorganisms,** as shown in Figure 13–1.

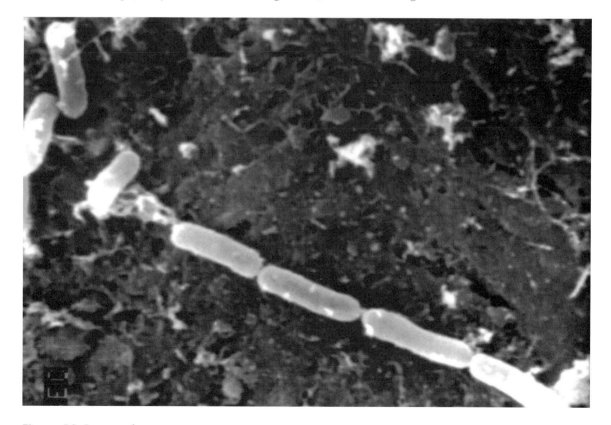

Figure 13-1 *Picture of a microorganism*

Bacteria, fungi, and other microorganisms are everywhere. They literally cover the earth. Most microorganisms are completely harmless and will not cause disease or illness. That's lucky, because it's impossible to rid the salon of all microorganisms. That is not the goal! Your job is to control the spread of a very tiny percentage of microorganisms. You must only be concerned about the ones that cause illness or disease in humans. Any microorganism that causes disease or illness in humans is called a pathogen (FT). Removing harmful pathogens and visible debris from implements or other surfaces is called **decontamination** (FT).

UNIVERSAL SANITATION: THE BEST DEFENSE

We have the finest medical system that has ever existed. We have the best-trained doctors, nurses, and technicians, the best hospitals, and the most technologically advanced equipment ever created. Researchers have learned more than ever about diseases. Science has developed better cures, and people are living decades longer thanks to the miracle of modern medicine. Then why are we, the modern generation, the most germ-paranoid culture of all time? It's easy to see why this is so. The media constantly bombard us with grossly exaggerated and often misleading stories designed to conjure up fears over the latest disease of the month! Reporters distort the facts and give opinions on subjects they don't really understand. You've seen these news stories and so have your clients. That's why the media sensationalize these stories, so that you will watch—and it works! This is the new reality that all salons must face. These stories generate irrational fears that harm your business. The professional nail industry has been a favorite media target in the past, and there's every reason to believe this will continue into the future. Potential clients see these stories and some become fearful of salon services. That hurts everyone in the professional beauty industry, including nail salons and spas.

When clients enter your salon they immediately begin to evaluate the cleanliness of the surroundings. Imagine walking into a new salon and seeing a pile of hair swept into the corner or finding your nail technician (and table) covered with nail dust. How would you feel being sent to a dingy or stale-smelling bathroom to wash your hands in a dirty sink? A concept called **universal sanitation** states that salons should always be clean, sanitary, and presentable (FT). Universal sanitation is achieved only when the entire salon is clean and sanitary, including employees, implements, machines, floors, trash cans, telephones, cash registers, doorknobs, bathrooms, waiting and eating areas, and so on. Universal sanitation is not a lofty or unattainable goal. It is an easy-to-achieve professional standard. Universal sanitation is important to any salon. It's also something to consider before accepting a position at a new salon. Does the salon practice universal sanitation and take it seriously? It's an important question to ask! It will be hard for you to maintain a professional working image while working in an unsanitary salon. Universal sanitation will increase your chances of being a success and ensure that you have happy clientele who will trust and respect your knowledge.

SANITATION: THE MOST IMPORTANT STEP

When it comes to ensuring your clients' safety and health, nothing is more important than sanitation. Sanitation is *not* the same as disinfection. In fact, they are quite different and should never be confused. Simply said, **sanitation** is the proper and thorough cleaning of an object or surface. We sanitize our dishes in a dishwasher. We sanitize our hands when we wash them. Sanitizing significantly reduces the number of pathogens and other contaminants to levels considered safe by health care professionals Ⓕ. Proper sanitation prevents the spread of pathogens. If a child gets the flu, we carefully wash the child's dishes to protect others in the family. Hot water and detergent wash the pathogens off, making the dishes safe for others to use. Proper washing removes up to 99 percent of all of the pathogens and other contaminants from a surface Ⓕ. This is why cleaning is so important in salons. There's nothing better than cleaning for controlling the spread of infections! For instance, scrubbing an abrasive file for only 10 seconds with liquid soap and warm running water will remove 99 percent of the contaminants from the surface. That's pretty good for a few seconds of scrubbing time.

After you finish sanitizing surfaces such as implements, tabletops, and doorknobs, they will still be contaminated with small amounts of microorganisms. It is very difficult to remove or destroy all microorganisms. Besides, we don't need to get them all. The vast majority are harmless. Also, medical research has proven that small amounts of pathogens will not usually cause illness. In most cases you must be exposed to very high concentrations of pathogens to become infected. In other words, it usually takes a lot of pathogens to cause an infection, usually five to ten thousand or more! So, now you can see why cleaning is so important in salons. It isn't necessary to eliminate all bacteria, fungi, and viruses— we only have to significantly reduce their numbers to keep them under control Ⓕ. You'll find that this is fairly easy to do if you follow and practice universal sanitation.

PROPER USE OF HAND SANITIZERS

Alcohol-based hand sanitizers are highly effective pathogen fighters, but they will not clean your hands. The only way to clean debris from your hands is to wash them with liquid soap and water. Even so, alcohol hand sanitizers are very useful in the salon.

Why put an alcohol hand sanitizer on clean hands? Clients love to use them after washing their hands. Also, you don't know what your client has touched between the restroom and your station. Besides, these products help calm their fears. So let clients see you using hand sanitizers and you'll build trust.

A good place to start is with your professional tools. Keeping your salon's implements and other utensils clean is the most important first step you can take. But please don't stop there. There's plenty more to do to ensure that your salon meets the standards of universal sanitation. For instance, make sure the bathroom and sink areas are kept clean and sanitary. These are common places for pathogens to spread from person to person.

THE WASH-'N'-RINSE SPRINT

Pathogens can grow in soap dishes and even on bars of soap. Toothbrushes, mascara brushes, and old cosmetic creams or lotions can all support the growth of pathogens. It's best to provide clients with a liquid soap and a soft, disinfectable scrub brush. Medical research has shown that liquid soaps are far more effective than regular bar soaps. Also, experts agree that regular hand washing can dramatically reduce pathogens on the skin. But studies show that most people wash their hands for only three to five seconds before rinsing. That's not nearly long enough!

Certain jobs can leave your hands heavily contaminated, such as changing a diaper or cleaning the trash basket or the bathroom. Under most other circumstances, hands can be thoroughly washed in 15 to 20 seconds. But after these types of jobs, take extra time (60 seconds) to thoroughly scrub your hands and nails. Pay close attention to the undersides of your nails and be sure to scrub them clean with a brush (Figure 13–2). But don't be too aggressive or damage the hyponychium or any other nail plate seals. Remember, it is important to thoroughly rinse your hands with lukewarm water. This is important because hot water can irritate skin. Be very sure to remove all soap residue, since it can cause skin irritation. Hands that feel dry, itchy, or tight after washing may be showing symptoms of irritation or allergy. Continued hand washing can cause the problem to worsen. To help prevent these problems, carefully rinse and dry your hands each time you wash them. If the hands are damp for long periods, that alone can cause skin irritation. Use a high-quality hand lotion, preferably dispensed by a pump or squeeze tube, to prevent dry skin. Shared jars of creams or lotion can be a breeding ground for pathogens. Pumps and squeeze tubes are much more sanitary. In the bathroom, pumps are the best choice. Also, take care to avoid excessive hand washing.

Even though your state rules require washing with liquid soap and water before every client, using a waterless (alcohol-based) hand sanitizer at the table is a great idea. There is nothing wrong with going over and above your state's regulations. What better way to impress clients?

It is possible to wash your hands too much. Skin irritation, itching, and dryness can also be caused by excessive hand washing (FT). Compulsive hand washers usually have very dry, chapped hands. Don't obsessively wash hands because you're afraid of "germs." This practice can damage the skin and increase your risk of developing an infection or skin disorder. Only wash hands when necessary,

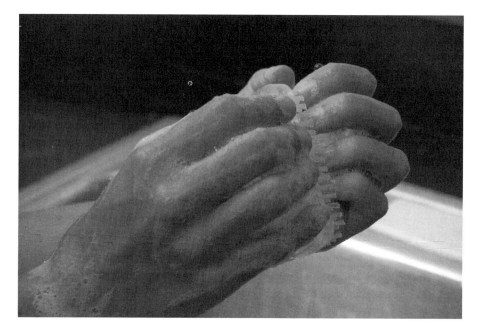

Figure 13-2 *Proper hand washing is extremely important for client protection*

that is, between clients, when leaving the bathroom, before and after eating, or when they are visibly dirty. It is important to wash between clients every time, no matter how busy your day. And when you wash your hands, wash them the right way.

DISINFECTION: THE ICING ON THE CAKE!

What about the approximately 1 percent of contaminants left on freshly cleaned (sanitized) surfaces? In most cases, they will not cause any problems. Floors, walls, trash cans, laundry hampers, and the like do not come in contact with the client's skin or nails, so the remaining low level of contamination cannot cause any problems. The surface is still clean and sanitary—that's good enough for these items! When more is needed, that's when disinfection becomes important. **Disinfection** is a process that kills the small number of pathogens remaining on a surface after sanitizing ⒡. In salons, this is best achieved with liquid disinfectants, such as alcohol, a 10 percent bleach solution, or professionally formulated disinfection products. As a nail professional, you will be expected to uphold the standards of your state or local regulations. But not all areas adhere to the same regulations, so check with your local state board or appropriate government offices to determine which of these disinfectants you may use in your salon.

Disinfectants ensure that all pathogens on a surface are destroyed and will not cause infection. Disinfectants are not for use on skin, hair, or nails ⒡. They

IT'S NOT THE CAKE!

Disinfection is not a replacement for cleaning. Remember, cleaning your work area and implements is the most important thing you can do to prevent the spread of diseases in the salon. You cannot disinfect a surface or object until it has first been properly cleaned. That's why disinfection is only the icing on the cake. Proper cleaning is the most important step by far!

are much too harsh and irritating, and they can also discolor natural or artificial nails. Never stick your fingers into disinfectant solutions or use them on your skin. **Antiseptic** solutions are designed for use on damaged or cut skin. Antiseptics slow down the growth of pathogens (FT). They are not powerful enough to completely destroy pathogens, but they are safer for skin contact and aid the healing process.

Disinfection products must pass a series of tests proving their effectiveness before receiving an **EPA registration number** from the Environmental Protection Agency. This number is proof of the product's effectiveness. To obtain an EPA registration number the product must prove that it is **bactericidal** (kills bacteria), **virucidal** (kills viruses), and **fungicidal** (kills fungi). Federal law requires that all disinfectants print their EPA registration number on the back of the label. Bleach, 90 percent ethyl alcohol, and 70 percent rubbing alcohol (isopropyl alcohol) do not require EPA registration since these were used as disinfectants before the category of EPA disinfectants was created. So they don't need a registration number to prove their effectiveness in a hospital setting.

STERILIZATION: NOT FOR SALONS!

A common myth says salon implements and tools should be sterilized. In general, the word *sterilize* is misunderstood and used incorrectly. For example, it's impossible to sterilize the nail plate or the skin. Sterilizing the skin would quickly kill it and damage the nail plate. **Sterilization** uses very high temperatures and pressurized steam to kill pathogens. To achieve these extreme conditions, hospitals use **autoclaves.** These devices are very expensive and difficult to use, and they're not needed in nail salons. Sterilization can also be achieved by using highly toxic and dangerous chemicals that are much too dangerous for salon use. Sterilization is identical to disinfection except in one area. Sterilization kills spores, a highly resistant form of bacteria. Some bacteria can become **spores** by quickly coating themselves with a waxy substance, much like a caterpillar spins a protective cocoon (FT). This is how some bacteria defend themselves from attack by disinfectants. Bacterial spores have very thick walls and need the most toxic disinfectants or the pressurized steam of an autoclave to destroy them. Luckily, spores aren't dangerous in the salon, so you don't need to worry about them. It's a different story for surgical wards and operating rooms. If a significant amount of spores get inside the body during surgery, a very serious infection could develop. This is why surgical instruments must be sterilized. But why aren't surgery room floors and tables sterilized? Because they do not come in direct contact with the patient, so disinfection is enough.

Obviously, it is foolish to suggest that salon implements must be sterilized! Salon implements are not used for surgery, so disinfection is more than enough to protect clients and ensure your salon provides safe services. Remember: if disinfection is good enough for a hospital, it is more than enough for a salon! Controlling pathogens in hospitals is much more difficult and important than it is for professional salons. The differences are obvious. Salons are hundreds, maybe thousands of times safer than hospitals. Why? Because salons deal with healthy people and hospitals treat very ill people. Clearly, they should be treated differently when it comes to disinfection practices.

WHY DISINFECT?

It is important to disinfect implements, tabletops, foot spas, and other such items. But before the disinfection process starts, you should know why you disinfect. The first and most important reason for salon disinfection is to give clients peace of mind and to assure them they are in good hands. Most clients will need this reassurance, since most don't realize how safe salons really are. The truth is that it is very unlikely a client will catch a serious illness or disease in the salon. And it is silly to suggest that salon services can kill people. But there are those who wrongly believe and incorrectly teach that HIV or tuberculosis could be transmitted by salon services.

Between 1983 and 2004 over 6 billion salon services were performed in professional nail salons without a single case of transmission of either HIV or tuberculosis by these services. Not even one! Why? These illnesses are not spread by salon services. It's never happened and probably never will. But even if it did, we'd know the odds were more than 1 in 5 billion! So why would some people claim that we need disinfectants to prevent HIV and tuberculosis in the salon? They argue that just because it hasn't happened doesn't mean it won't happen someday. They've been making this same argument for over 20 years and it still hasn't happened. Why should a salon use products to protect against something that has never happened? HIV, hepatitis, or tuberculosis cannot be spread by manicures, pedicures, or other nail services (FT). Obviously, this is *not* the real reason for disinfection. Anyone who claims otherwise is not telling you the truth. The truth is that salons are safe. Your job as a professional is to keep them safe. Don't disinfect to save lives—that's complete nonsense. Disinfect to protect your clients from nail and skin infections or colds and flu. These are the issues that challenge nail professionals.

If you learn nothing else from this book, please remember this: it is your professional responsibility to protect your clients by practicing proper sanitation and disinfection, all the time and to the best of your ability. Every nail infection is a black eye for our industry. Every skin infection is a blow to our image as professionals. When you are granted a nail license by your state, you will be making several promises in return for the privilege of serving as a nail professional. One of those promises is to safeguard the health of your clientele. If you neglect this promise, you may endanger your clients, ruin the reputation of your salon, lose your professional license, and risk being sued. Sanitation and disinfection are serious responsibilities, so take them seriously!

IT'S A RISKY WORLD

What is universal sanitation really designed to prevent? In the following section, you will learn about some of the possibilities that can occur if proper care isn't taken. You will also learn what is not spread by salon services. But first, let's start with the most common problems.

Bacterial Infections

Bacterial infections of the nail plate and the surrounding skin are by far the most common infection resulting from a nail salon service. These infections may appear as light yellow to dark green stains on the surface of the intact nail plate (see Figure 5–1). If the nail plate separates from the nail bed (see Figure 4–3), a bacterial infection may occur under the plate. Painful swelling, continual warmth, and redness or tenderness of the skin surrounding the nail plate may also be signs of bacterial infections (see Figure 5–6). Bacterial infections may also be found on the leg after a pedicure. Clients usually shave before the pedicure, even though it is best not to do so. Tiny razor nicks in the skin provide a perfect opportunity for a bacterial infection, especially if the foot bath is not properly cleaned and disinfected. Recommend that your clients shave the night before their appointment to reduce the risk of infection.

BILLIONS TO ONE?

It seems silly to suggest that salons should protect against diseases that are not spread by salon services. That's the case with illnesses such as HIV and tuberculosis. According to the odds, clients are more likely to be struck by lightning, die from a bee sting, or be killed in an accident on their way to your salon than to catch either disease from a salon service.

Don't be fooled. Salon services are relatively safe, especially when compared to driving a car or even walking in a crosswalk.

Fungal Infections

Fungal infections can make the nail plate thicken, crumble, and discolor. The nail plate's color can range from whitish to yellow to brown or black. Fingernails may develop fungal infections, but the vast majority of these are found on toenails. These type of infections are difficult to spread, and clients usually become infected outside the salon. Still, nail professionals must take care to prevent transmission to other clients. Fungal skin infections can also occur on the bottoms of the feet and between the toes, as in the case of athlete's foot (see Chapter 5). Ringworm is another example of a fungal skin infection that may be transmitted during salon services.

Viral Infections

Warts on hands and feet are commonly seen in the salon setting. They are most often found on the bottom of the feet (plantar warts) or the skin around the nail plate. The viruses that cause warts are highly contagious. Warts vary in color from flesh tones to dark brown-black. Salon professionals should take great care when working near anything they suspect could be a wart. Cutting or scratching a wart may cause it to spread to other parts of the body or to another person. Colds, flu, chicken pox, mumps, and measles are all viruses and can also spread by casual contact, such as coughing or sneezing.

NOT SPREAD BY SALON SERVICES

Mold and **mildew** are terms that are sometimes incorrectly used to describe infections of the nail plate, but neither of these infect the nail plate. **HIV** is the virus that causes acquired immune deficiency syndrome (AIDS). HIV is not spread by salon services and never has been. This is not how HIV is transmitted. **Hepatitis** is a virus that is about 100 times more infectious than HIV. In the 1980s some suggested that hepatitis could be spread by salon services. It is now known that this does not occur. In the salon hepatitis could be transmitted only under extremely rare and unlikely circumstances, so it should not be considered a significant risk there. **Tuberculosis** is a bacterial infection of the lungs and is spread only by coughing. Tuberculosis is not transmitted by any salon products or services. In short, salon services do not transmit life-threatening diseases. If anyone tells you differently, they're not telling you the truth.

FEAR-BASED MARKETING

Everyone knows that sex sells . . . but not as much as fear sells. Fear is a powerful emotion that motivates people to do (and buy) things they normally wouldn't. Using fear as a sales tool is expected for burglar alarms and flood insurance, but for nail salon products? How did this happen? As the professional nail salon industry grew during the 1980s, the Nail Manufacturers Council (NMC) began to focus on sanitation and disinfection issues in the nail industry. The NMC is a group of leading manufacturers of nail products who come together to work for the betterment of the industry. One of their main goals was to raise standards and improve the image of the professional salon by focusing on sanitation and disinfection education.

Unfortunately, some marketers saw this as an opportunity to sell their disinfection products. They began to emphasize the supposed threat of HIV, tuberculosis, and hepatitis in nail salons and started to use fear of these diseases to scare nail technicians into using their products. Fear-based marketing techniques really do work! These marketers succeeded in scaring many nail technicians into disinfecting, but they damaged our industry's reputation in the process. How? Nail technicians became frightened they might accidentally give their clients some horrible disease. So they warned clients they would have to disinfect to avoid giving them some horrible disease. No surprise that they frightened their clients! Then the fear-based marketers went to the media and the state boards and frightened them. Now everyone's frightened about something that's never happened!

Our industry has been tainted with irrational fear, and we are victims of unjustified negative criticism. That's the danger of fear-based marketing. That's why we should resist it whenever and wherever we can! If someone tries to scare you into buying a product, you should ask yourself why. If it's such a good product, it should be sold based on its benefits! Why create exaggerated or irrational fears? It doesn't matter if it's a nail enhancement product, an abrasive file, an adhesive, or a lotion or cream. It is wrong to use fear to sell professional beauty products and services.

Our industry is about feel-good products and services. Salons are safe havens for clients who want to feel good. It is important that our industry not forget this. So the next time someone tries to scare you into buying a product, resist this marketing ploy and don't let irrational fear influence you. Tell your customers that salons are safe, and so are salon services when performed correctly by a trained professional. Show them how your professional training and education will ensure their safety and health. And be leery of any marketing campaign or education that is designed to frighten you or tell you about the evils of a competitor's products. In short, reject fear-based marketing! It's bad for everyone and it hurts our industry (*FT*).

BENEFITS? WHAT BENEFITS?

By using proper sanitation and disinfection, you're doing more than controlling pathogens. You're helping raise the standards of your profession. Everyone benefits from universal sanitation. It's a standard of excellence that all should strive to achieve. Clients expect more than just beautiful hands and feet. They expect your best practices, attention, and skill. They also expect you to educate them about their nails. The more you know, the more you can teach and help them.

When you talk to your clients, address their fears with the facts. Educate them with the truth! Then prove to them that you are following the proper procedures to ensure their safety. That's the best way to handle these important issues.

THE DISINFECTANT DILEMMA: WHAT TO USE?

Alcohol and Bleach

Bleach, 70 percent isopropyl alcohol, and 90 percent ethyl alcohol are very powerful and highly effective disinfectants. For example, flushing a 10 percent solution of bleach through the piping of the throne-style pedicure chairs for at least 15 minutes is considered to be one of the best ways to control pathogens. But bleach has a strong odor, can discolor some materials, and has almost no cleaning (sanitation) power, so its usefulness is somewhat limited. Alcohol can be an extremely useful disinfectant if implements are completely immersed for 15 minutes. Just wiping alcohol across the surface of an implement will not disinfect it. Proper disinfection can be achieved only by completely immersing the clean implements into the solution. After disinfecting, alcohol will evaporate from the implements, but bleach must be rinsed away with clean running water. Also, alcohol must not be diluted with water or it will lose effectiveness.

Every alcohol is different, so don't lump them together as if they were all the same. Methyl alcohol is also called wood alcohol, because it was originally obtained from wood, but is now manufactured in a different way. This type of alcohol is poisonous and causes blindness if ingested. Ethyl alcohol or grain alcohol is obtained from grain and is not nearly as poisonous. In fact, it is the same alcohol found in vodka, beer, or wine. Isopropyl alcohol or rubbing alcohol is the type most commonly used in salons. Isopropyl alcohol is very poisonous to drink but is a great disinfectant when correctly used.

Each of these is a highly flammable, strong-smelling, colorless liquid. At concentrations above 50 percent they are very drying to the skin and hair. But this is not true of all alcohols! In fact, very few alcohols are drying to skin. Cetyl alcohol and stearyl alcohol are pure white, waxy-feeling solids. They are not flammable, have no odor, and are nontoxic if ingested. Neither of these alcohols will dry out the skin; in fact, they are both excellent skin and hair conditioners. Don't be fooled by the name. Just because it's an alcohol doesn't mean it's drying to the skin.

Quaternary Ammonium Compounds

Quaternary ammonium compounds (quats) are the most commonly used type of salon disinfectant ⓕⓣ. In general, quats have the advantage of being safe, fast-acting, and very good cleaning agents. They are very effective in products designed for cleaning tables, chairs, countertops, cushions, mats, register keys, telephone receivers, and other surfaces. Most quat disinfectants are blends of different types of quats. Blending several types of quats into one formula will dramatically increase effectiveness. Quats are the most cost-effective of all professional salon disinfectants. Most quats are effective after 10 minutes of immersion. (Of course, it is important to read, understand, and follow manufacturer's instructions when using any type of disinfectant system. Instructions can change, so you should periodically reread labels and MSDSs for products you've used before.) You should not leave metal implements in the solution for longer than 10 minutes. Most disinfectants contain corrosion and rust inhibitors, but immersing implements for too long can dull sharp edges or pit metal surfaces. Implements should not be stored overnight in disinfectant solutions. Overall, quats are one of the best choices for salon disinfection.

Phenolics

Like quats, **phenolics** have been used for many years to disinfect implements. They too can be safe and effective if used according to instructions. Phenolics can soften and damage some rubber materials and certain plastics. Care should be taken to avoid skin contact with all disinfectants, especially those made with phenolics. The liquid concentrate can cause serious skin irritation and is corrosive to the eyes. Avoid uncontrolled spraying of phenolic disinfectants. Inhalation of the mists can be very irritating to the sensitive lining of the nose, throat, and lungs. Phenolics are very effective, but they're the most expensive of all professional salon disinfectants.

STEPS OF PROPER SANITATION AND DISINFECTION

The first step is to place the disinfection solution into a container with a lid. In the early days of the nail industry these containers were incorrectly called "wet sanitizers." Of course their purpose is not to clean but to disinfect. The correct term for the container used to disinfect your implements is **disinfectant container.** But before you can disinfect, you must carefully scrub implements, abrasive files, and other tools with a clean brush, liquid soap, and running water. Scrub away all visible or sticky debris and completely rinse away all traces of soap. Hot water can be irritating to skin and will not get the implement or files any cleaner, so use lukewarm water. After rinsing, pat dry on a clean towel. Then completely immerse the implements into the container of clean disinfectant solution. Make sure to avoid skin contact with the liquid disinfectant solution. After soaking for the required time, carefully remove the implements. Immersion time will depend on the manufacturer's instructions. Some disinfectants must be rinsed off before drying. Other types of disinfectants do not require rinsing. As always, exactly follow the manufacturer's instructions when using any disinfectant.

After disinfection, store implements and tools in a place where they can be kept sanitary. If they become contaminated again with dust or other debris, repeat the sanitation and disinfection process. The best way to prevent implements

CUSTOM IMPLEMENTS: A GOOD IDEA?

Some clients prefer to have their own implements and abrasives dedicated for their personal use. This is not necessary if proper sanitation and disinfection are used. But for the client who insists upon taking this extra precaution, here are a few guidelines to remember.

Custom tools and implements must be clean and disinfected after each use, even though they are used on only one client! Also, never allow clients to take the implements home with them. You never know what a client will do with the implements or how they will be used (for example, clipping the family dog's nails), so make sure you keep them properly stored at the salon.

Not all state rules allow the use of custom implements. Check your regulations to be sure.

from becoming recontaminated is to wrap them in a clean towel and store in a dry location. Never store implements in an airtight container or bag. Some pathogens can grow rapidly under these conditions. This is especially true for abrasive files, since they are absorbent and can retain moisture.

What's the best way to clean and disinfect surfaces that cannot be immersed in disinfectant, such as tabletops and doorknobs? First, clean the surface with a suitable cleaner. Use one that's compatible with the surfaces you are cleaning. Second, spray with an appropriate disinfectant. Use one designed for large surfaces, such as a 10 percent bleach solution or pine-oil-based products. You can also purchase professional disinfectants designed for cleaning large surfaces. To properly disinfect, evenly wet the cleaned surface with the disinfectant and allow it to remain wet for ten minutes before wiping dry. Also, be sure to avoid coming into contact with or inhaling any mists that result from spraying. You should wear cotton-lined rubber or nitrile gloves to prevent overexposing your hands to the disinfectant. Ask the manufacturer or distributor to provide you with the Material Safety Data Sheet for all cleaners and disinfectants that you use in the salon. The MSDS is a storehouse of valuable safety, first aid, storage, and disposal information about the product. You should request MSDSs for all your professional products, especially cleaners and disinfectants.

Sanitizing and Disinfecting Implements

Before your service begins, you should perform the following steps:

- Thoroughly wash implements with soap and warm water (Figure 13–3a).
- Rinse away all traces of soap with clear, lukewarm running water, then dry with a clean or disposable towel (Figure 13–3b).
- Completely immerse implements in an EPA-registered, hospital-level disinfectant for the required time (Figure 13–3c).

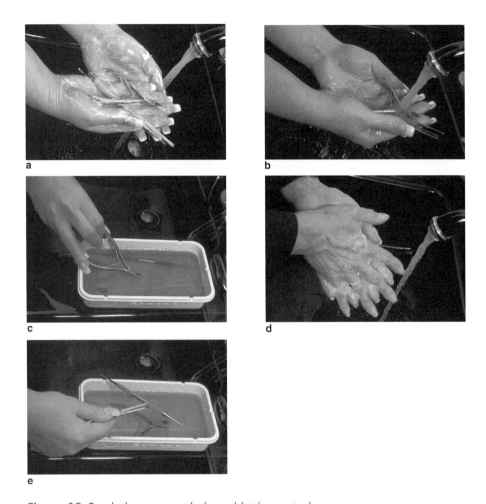

Figure 13-3 *Take the time to properly clean and disinfect your implements*

- Wash hands with soap, rinse well, and dry with a clean or disposable towel (Figure 13–3d).
- Remove implements from disinfection solution with tongs, rinse well in water if required, and wipe dry with a clean or disposable towel (Figure 13–3e).

Follow your state regulations for storage of sanitized manicuring implements.

DEALING WITH NAIL INFECTIONS AND BLOOD

State regulations have requirements for dealing with infections and blood. Clients with open or oozing sores should not receive any services on or near the affected areas. The sores could be infected with pathogens and transferred from person to person if care is not taken. Blood can carry infectious pathogens, so nail professionals must understand how to deal with cuts and other wounds. Many regulations and guidelines have been written about dealing with blood spills. Most of these deal with the health care and hospital setting, where workers can encounter large amounts of blood. The nail salon is an entirely different situation, but salons can adopt some of the procedures used in hospitals. First, avoid touching the wound or blood. It's unlikely that you can catch a disease simply by touching infected blood, but there is a possibility that a contaminated implement could transmit an infection, even though it is unlikely. Properly cleaning and disinfecting the implement will completely eliminate that risk.

Cutting a client's skin with an abrasive file creates a different type of situation, however. Once blood is drawn, the rules change. Remember, abrasive files are designed for use on healthy nail plates surrounded by intact skin. Abrasive files made with absorbent materials are more difficult to properly clean when they come in contact with blood. So to ensure the client's safety, abrasive files that are made from absorbent materials and come in contact with blood must be sealed in a plastic bag and thrown into the waste receptacle. Also, remember that when you empty the waste receptacle, be sure to twist or tie the outer bag before throwing it away, as an added safety precaution. Other salon items made from absorbent materials, such as towels, robes, slippers, and other objects, should be machine-washed in hot water, using bleach where possible.

WHAT ABOUT BRUSHES?

Several types of brushes are used in professional nail salons. In some cases, these brushes must be cleaned and disinfected between each client; in other cases, this is not necessary or recommended. For instance, if you use a brush to apply nail oil to a client's natural nail, the brush should not be placed back into the original product container or used on another client. This practice can transfer pathogens into the product and lead to contamination. Droppers are a much better option for applying nail oils.

Not all brushes can transmit infections. Why disinfect a brush used to apply 70 percent isopropyl alcohol to the nail plate? It would make no sense. The brush was used in alcohol, which is the disinfectant. Pathogens cannot grow in alcohol. Pathogens cannot grow in acrylic monomer liquids, UV gels, primers, nail polish, nail dehydrators, and other solvent-based products, either. These products have several things in common. None of them contains significant amounts of water. Pathogens need water to live and grow. Pathogens also need food. None of these products can act as food for pathogens. Also, many types of pathogens would break apart and dissolve in these products. For these reasons, such products are considered to be **self-disinfecting.** This is why brushes used to apply such products cannot transfer pathogens from client to client. For all practical purposes, they are disinfected each time the brush is returned to the product. Therefore, these types of brushes do not require disinfection when used according to manufacturer's instructions ⒡.

> ## RISKY ABRASIVES?
>
> Abrasive files designed for use on fingernails, toenails, and feet are extremely safe to use. The truth is, they are highly unlikely to transmit an infection or disease when properly used. How can you ensure they are safe? It's actually very simple and easy. Here's how:
>
> 1. These tools are designed for use on intact, healthy skin and nails. If they are used on infected skin or nails, they should be disposed of immediately.
> 2. After each service, the file must be scrubbed with liquid soap, rinsed clean, fully immersed for the required time in a disinfectant solution, dried, and properly stored. This will virtually eliminate the risk of spreading an infection or disease with an abrasive file.

Here are a few examples. Nail polish brushes may be used without sanitizing or disinfecting. If they become clogged, use an oil-free polish remover to clean the brush. Brushes used to apply artificial nail products should be cleaned in the same product that is being applied to the nail—monomer brushes in monomer, gel brushes in gel. Of course, all brushes must be properly stored to prevent contamination, especially from dust, lint, or other debris. Artificial nail enhancement brushes should not be washed with soap and water or placed in disinfectant solutions. This practice can harm the brush, contaminate the enhancement products, and lead to service breakdown. This practice may also cause irritation or allergy. Trace amounts of disinfectant solution absorbed by the brush could cause sensitive clients to develop irritations or allergy of the nail bed or tissue surrounding the plate.

Take these steps and both you and your clients can enjoy peace of mind.

WHY WE DO IT

You have learned that the risks of transmitting disease or infection in the salon are very low, but what is sanitation and disinfection supposed to prevent? Common salon problems are bacterial infections of the nail plate and surrounding skin folds, warts, and fungal foot infections. That's about it. Skin infections of the legs after pedicures are rare but do happen. Cold and flu are also spread in the salon. These are the main things in the salon that we are trying to prevent with cleaning and disinfection! Prevention of these problems is the goal of universal sanitation in the salon.

FROM STORAGE TO DISPOSAL

When it comes to proper storage and disposal of cleaning agents or disinfectants, it is important to read, understand, and follow the manufacturer's directions, warnings, and other instructions (such as on the MSDS). Always store cleaning and disinfectant products in their original containers. Use a permanent marker or label to clearly mark the contents on spray bottles and other containers. Make it a practice to never have an unmarked container in your salon. Proper labels are important both for safety reasons as well as to enhance your professional image.

In general, disinfectant solutions should be changed each day or whenever they become cloudy or contaminated. Pathogens can grow inside disinfectant solutions that are heavily contaminated, so it is important to change them often. Certain salon disinfectants are safe to rinse down the drain (along with plenty of water), while others should not be disposed of in the sink. What it comes to bleach and alcohol, the sink is the best way to dispose of them. When disposing of disinfectants, make sure to wear safety glasses to protect your eyes from splashes. If you are planning to dispose of other disinfectants down the drain, please check to see if it is safe for the environment. Never dump disinfectant solutions down the drain unless the manufacturer's label or other written directions say that you can.

DISINFECTANT SAFETY

All disinfectants can be hazardous if improperly used. Disinfectants must not be treated too lightly. They are powerful, professional-strength tools. All disinfectants are poisonous if ingested. Especially in concentrated form, many can cause skin or eye damage (Figure 13–4). Never pour any disinfectant solution over your hands. This foolish practice can cause skin irritation and other problems. Carefully weigh and measure disinfectant solutions when mixing. This will ensure peak performance. Store disinfectants properly, use caution, and keep away from small children.

Formalin is another name for formaldehyde. Formalin tablets and solutions should not be used as disinfectants. Inhalation of formalin vapors can cause allergies of the respiratory system, resulting in symptoms such as coughing, wheezing, and a sensation of tightness in the chest. Vapors can also cause asthmalike symptoms in some people and may be very irritating to the eyes, nose, and throat. The same is true for **glutaraldehyde,** another disinfectant that should never be used in the salon for any purposes. Neither of these disinfectants is safe or appropriate for salon use. Skin contact with the liquid or inhalation of vapors can cause serious allergic reactions and breathing difficulties. They can be highly irritating to eyes, nose, throat, and lungs and may cause skin irritation, dryness, or rash. Symptoms may appear after several months of use and usually worsen with continued exposure. Long-term exposure can lead to chronic health problems. Avoid using either of these because of their potential toxic effects on salon workers. The

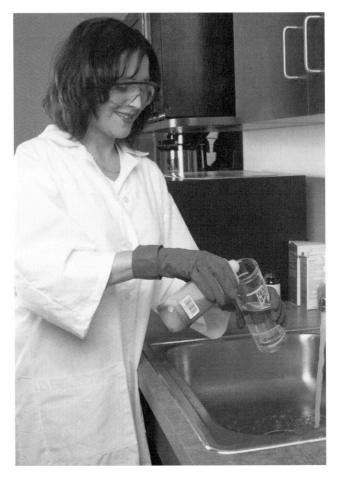

Figure 13-4 *Always wear safety glasses and gloves when mixing products, especially disinfectants*

only appropriate use for these disinfectants is in high-risk medical facilities such as emergency rooms, intensive care wards, surgery, and so on.

Please, don't let these words of warning prevent you from regularly using disinfectants. If used correctly, professional salon disinfectants are safe. In fact, the consequences of not using them are far more serious. Use them wisely, use them correctly, and disinfectants will work for you.

YOU REGISTERED YOUR WHAT?

Ultrasonic cleaning baths are sometimes sold in combination with disinfectant products. These units use high-frequency sound waves to create bubbles that provide limited cleansing action. These devices are not required equipment and they do not increase the effectiveness of salon disinfectant solutions, but they do provide improved cleaning action.

Implements and abrasives should be scrubbed clean (using a brush) before being immersed in disinfectant solution. This is one of the most effective steps in the entire process. Proper scrubbing is needed to ensure proper disinfection, and it should not be ignored or replaced. Ultraviolet (UV) sanitizers make useful storage containers, but they cannot properly disinfect salon implements. But once the implement is properly disinfected, it may be stored inside a UV sanitizer. Using a UV sanitizing cabinet for storage is a great way to impress your client. Steam sanitizers, originally designed for toothbrushes, are not effective in the salon. These devices cannot properly clean and disinfect your implements. Electric or bead sterilizers should not be used in the salon. They cannot sterilize or disinfect implements and provide no benefits to you or the client. In fact, they can be unsanitary.

Any of these devices can be registered with the FDA. This is not the same as FDA approval. In fact, such registrations mean very little! The FDA does not give approvals for any cosmetic products, tools, or devices used in beauty salons or for cosmetic purposes. The FDA only approves foods and drugs. When it comes to the cosmetic industry, the FDA only disapproves when it doesn't like something. Registration with the FDA simply means information about a product is on file with the Food and Drug Administration. The registration is no big deal and relatively easy to get, so don't be impressed by such claims. It does not mean the device will work as promised.

BASIC CHECKLIST

Deciding which sanitation and disinfection products are best for your salon can be confusing. There are many choices, so shop around and compare. Take the time to learn about several different systems before you decide. Then you'll be better able to choose what's best. Here are the basics that you'll need:

1. A disinfectant solution for implements and a disinfectant surface cleaner for tabletops and other surfaces that cannot be immersed.

2. A folder to hold manufacturer's instructions, MSDSs, state regulations, and other information.

3. A disinfectant container for immersing implements.

4. A pair of tongs to immerse and remove implements.

5. A pair of cotton-lined rubber or nitrile gloves, safety glasses, and a funnel for pouring, mixing, and transferring disinfectant solutions.

6. Permanent markers and labels for identifying contents of spray bottles and other containers.

7. Brushes for scrubbing and towels for blotting implements dry.

8. Sanitary containers or towels for implement storage.

PUT YOUR BEST FOOT FORWARD

Today, clients are more concerned than ever about health and safety issues. Just think about what they see when they walk into a salon. Will they find dusty tables and carpets or dirty abrasives? Pretend for a moment that you are the client. What would you think if you walked into a poorly maintained or unsanitary salon? Instead of ignoring the issue, face it squarely. Take the time to explain to clients that salon services are safe. Tell them that you use sanitation and disinfection procedures to ensure their safety and well-being. After you reassure them with the facts, it is time to practice what you preach. Show your clients that you're a stickler for cleanliness and you will always have a full book and command the highest prices. Here are some things you should do in your salon that will impress and protect your clients.

- Keep all floors swept clean and mopped as needed.
- Keep work areas and tables free of dusts, and vacuum carpets often.
- Deposit all waste materials in a metal trash can with a self-closing lid.
- Keep windows, screens, curtains, ceiling fans, and vents clean and dust-free.
- All work areas must be well lighted and well ventilated.
- Salons must have both hot and cold running water.
- Restrooms must be clean, tidy, and properly functioning.
- Provide toilet tissue, paper towels, and liquid soap.
- Wash hands after using the restroom and in between clients.
- Use alcohol hand sanitizers and provide them for your clients.
- Provide disposable drinking cups in a sanitary cup dispenser.
- Clean sinks and drinking fountains regularly.
- Properly clean and disinfect all implements, tools, and abrasive files.
- Use tongs to handle implements during disinfection.
- The salon must be free from insects and rodents.
- Salon should never be used as cooking or living quarters.
- Food must never be placed in refrigerators used to store salon products.
- Eating, drinking, and smoking are prohibited in chemical workplaces, including salons.
- Empty trash cans regularly throughout the day.
- Always wear clean, freshly laundered clothing.
- Bathe every day before coming to work and use deodorant.
- Brush your teeth regularly and check your breath, especially after smoking.

- Each client should receive freshly laundered towels.
- Use clean cotton balls, pads, or sponges in your services.
- Remove products from containers with a clean spatula, not fingers.
- Makeup, lipstick, cosmetic puffs, pencils, and brushes must never be shared.
- Properly mark, seal, and store all containers.
- Wash your hands before and after performing services, before and after eating, and after smoking.
- Keep the outside of all containers clean and labels legible.
- Properly store dirty or soiled linen until it is machine-washed in hot water.
- Avoid touching your face, mouth, or eye area while performing services.
- Do not allow pets or other animals in the salon, except for trained Seeing Eye dogs.

FAST TRACK (FT)

(FT) Microorganisms that cause disease or illness in humans are called pathogens.

(FT) Decontamination is the removal of pathogens and visible debris from a surface.

(FT) With universal sanitation, salons are always clean, sanitary, and presentable.

(FT) Sanitizing significantly reduces the number of pathogens or other contaminants.

(FT) Proper washing removes up to 99 percent of pathogens/contaminants from a surface.

(FT) We can't eliminate all bacteria, fungi, and viruses, only keep them under control.

(FT) Skin irritation, itching, and dryness can be signs of excessive hand washing.

(FT) Disinfection kills the small number of pathogens left after sanitizing.

(FT) Disinfectants are not for use on skin, hair, or nails.

(FT) Antiseptic solutions slow down the growth of pathogens on skin.

(FT) Spores are coated with a waxy, protective substance and are waiting to become bacteria.

(FT) Neither HIV, tuberculosis, nor hepatitis is spread by manicures and pedicures.

FT Reject fear-based marketing! It's bad for everyone and hurts our industry.

FT Quaternary ammonium compounds (quats) are the most commonly used type of salon disinfectant.

FT Brushes used to apply self-disinfecting products don't require disinfection.

Review Questions

1. Besides pathogens, name something else that's considered a contaminant in salons.

2. Up to what percentage of contaminants are washed from a surface by proper sanitation alone?

3. How long should you wash your hands if they become heavily contaminated?

4. Give two reasons why it's so important to rinse your hands thoroughly and use lukewarm water.

5. Why are pedicure clients with freshly shaved legs more susceptible to skin infection?

6. _____, _____, and _____ are three highly effective disinfectants that do not require EPA registration numbers.

7. Quats are both good disinfectants as well as good _____.

8. If you cut a client's skin with an abrasive file, what two things should you do?

9. Why are monomer liquids and nail polish considered to be self-disinfecting?

10. Name two disinfectants that are not safe for use in the professional salon.

11. Give an example of a brush used in a salon service that must be disinfected.

12. Give two examples of a brush used in salon services that do not require disinfection.

13. Does an FDA registration ensure that a product will work as promised by the manufacturer? Explain your answer.

14. If an alcohol hand sanitizer is used, are your hands clean? Explain your answer.

15. Is HIV, hepatitis, or tuberculosis transmitted by salon services?

Chapter 14

Every Breath You Take

Objective

In this chapter you will learn how to evaluate the air quality in your salon. You will gain an understanding about the causes of poor air quality and discover some easy solutions. You'll also see that by knowing the proper steps to take, it's easy to protect yourself and improve the quality of the air you breathe.

ODORS, ODORS EVERYWHERE

Our nose serves two important functions. We smell and inhale air through the nose. Why do we smell? A small group of special cells in the upper part of our nasal cavity can detect seven basic odors. Every smell is a combination of these basic odors. They are camphor, musk, peppermint, ether, floral, pungent, or putrid *(FT)*. Our nose contains about 25 million of these smelling cells in each nostril, and all of them send messages directly to the brain through the **olfactory nerve.** This is how the brain gets information through the nose. Sinus inflammation or blockage, as with a common cold, dulls the sense of smell. Also, the sense of smell is weaker in a person who smokes, which explains why smoking affects the sense of taste.

Approximately 75 percent of our sense of taste actually comes from our nose and the odor of the food. As vapors pass by these smelling cells, they bind together like a key fitting into a lock. The smelling cells identify the shape and size of the vapor molecule. That's right—odor is dependent on shape and size. If you've ever fumbled with your key chain in the dark, you can understand that a small difference in an object's shape can make a big difference in the way it works. The same is true for vapor molecules. If a molecule is too large, it will have no odor. Wedge-shaped molecules smell like peppermint, tadpole-shaped molecules smell of flowers, musky odors are shaped like necklaces, ether odors are like shoestrings, and camphor (mothball) vapors are shaped like footballs. The brain uses this information to create the sensation that we call odor.

Why use ventilation? Most people wrongly believed that ventilation is used to reduce odor. The odors aren't dangerous and are not what must be eliminated. Odor doesn't determine the safety of a chemical *(FT)*. Many people mistakenly believe that anything with a sweet, pleasant aroma must contain only good and wholesome ingredients, which is of course untrue. But who would think a salon needed ventilation if the room smelled nice? It is our animal nature to be attracted to nice smells and to be suspicious of strange or funny odors. We assume bad-smelling chemicals must be dangerous. Nothing could be further from the truth! Smells are caused by vapors stimulating special odor-detecting cells in our nose *(FT)*. Do your kidneys, blood, or liver really care what a product smells like? Of course not! There's no way your nose can tell if a vapor could cause liver damage. That's not how the body works. Even so, odors are very useful if used correctly. Our nose is a highly sensitive vapor detector. It can detect a smell when there is only 1 vapor molecule per 1 million molecules of air (1 ppm). Odors can help determine if the salon environment needs improving. But there is a lot more to know before we can do this correctly.

HOW'S THE AIR IN THERE?

The quality of indoor breathing air has become a very hot topic in the last decade. Some think this is a modern-day problem, but it isn't. Indoor air quality has been an important problem for many centuries. Until the 1900s, oil lamps, coal heaters, wood stoves, and candles created fumes, a mixture of tiny, solid particles suspended in gases, as well as other serious air quality issues for both homes and businesses. Electric lights, fans, and central air-conditioning have alleviated many of the problems of the past, but they have created some new ones that we must deal with. **Sick building syndrome** is a well-known issue. It occurs in offices and buildings across the country. Occupants of affected office buildings complain of sore eyes, fatigue, dermatitis, headaches, nausea, coughing, or frequent lung and throat irritations. Usually the symptoms diminish or disappear when they leave the office.

Indoor air quality problems can be caused by many things. Poor or improperly maintained ventilation is often the reason. What's causing these problems? Excessive levels of carbon monoxide, airborne wood dusts, airborne molds, particles from ceiling insulation, and solvent vapors are just a few common examples. Building materials and carpeting are often blamed for poor air quality. It is well known that both can slowly release solvents into the air. But over the last 10 years inspections by the National Institute for Occupational Safety and Health (NIOSH) has uncovered some surprising facts. They discovered that 52 percent of these issues were caused by inadequate ventilation. Only 4 percent of the air quality problems were caused by building construction materials, carpeting, and so on. A large percentage of the contaminants were brought into the building. For example, about 16 percent of the air quality problems were created by things such as photocopiers, fax machines, cleaning supplies, solvents, and office supplies. This same issue faces salons today. Contamination created inside the salon must be controlled to maintain proper air quality.

HOW'S YOUR SALON AIR?

Although salons face many of the same issues found in high-rise office buildings, their situations are quite different. Salons have special and unique ventilation requirements. Unfortunately, most salon ventilation systems are identical to the standard systems found in offices. This type of system is called **general ventilation.** These systems are designed to exchange old, stale air with new, fresh air while controlling the room temperature. These systems are useful and will improve air circulation and quality, but they are not nearly enough for salons. General ventilation is a basic requirement for all workplaces, but salons need more (FT). Since salons use professional products on a regular basis, their ventilation systems must be upgraded to ensure safe air quality. Professional products and services generate vapors, mists, and dusts that must all be properly controlled. Luckily, it's easy to maintain a healthy air quality in salons if the right steps are taken. How do you know when there's an air quality issue in your salon? The best way is to have an air quality specialist test and evaluate your salon air. But until then, the following checklist will help you do a self-rating of your breathing air quality.

- Do strong product odors linger for more than ten minutes after use?
- Do strong odors travel far away from the source, such as into other rooms?

- Can you still smell product odors when you open the shop in the morning?
- Do the walls ever "sweat" with moisture or the windows become foggy?
- When someone opens the door or window, does the air rush in or rush out?
- Does the air coming from ventilation ducts smell stale or musty?
- Have the walls become dingy, stained, or discolored?
- Do clients often complain of strong or offensive odors?
- Do you ever open a window or door when odors become too strong?
- Do you regularly service and clean the ventilation system?
- Do employees often complain about headaches, nausea, sore throats, coughs, blurry vision, watery eyes, insomnia, irritability, drowsiness, dizziness, runny or bloody noses, sneezing, tingling toes or fingers, chest aches or pains, shortness of breath, loss of coordination, or loss of appetite?
- Do you find that strong or offensive odors don't bother you anymore or that you just don't notice them?
- Do you often get funny tastes in your mouth or does food seem to lack flavor?

The last two points may seem unrelated to the ones preceding them, but these are both important early warning signs of overexposure. Some nail technicians consider themselves lucky because they don't notice product odors. They're not lucky if they are suffering from **olfactory fatigue** (FT). This condition occurs when the **olfactory glands,** a concentrated area of olfactory nerves in the nose, get tired of overwhelming smells. When this happens, the nose just quits smelling the odor! Over time this can result in permanent damage and may drastically reduce your ability to smell (FT). Once this happens, you will also lose the ability to properly taste food. Imagine chocolate ice cream tasting bland and boring for the rest of your life!

If you answered yes to any of the above questions, then your ventilation may need attention or improvement. But if the purpose of ventilation is not to control odors, then why go to the trouble of using it? In Chapter 11 you learned that there are three types of air contaminants in the salon: vapors, mists, and dusts (FT). Proper ventilation is designed to control all three and reduce the risk of overexposure. Vapors come from the evaporation of liquids (FT). Mists are fine droplets of liquid created by aerosol and pump sprayers (FT). Dusts are particles ranging from very large (pinhead size) to nearly invisible, microscopic particles (FT). Luckily, these air contaminants are easily controlled. It is possible to "breathe easy" in the salon and ensure that everyone's health is protected.

BREATHING ZONES

Everyone is concerned about the environment, especially the air. Protecting the quality of our planet's air is vital. Still, there is one place on earth that is more important to you than any other. That special place is called your **breathing zone.** Your breathing zone is an invisible sphere about twice the size of a basketball ⒡. It sits directly in front of your mouth. You can't see it, but it is always there. When you turn your head or leave the room, your breathing zone moves with you. Every single breath you take throughout your life comes from your breathing zone. Fewer things have a greater impact on your health than what occurs in this small area. There is nothing more important than protecting this precious space. This is the true purpose of ventilation! ⒡

Fact: Proper Ventilation Should Protect Your Breathing Zone

Problems can occur when nail technicians inhale excessive amounts of certain vapors. These vapors come from the evaporation of liquids used in the salon. A common myth is that some liquids do not evaporate. This is false! All nail products in liquid form will evaporate and contribute to the total vapors in the air. Odorless monomers and UV gel oligomers are good examples. The lower odor of these products doesn't mean they don't evaporate. They are low-odor because you can't smell the vapors unless you really try. Proper ventilation is still required, odors or no odors ⒡. Also, all artificial nail products generate dusts that must be controlled with proper ventilation ⒡.

Ventilation isn't just for vapors and mists. All vapors, with or without odors, must be controlled. The same is true for pleasant fragrances. Spraying perfumes or using aromatherapy or scented nail products to deal with vapors will only make matters worse ⒡. Covering odors with even more odors isn't the answer. This can actually increase your risk of inhalation overexposure. Is it safer to close your eyes while crossing the street? Just because you don't see the cars doesn't mean they aren't there.

What can nail technicians do to lower their exposure to vapors? Luckily, some of the most effective ways to eliminate vapors are the easiest and least expensive. Here are four easy ways to dramatically improve your salon's air quality.

1. Keep All Products Tightly Sealed When Not in Use

Any liquid or gel product will create vapors. It may seem more convenient to leave the cap off the product while you're working, but it will certainly increase your risks. Make sure to keep all product containers tightly closed when you are not using them ⒡. As vapors escape from the product into your air, they can enter your breathing zone. This can lead to inhalation overexposure and eye, lip, or nasal irritation. The longer you leave your product open, the greater chance of lowering its effectiveness and shortening its shelf life. Open your containers only when needed and then quickly reseal them. Open product containers can lower air quality and drastically increase the danger of accidental spills.

This is especially important for products that contain rapidly evaporating ingredients, such as monomers, nail polish, topcoats, base coats, hardeners, removers, primers, and so on (FT). Rapid evaporation leaves slowly evaporating ingredients behind. That is why nail polishes thicken in the bottle. Evaporation is more important with bulk containers. For example, you should only fill dappen dishes from a small (4-ounce) container of monomer liquid.

What could happen if you refill each time from a 16-ounce container? Every time you open a bottle, rapidly evaporating ingredients escape. If you open a 16-ounce container many times a day, after a while evaporation will slowly change the chemical composition of your monomer liquid. These changes will lower the effectiveness of the product and lead to service breakdown. The first ounce you remove from a bottle will be different from the 8th ounce and much different from the 16th. Ideally, you should fill 4-ounce containers from the larger size (FT). Then use a clean eyedropper to fill your dappen dish from the smaller container. Open product containers as little as possible and don't leave them open for long. This will help maintain the quality of your products. You'll see fewer product-related service breakdowns if you do.

2. Use a Small, Covered Dappen Dish to Hold Your Monomer

Avoid using large jars or containers to hold your liquid monomer. Choose a small, covered dappen dish instead (FT). If you spread any liquid out over a larger surface, you'll have much greater evaporation and create a greater risk of inhalation overexposure. Dappen dishes with larger openings create more vapors (FT). You'll be surprised at how much more! A dish with a 1-inch opening creates 4 times more vapor than a dish with a ½-inch opening. A 1½-inch opening creates 9 times the vapor. A 2-inch opening creates 16 times more vapor, and a 3-inch opening creates 36 times more vapor. To minimize evaporation, you should use a dish with the smallest opening that is feasible. Also, a large marble makes a great cover for monomer dappen dishes (Figure 14–1). Never use a dappen dish without a lid—if a large marble won't cover the opening, you need a smaller dish. As soon as you finish applying the enhancement product, cover your dappen dish to prevent evaporation of monomer vapors into the salon air.

3. Empty Waste Containers Often Throughout the Day and Before Going Home

You'd be surprised at the amount of vapors that come from the waste can. Don't just wipe up a spill with a paper towel and then throw it into an open trash container. Those vapors will soon be invading your breathing zone and drifting through the salon. Metal waste cans with self-closing lids are excellent for controlling vapors. Remember to empty your trash several times each day and before

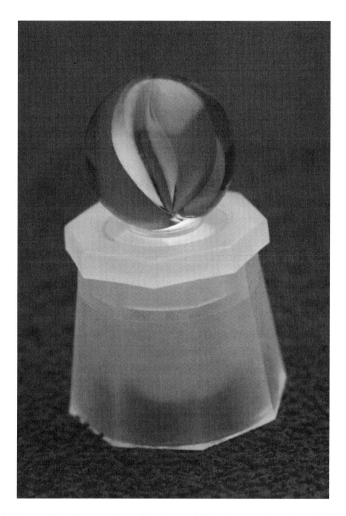

Figure 14-1 *A marble makes a good cover for a dappen dish, but be sure to keep the marble clean and free from product residue to avoid skin contact*

you leave at night ⒻⓉ. Otherwise, vapors will leak out overnight and will be there to greet you in the morning. In general, good housekeeping is an important safety tool and will help reduce the amount of monomer vapors in the salon air.

4. Don't Wipe Monomer Brushes on Your Table Towel

Most nail enhancement monomers are very volatile and evaporate quickly. Wiping your brush on a table towel puts monomer vapors into the air. It's better to wipe your brush on a disposable pad. When you have finished applying the product, throw away the monomer-soaked pad. Plastic-backed pads can help prevent skin overexposure of the fingers. Also, be very careful not to put your arm in the area where you wipe your brush (FT).

These four simple steps can greatly improve the quality of your salon air, but there is more you must do to finish the job. Your salon still must be properly ventilated. These steps are so important because they make it easier for your ventilation to work properly. The fewer vapors there are in the air, the fewer that must be removed.

WHAT TO AVOID

Much of what nail technicians were told in the past about ventilation was incorrect. With so much misinformation, it's not surprising that nail professionals are confused. Let's explore some of the myths about ventilation. Then making the proper choices will be much easier.

Myth #1: If You Need Ventilation, Just Open a Window or Turn On the Fan

Open doors and windows, air conditioners, and fans are not ventilation—they are circulation. These methods circulate the vapors around the room so everyone can breathe them equally! High-quality, efficient ventilation systems do not just spread vapors around the room.

Myth #2: You Should Choose a Ventilation System That Purifies the Air

It is impossible to cost-effectively purify the air in the salon. Home or office systems that claim to purify the air are making greatly exaggerated claims. Sure, they remove some impurities . . . but not all impurities, not even close! But that's not the goal of proper ventilation. Yes, there are systems that remove all impurities from the air, but they're not sold to salons. The space shuttle has an air purification system for the astronauts. But you can bet that NASA didn't pay $800 (or even $8,000) for the system! It is impossible to purify the air in a salon environment. Don't even try! Luckily, it isn't necessary to purify the air. Remember the overexposure principle? You need only to lower your exposure to safe levels to have safe breathing air. Never buy a device hoping that it will purify the air. You will be disappointed.

Myth #3: The Ventilation System Must Be Doing Its Job if You Can't Smell Any Odors

Many devices sold to nail salons claim to "eliminate odors." As you have learned, eliminating odors doesn't mean the air is safe. You will learn later that some systems actually increase your risk of inhalation overexposure while they remove odors. Other systems simply conceal odors without improving air quality.

Remember, vapors, dusts, and mists are what needs to be controlled, not odors. Use proper ventilation and odors will disappear with the vapors. All salons need proper ventilation, even if you only do manicures and pedicures. Even if your salon smells fresh and sweet, you need proper ventilation.

WHAT'S UP NEXT?

In this chapter, you learned the what and why of proper ventilation in the salon. In the next chapter, you'll learn how to make ventilation work in your salon.

FAST TRACK (FT)

(FT) Every smell is a combination of seven basic odors.

(FT) The odor of a chemical doesn't determine its safety.

(FT) Smells are vapors stimulating special odor-detecting cells in the nose.

(FT) General ventilation is a basic requirement for all workplaces, but salons need more.

(FT) Nail technicians can't smell strong odors if suffering from olfactory fatigue.

(FT) Olfactory fatigue may permanently affect the sense of smell and taste.

(FT) The three types of air contaminants are vapors, mists, and dusts.

(FT) Vapors come from the evaporation of liquids.

(FT) Mists are fine droplets of liquid created by aerosol and pump sprayers.

(FT) Dusts range from pinhead size to nearly invisible particles.

(FT) Your breathing zone is an invisible sphere twice the size of a basketball.

(FT) The true purpose of ventilation is to protect your breathing zone.

(FT) Proper ventilation is still required, odors or no odors.

(FT) All artificial nail products generate dusts that must be controlled with proper ventilation.

(FT) You can't improve air quality with nice-smelling odors that cover the bad-smelling ones.

(FT) Keep all products tightly sealed when not in use.

(FT) It is especially important to keep covered all products that contain rapidly evaporating ingredients.

(FT) Fill dampen dishes from a small (i.e., 4-ounce) container of monomer liquid.

(FT) Use liquid monomers in a small dappen dish with a lid.

(FT) Dappen dishes with larger openings create much more vapors.

(FT) Empty your waste container often.

(FT) Avoid putting your arm in the area where you wipe your brush.

Review Questions

1. _____ is a condition where your nose can no longer smell certain strong odors.
2. Your _____ is an invisible sphere about twice the size of a basketball.
3. Never use a _____ without a lid.
4. How are fumes different from vapors?
5. If you no longer smell strong odors in the salon, you may be suffering from _____.
6. Should you try to purify the air in the salon?
7. Why can't we smell certain types of vapors?
8. What two important factors help the brain determine the odor of a vapor molecule?
9. Why should you wipe your brush on a disposable pad instead of your table towel?
10. Why is it important to empty the salon's waste cans throughout the day?
11. If the air smells funny in the salon, why not just use aromatherapy oil or perfume?
12. Why not use a wide-mouth dappen dish to hold your monomer liquid?
13. Is it all right to fill your dappen dish from a 16-ounce bottle of monomer liquid?
14. Name three disadvantages of leaving caps off of your products for too long.
15. Which is it more important to remove from the salon air, vapors or odors?

Chapter

15

Clearing the Air

Objective

This chapter covers the various types of ventilation equipment available to salons. You'll learn how to select and use the best equipment for improving the quality of your salon's air. You'll discover what works and what doesn't work for salons and how to avoid inhalation overexposure to vapors, mists, and dusts.

USE ADEQUATE VENTILATION!

You see this phrase in many places. But what is adequate ventilation, anyway? How do you know if your salon has it? What will happen if you don't? In this chapter you will learn what proper ventilation is and isn't. You will also see that proper ventilation offers great advantages and benefits. The greatest of these is peace of mind. Ventilation will help you prevent inhalation overexposure, as you learned in the last chapter. But before you can understand how proper ventilation works, you'll need to learn some basics.

HEPA FILTERS

Dusts come in the doors and windows along with pollen. These can lower the quality of air in the salons. Probably most dust particles in nail salons are created while filing artificial nails. Microscopic dust particles are found anywhere that hand abrasives or electric files are used. **HEPA filters** are very-high-efficiency particle filters *(FT)*. They are often sold as room air cleaners for homes. But commercial-quality devices are available. Advertisements for such devices claim they are up to 99.93 percent efficient and capture even the tiniest particles. These claims are valid for true, high-quality HEPA filters. But HEPA filters can only control dusts, pollens, and fumes such as cigarette smoke. They have no effect on vapors or gases *(FT)*. **Room air cleaning units** use HEPA filters in combination with powerful air blowers that draw air through the filters. Most are excellent at controlling air contaminants in the home but have limited usefulness in the salon setting.

Ventilation must protect your breathing zone. The best HEPA filter, costing $100 or more, can't protect your breathing zone from dusts as well as a simple 50-cent dust mask! Why? HEPA filters are designed to be placed on the floor near your nail station. But the highest concentration of dusts in the room is found between the nail technician's mouth and the client's hand—in other words, in your breathing zone! HEPA filters will do an excellent job of controlling dusts in the room air, but dust masks have a huge advantage. Dust masks filter your breathing air as it goes into your mouth and lungs! Nothing could be better or more effective. In the long run, dust masks are the best way to reduce exposure to dusts. HEPA filters can be useful in the salon, but they can't replace dust masks. Use both for optimal dust control and protection.

Although HEPA filters are extremely good at capturing dusts, they have absolutely no effect on vapors. Vapor molecules are hundreds of times smaller than the tiniest dust particles. Vapors whiz right through a HEPA filter as though it wasn't even there. To address this problem, some HEPA filters are used in combination with high-quality activated charcoal filters to improve their effectiveness as room air cleaners, as described below *(FT)*.

WHAT IS ACTIVATED CHARCOAL?

Activated charcoal (also called activated carbon) is very different from the charcoal used in barbecue grills. A very special process is used to give this charcoal an incredible ability to absorb contaminants from water or air. Activated charcoal does not absorb all impurities. What it can absorb depends on whether it's being used to clean water or air. Activated charcoal is used in fish tanks to remove impurities from the water, such as organic debris from decaying food and wastes. Activated charcoal is also used in commercial air cleaners to absorb chemical vapors directly from the air.

Barbecue charcoal is made by burning materials such as wood, nutshells, or coconut husks. This charcoal can only become activated after treating it with high-pressure steam in an oxygen-free chamber that is heated to 1,800°F (980°C). This unique treatment creates an extremely porous and super-absorbent material. During treatment, each charcoal granule becomes riddled with hundreds of thousands of extremely tiny crevices and microscopic channels. This is how contaminants are absorbed and become trapped, as seen in Figure 15–1. Each granule becomes a "chemical sponge," mopping vapors from the air (FT). Technically, the term for this is *adsorption*—collecting gas or liquid molecules on their surface—but here we'll use the less technical term *absorb*.

Activated charcoal can absorb many types of chemicals, but not all. Some contaminants are strongly absorbed, while others are weakly absorbed and some are not absorbed at all. Manufacturers address this problem by selling special grades or blends of activated charcoal. This charcoal is treated with special additives to improve efficiency or to absorb a broader range of chemical vapors. You will soon see how activated charcoal can be combined with HEPA filters to create the best air cleaning solutions for salons.

WHICH ONE WORKS?

Some types of dust masks are better designed that others. Some are inappropriate for salon use. For example, avoid using flimsy surgical-type masks designed for medical professionals. These don't fit very well and provide only minimal protection. If the mask does not fit well, your protection will be lowered. Be sure to look for masks that are N95-certified, as described in Chapter 11. These masks will block 95 percent of the tiniest dust particles. You can even find a mask with a small valve that allows you to exhale but won't let you breathe in any dust. These one-way valves will prevent moisture from building up inside the mask and will increase comfort.

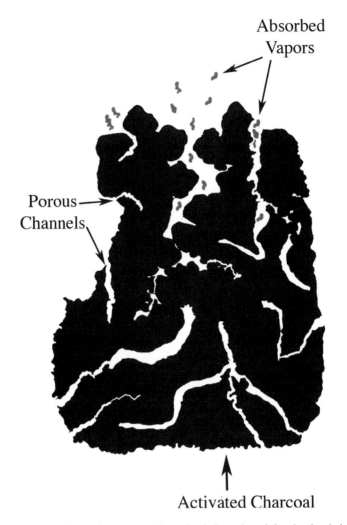

Figure 15-1 *Chemical contaminants being absorbed into channels found within the highly porous activated charcoal particle*

VENTILATED NAIL TABLES

Most ventilated nail tables rely on a ½-inch (12-millimeter) tray filled with a small amount of activated charcoal to absorb vapors. Good in theory, but in practice these thin, loosely filled trays have very little effectiveness. They will only give you a false sense of security. There are a few other problems with ventilated nail tables. Activated charcoal is like a chemical sponge, absorbing vapors from the air. But like a sponge, activated charcoal soon becomes completely saturated and ineffective. Nail table filters are usually lightweight and loosely filled with activated charcoal. You can even see through many of them. Monomer vapors are not easily absorbed by activated charcoal, especially with these flimsy filters. Such filters are practically worthless, even if replaced every few days. Activated charcoal filters cannot be reused or cleaned. Shaking out the collected nail dust does not remove the absorbed chemicals. Once an activated charcoal filter has been used up, it must be thrown away.

After the contaminated air passes through the charcoal filter tray, it is blown back into the salon. The remaining, unabsorbed contaminants are simply pushed from the table and back into the salon air. Blocking the air intake on the table will further reduce its effectiveness. Never place anything over the intake vent on the table, especially a towel! The towel will block the flow of air. You may as well turn off the fan inside your table. If you use a ventilated table, never block the flow of air into this vent.

With all these drawbacks, does this mean you should throw out your ventilated table? Not necessarily! These tables can be modified and made much more effective. There are two routes you can take to improve the efficiency of ventilated nail tables.

1. Use a Supplementary Air Blower to Expel Contaminated Air

The easiest solution for improving the effectiveness of ventilated nail tables is to use an **outdoor venting system.** These systems vent the air outdoors instead of back into the salon. Simply connecting a tube or duct to the table's exit vent and directing the vapors outdoors is not enough. The fan that comes with most ventilated tables is not powerful enough to do the job. It is better to purchase a more powerful air blower that can be mounted outside the salon. **Air blowers** are designed to pull air through the table and down the ventilation duct and then expel the contaminated air to the outdoors. If the tube between the table and the outside blower is too long, it will be harder for the blower to work efficiently. In this case, a bigger air blower is needed to compensate for longer distances. You should consult with a local ventilation company or expert to determine the appropriate-sized blower and duct configuration. Local **heating, ventilating, and air-conditioning (HVAC)** companies and experts can be found in the yellow pages. Not only can HVAC professionals help decide which system is best, they can install and maintain it as well.

Outdoor venting systems can also be combined with HEPA filters and activated charcoal (Figure 15–2) to clean the air as it exits the salon. This option is especially useful if you have nearby neighbors who complain of odors coming from the salon.

2. Filter Air Through a HEPA Filter, Followed by a 3–4-Inch (18–20-Millimeter) Bed of Activated Charcoal

Although salon air cannot be purified, it is possible to clean the air by removing enough contaminants to prevent overexposure. Remember, the goal is to lower

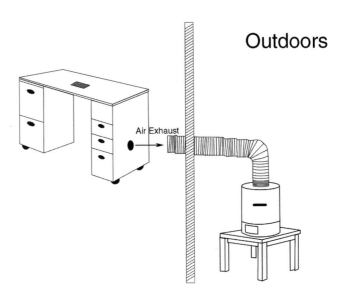

Figure 15-2 *This venting system design draws air through the nail table, filters it, and expels it outside*

the concentration of vapors, mists, and dusts to safe levels. This can be done with a properly designed activated charcoal system. As stated above, activated charcoal can work with an outdoor venting system to remove odors that your neighbors may find offensive. But these systems have two other important uses. First, some salons have no outside access for vents. Second, some nail technicians prefer to purchase systems that they can take with them when changing salons. In these two cases, the best choice might be a combination air blower/HEPA filter/activated charcoal system. Such air cleaners are commonly sold for use in homes and offices. But systems designed for homes or offices are not very useful in salons. Salons should consider only commercial-grade, high-quality units. Commercial-grade units use larger, ultra-quiet air blowers and much better filters. Overall, they are more efficient. These units hold between 18 and 125 pounds (8 and 57 kilograms) of activated charcoal, depending on their size. A properly designed system will draw salon air through a thick bed or filter (3–4 inches or 18–20 millimeters) containing activated charcoal. The extra thickness will allow the large majority of the vapors to be absorbed. This will clean the air well enough to be returned to the salon.

Whichever system you choose, it must be easy to refill with fresh activated charcoal, and you should do this regularly. Under normal circumstances, the activated charcoal bed or filter should be replaced every three to five months, depending on thickness and usage. Do not use these filters for too long ⒻⓉ. Remember, activated charcoal is like a chemical sponge. Like a sponge, the filter will quickly fill up after three months of heavy use or five months of occasional use. *Important:* Using activated charcoal filters for too long a period can create two problems. First, air contaminants will not be absorbed and air quality will be lowered. The longer the filter is used, the harder it will be to absorb vapors. After a while, the filter will become saturated and stop absorbing vapors. Second, completely saturated filters can create a fire hazard, since many of the absorbed vapors are flammable (FT). Therefore, it is best to change these filters often. Check with the manufacturer of the filter for more information and guidance.

What's the cost of changing these filters? The average salon can expect to spend on average about $3–4 per week on filters, depending on the size and number of units. Some may think the cost for activated charcoal filters is high, but their value is high as well if the units are properly maintained. If not, it's just a waste of electricity. And as stated above, it could create a fire hazard.

Air blower speed is another important consideration. These units usually have three speeds, low, medium, and high. At higher speeds, air rushes by too quickly for the activated charcoal to absorb vapors. Also, these units are much louder when they run at high speeds. Choose slower speeds for more efficient absorption and quieter operation.

HEPA filters are often used in combination with activated charcoal. Dusts can pose big problems for activated charcoal systems. Dusts can clog up an activated charcoal bed or filter, preventing it from absorbing vapors and reducing the filter's effectiveness. To avoid this problem, the best systems use a pre-filter to keep dusts out of the activated charcoal. HEPA filters are not the only type of pre-filter. **Microfilters** are highly efficient air filters, but they do not meet the high standards set for HEPA filters. Even so, microfilters are still extremely efficient. For some applications they are the most effective choice (FT). For example, they make excellent pre-filters for air conditioners and heating systems. Microfilters are used to make high-efficiency disposable dust masks and vacuum cleaner bags.

Two types of activated charcoal systems are useful in salons. The first type is the most common but not the most effective. This system works by pulling contaminated air from the surrounding area and returning clean air to the room. These are called room air cleaning units (FT). High-quality room cleaning units always come with a HEPA pre-filter. Don't purchase one without it (see Figure 15–3). These units are designed to pull air through vents in the bottom and expel clean, filtered air out the top or sides.

Room cleaning units come in a range of sizes. The size of the system you'll need is based on the square footage of the room. This is an extremely important factor. Each unit comes with a recommended room size. That recommendation is based on a unit running at its highest speed. It is not uncommon for these room sizes to be overstated and overly optimistic. Slower fan speeds are preferable, so choose a system design for a room that is larger than your salon. Suppose you purchase a commercial-grade system that will handle a 400-square-foot (37-square-meter) area with a 10-foot (3-meter) ceiling. A salon between 300 and 400 square feet should have two units, located in different parts of the salon. A salon with 400 to 600 square feet (37 to 55 square meters) should have three units.

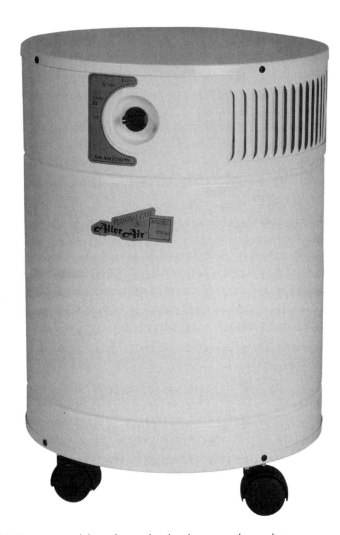

Figure 15-3 *An activated charcoal system based on the room air cleaning design*

Have 14-foot (4-meter) ceilings? You'll need an extra unit. All units should be set to run at slow speed. Your air quality will be much better and clients will not be disturbed by the racket these units can create at higher speeds.

Room air cleaning units will help improve air quality in the salon when used correctly. But they have one major drawback. These units pull air from the room, not your breathing zone, where the highest concentration of dusts and vapors are found. Room air cleaning units sitting 10 feet (3 meters) from your station are not actively protecting your breathing zone. Yes, there is value to cleaning the room air, but it's better to attack the problem at the source. This is why it is important to put these units as close as feasible to the nail stations. When used properly, room air cleaning units can help improve salon air quality, but they are not as effective as the local exhaust systems described below.

LOCAL EXHAUST

The most complete and effective solution for improving salon air quality is called **local exhaust.** The idea behind local exhaust is simple. Local exhaust systems capture and control vapors, dusts, and mists right at the source. This way, they never escape into the salon air. Ventilated nail tables are one type of local exhaust system. But they need some modification to be effective. Ideally, the vapors from the ventilated table should be expelled outdoors. But there's another way to modify ventilated nail tables. What about salons without any convenient outside access for ducts or vents? In this case the best solution is to replace the outside ventilation system with a combination HEPA filter/activated charcoal system. These systems are nearly identical to the room air cleaning units discussed above. There's only one important difference. These systems are designed to draw air through the ventilated table instead of from an open room. Passing the contaminated air through a 3- to 4-inch (18- to 20-millimeter) thick bed or filter of activated charcoal will absorb most air contaminants. If the bed or filter is changed often, air quality will improve significantly and the risk of inhalation overexposure will be reduced. If enough of these systems are used properly in the salon, air quality will dramatically improve. Even so, these room air cleaning units are not the most effective solution for controlling air contaminants.

The most effective type of local exhaust uses a bendable or movable hose or tube to capture vapors, dusts, and mists (see Figure 15–4). These movable tubes work with either an outdoor venting system or a HEPA filter/activated charcoal system. The movable tube can be placed where needed—directly over your dappen dish, beside your electric file when rebalancing, between your face and the artificial nail while you sculpt. This movable ventilation tube collects contaminants as they enter your breathing zone. In this way vapors, dusts, and mists are captured at the source and can never escape into the salon air or become inhaled. Another solution is to drop a 3- to 4-inch rigid, hollow tube directly from the ceiling. The opening of this tube should hang just above eye level, directly over the center of your table. Of course, a movable tube that can be positioned where needed is superior. The ideal salon ventilation is a movable-tube local exhaust system combined with outdoor venting. Now you can see why this is the preferred system. Local exhaust protects your breathing zone but also keeps the rest of the salon air clean as well. And with outdoor venting, you don't have the worry or

CHANGING TIMES

How often should you change your activated charcoal filter? That depends on thickness, packing density, fan speed, room size, how often it was used, and several other factors. In general, expect to change your activated charcoal filters three or four times a year on average. HEPA filters can last up to a year. For more detailed information, you should ask the manufacturer.

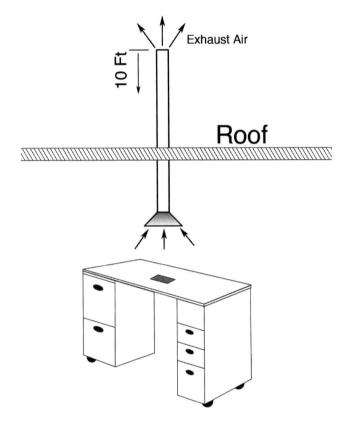

Figure 15-4 A typical design for a local exhaust ventilation system that expels air to the roof (the duct could just as easily be directed through a wall or window)

expense of filters. Local exhaust systems can also be used together with commercial room air cleaning units. This would be a very powerful solution to just about any salon air quality problem. There's not a better combination.

DUCTS, BLOWERS, AND MAINTENANCE

Depending on your situation, an HVAC professional may be able to link a local exhaust system into the existing general ventilation system. But most of the time, ventilation ducts must be installed through the ceiling to the roof. In most cases installing ducts will be the best solution. If you already have ducts to the roof, make sure the outlet is at least 10 feet (3 meters) higher than the roof or any air intake vents within a 50-foot (15-meter) circle *FT* . This is a very important requirement! If the exhaust vent is too close, vapors could be sucked back into the building. What could be worse than to get rid of the vapors, only to pull them back inside? When neighbors complain they can smell vapors from your salon, this is often the reason.

Pay close attention to the location of any vents that penetrate through a wall or window. Extend the exhaust pipe away from the building to make sure that vapors are not pulled back into the building. Take precautions to ensure that vapors will not be drawn into nearby homes or businesses, either. Even though there is no risk of overexposure in adjacent buildings or offices, strange odors can make people fearful and paranoid. The media has trained us to imagine the worst when it comes to "chemicals," so expect that this is exactly what you're neighbors will do. It's best to avoid the situation.

Ventilation ducts move fresh air in and out of the salon. They must be kept clean. Dusts, molds, bacteria, and construction materials can accumulate in ducts. This can increase your energy bill and lower the quality of your air. If the air coming from the vents smells stale or musty, it needs cleaning. Ventilation ducts should be inspected once each month as part of a regular maintenance program. The inefficiency of ventilation systems can be monitored fairly easily. **Smoke powders** are extremely fine, white powders used for testing ventilation (Figure 15–5). The smoke powder rides on air currents, tracking the flow of air.

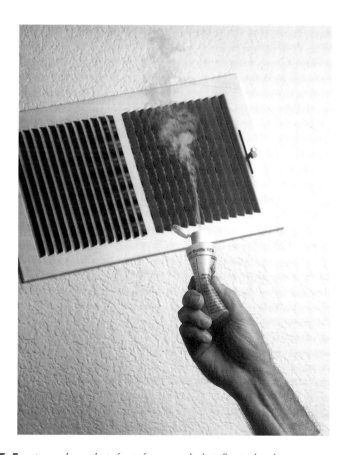

Figure 15–5 *Using smoke powder in front of a vent to check air flow in the salon*

There are many types of smoke powder products. They are available in bottles, pencils, and tubes. They can be used to track the movement of air through the entire salon and near each vent. For example, releasing a few small puffs of smoke powder near a nail table will show how well the air is moving around the station. If the smoke powder stays suspended in one spot for several seconds, the ventilation may be poor in that area. The smoke powder should disperse in seconds if there is adequate ventilation. Smoke powder released near a nail exhaust vent should be pulled in at a vigorous rate. Smoke powder released into the breathing zone is also a useful way to evaluate local ventilation. Ideally, the smoke powder should be quickly pulled into local ventilation tubes or ducts and away from your face.

Besides checking for cleanliness, make sure the system's fans and belts are in good working order. Inhalation allergies, chronic bronchitis, asthma, and other related illnesses are worsened by poorly maintained ventilation systems. If moisture leaks into the ducts or air blowers, have them immediately cleaned and repaired; otherwise molds and bacteria can begin to grow. Studies show that about 5 percent of ventilation problems involve mold or bacterial contamination in ducts or equipment. Never spray water into ventilation ducts. Also, keep the salon humidity at or below 55 percent (*FT*). Use a dehumidifier if necessary, especially during the summer months. This will help control the growth of bacteria and fungi that can lower the quality of salon air and aggravate breathing problems (*FT*).

WHAT WORKS BEST?

What is the best ventilation system for salons? The answer to this question often depends on the particular salon or situation. Is a salon large and expansive or a small room with one nail station? Is there easy access through a wall or window or to the roof? Will the system be mounted permanently or should it be portable? Does the salon need ventilation for one, two, or many stations? There are a lot of choices for salon professionals to make. To help simplify things, here is a brief overview of the various ventilation systems. You will notice they are ranked with the most effective at the top of the list. Of course, it's always better to seek out and follow the advice of a professional HVAC expert, who can help decide what's best (*FT*).

Here is an overview of the best choices for nail salons:

1. *A movable-tube local exhaust system linked to an outdoor venting system.* This is the best choice overall, especially for linking several stations into one exhaust system (*FT*). Such systems can be very cost-effective to build and run, even for single-table units.

2. *A ventilated nail table linked to an outdoor venting system.* This is great for a salon that already has ventilated tables and can install ducts.

3. *A movable-tube local exhaust system vented through a 3- to 4-inch (18-20 mm) HEPA filter/activated charcoal system.* This is the best solution for

nail technicians who want a portable system. But these systems are usually more costly than outdoor venting.

4. *A ventilated nail table vented through a 3- to 4-inch HEPA filter/activated charcoal system.* This is great for a salon that already has ventilated tables and has no outside or roof access for ventilation ducts. Microfilters combined with a thick bed of activated charcoal can also be highly effective.

5. *A commercial-grade, high-quality HEPA filter/activated charcoal room air cleaner unit containing at least 18 pounds (8 kilograms) of activated charcoal.* Even more charcoal is better. These work well in conjunction with local ventilation. Used correctly, they can make a great improvement in air quality. But they are not nearly as effective as local ventilation.

WHERE TO GET IT

There are several important sources of ventilation equipment that are useful for nail technicians in salons. The following companies are excellent sources. They can answer questions and provide ventilation equipment, parts, and supplies.

AllerAir designs and manufacturers high-efficiency air cleaning systems that really work. They make several systems that are very useful in salons. If you have a unique or difficult situation in your salon, their team of HVAC experts can also custom-design ventilation solutions. An excellent source for your ventilation needs. Their Web site is at www.allerair.com, or call 1-888-852-8247.

Lab Safety Supply sells many types of safety equipment, including local exhaust systems, ventilation equipment, smoke powder, N95-rated dust and mist masks, spill cleanup kits, waste receptacles, first-aid kits, ergonomic wrist supports, air testing devices, nitrile gloves, and comfortable safety eyewear. Ask for a free copy of their latest general catalog. On their Web site you can find specifications for modifying nail tables with outdoor exhaust systems. Their Web site is at www.labsafety.com, or call 1-800-356-2501.

Graniger is a distributor of air blowers, ducts, tubing, and other supplies needed for constructing, repairing, or improving ventilation systems. Their Web site is at www.grainger.com, or call 1-888-361-8649.

The Thomas Register is an online search engine that will help you find companies that make any type of ventilation equipment, materials, or supplies: www.thomasregister.com.

Or you can ask a local professional HVAC company to custom-design a system to meet your salon's needs. Custom systems can be built fairly inexpensively. If a complete system is purchased, a ventilation professional may still be needed to install and test the equipment. Also, you will need a professional to ensure that the ventilation is working properly and to perform air quality testing in the salon to ensure that the ventilation system is performing at its best.

AIR BALANCING ACT

Incorrectly installed or inappropriate ventilation systems can upset the **air balance** in the salon. If you pull too much air out of the salon, it will create a **negative air balance.** This means the air pressure inside the salon or room is less than the pressure outside. When doors are open, outside air will rush into the salon, bringing in contaminants—pollen, dusts, smoke, pollution. If air-conditioning or other equipment is pumping too much air into the salon, then a **positive air balance** is created. The amount of air inside the salon is greater than the amount outside. This forces air to flow out of the salon. Positive air balances can be very costly. A positive air balance pushes heated or cooled air out of the salon, and that's expensive! It's like leaving a window open somewhere in a house with the heater set on high. Sometimes nail stations are located in a separate room inside the salon. If there is positive air pressure in that room, vapors and their odors will be pushed from the nail area into other rooms or other parts of the salon. If others in your salon complain about offensive odors, oftentimes a positive air balance is to blame. HVAC experts have techniques and special equipment for supplying extra air to maintain a proper air balance in the salon.

Other factors can also allow vapors and odors to spread through the salon or into neighboring businesses. If neighbors or others complain of odors, HVAC professionals can help track down the source of the vapors. For example, they will check to ensure that light switches and electrical outlets are airtight, seal spaces between shared utility pipes, look for open seams in adjoining walls or ceiling, and so on.

LEAKY VACUUM CLEANERS

Most vacuum cleaners don't do as good a job as you may think. They may pick up the dusts, but they're not very good at holding on to them. A standard house vacuum cleaner leaks a lot of dust, mostly because of the dust bags. These vacuums are great for picking up dirt, hair, small pieces of paper, and other such debris. But they don't handle the tiniest dusts very well. Some vacuums are specially designed to have both leakproof seals and collection bags. They are called **HEPA-rated vacuum cleaners.** In Europe they are called **Class S vacuum cleaners.** To get a HEPA or S rating, a vacuum cleaner must prove it will contain 99.97 percent of the captured dusts. In other words, for every 10,000 dust particles collected, only 3 particles would escape back into the room. These vacuum cleaners use HEPA filters to prevent tiny dusts from escaping, as well as leakproof dust collection bags (FT). Some HEPA vacuum cleaners are designed for home use but are of lower efficiency and quality. The better units have both a filter and indicators that tells you when to change the bag and the filter. Salons should only use commercial-grade vacuum cleaners capable of filtering at least 100 cfm (cubic feet per minute) or 2.8 m³/min. (cubic meters per minute) of air. The very best units exceed 130 cfm (3.7 m³/min) but can cost $900 to $1,000. They're worth it, though, if you want the very best in dust control.

HUMIDIFIERS AND DEHUMIDIFIERS

Controlling salon humidity is very important. **Humidity** is a measure of air wetness. A humidity of 100 percent means that the air is completely saturated with moisture. A level of 30 to 55 percent humidity is the best range for indoor air. Below 30 percent humidity the air is considered to be very dry. Determining the humidity in your salon is simple. Humidity measurement gauges can be purchased at most garden, pet, or home improvement stores or on the Internet. The amount of water vapor contained in the air changes all the time. On some days the salon may feel very humid; other days the air will feel very dry. In humid parts of the world the air usually contains a large amount of water (above 75 percent); conversely, in the dry desert regions of the world the air barely has any water. The average air humidity in the Sahara Desert is about 20 percent. But you don't have to live in a desert to suffer from the effects of dry air. The amount of water in the air depends mostly on temperature. Warmer air holds more water; colder air cannot hold as much water. That's why a cold window fogs up when warm, moist air touches it.

Draw cold air through a heating system and it will make the air even drier. Heating systems can remove more than half of the moisture from incoming air. Dry air is like a sponge, absorbing moisture wherever it can find it. Some typical signs of overly dry air are static electric shocks when you touch doorknobs or other people, plants that need frequent watering, dry or itchy skin, cracked lips, raspy throats, sore or irritated eyes, and frequent nosebleeds. During the winter months, salon humidity can drop to 18 percent. Dry air can dehydrate delicate body tissues such as your skin, eyes, throat, and nasal passages. Other health problems that can arise from dehydration include joint and muscle pain.

Common infection-causing bacteria die up to 20 times faster when the relative humidity is lowered from 70 percent to 45 percent. Mold and mildew are less likely to grow if the humidity is kept below 55 percent. For these reasons, it is recommended that the ideal salon humidity be maintained between 30 and 55 percent.

If the salon humidity is too high, a **dehumidifier** can be used to pull moisture from the air. Water is collected in a container, decreasing the salon's humidity. These containers must be emptied and cleaned each day. The dehumidifier and collection container must be cleaned and disinfected weekly.

A **humidifier** is designed to evaporate moisture into dry air and increase the humidity. They must also be cleaned weekly to prevent the growth of bacteria and mold. A condition called **humidifier fever** or **humidifier lung** is caused by improperly cleaned and maintained humidifiers. This condition can mimic asthma or pneumonia. Typical symptoms are flulike, with fever, chills, loss of appetite, headache, and cough. Proper cleaning and maintenance is a must with humidifiers. Consult with the device's manufacturer for more information on how to properly maintain and use them in your salon.

OZONE GENERATORS

Some devices are marketed as "controlling odors." One type generates and releases a chemical called ozone. Ozone-generating devices are sometimes sold using deceptive marketing techniques to fool nail technicians (and others). Advertisers will even hide the fact that they are selling ozone generators by calling it "activated oxygen," "allotropic oxygen," or "triatomic oxygen." Each of these misleading names is designed to fool the unsuspecting. These advertisers and marketers claim that ozone will eliminate all odors while vapors are changed into harmless carbon dioxide, air, and water. These deceptive advertisements also boast that ozone changes hundreds of "dangerous chemicals to a harmless state." This is a completely bogus claim, but wouldn't it be wonderful if this was really true? Factories would simply mount ozone generators on their smokestacks and our nation's air pollution problem would instantly disappear. Of course, this is just as silly as it sounds. In the salon, ozone doesn't eliminate vapors. Here's the trick: ozone only converts the vapors into different substances, usually with a lower or different odor. These new vapors can be even more harmful to breathe.

The picture gets worse! Ozone is also a major component of smog. Even at very low concentrations, ozone can be hazardous to health and may cause eye, throat, and lung irritation and aggravate asthma. These devices are not useful in the salon environment (or homes or offices, for that matter). Users of these devices will often report they have a funny, metallic taste in their mouths or smell an "electrical burning smell" (ozone) in the air. Beware! Avoid any air cleaner or ventilation device designed to generate ozone. Even at extremely low concentrations, ozone can lead to serious respiratory problems. Never use ozone generators for any purpose in the salon. They will not improve the quality of salon air. Ozone air cleaners will only make matters worse, not better.

Here are a few excerpts from the U.S. Environmental Protection Agency (EPA) Web site concerning air cleaners that generate ozone:

- "When inhaled, ozone can damage the lungs."
- "Healthy people, as well as those with respiratory difficulty, can experience breathing problems when exposed to ozone."
- "Manufacturers and vendors of ozone devices often use misleading terms to describe ozone. Terms such as 'energized oxygen' or 'pure air' suggest that ozone is a healthy kind of oxygen. Ozone is a toxic gas with vastly different chemical and toxicological properties from oxygen."
- "Ozone has little potential to remove indoor air contaminants."
- "Several brands of ozone generators have [an] EPA establishment number on their packaging. This number helps the EPA identify the specific facility that produces the product. The display of this number does not imply EPA endorsement or suggest in any way that the EPA has found this product to be either safe or effective."

In short, avoid any air cleaning devices that generate ozone, activated oxygen, allotropic oxygen, or triatomic oxygen ⒻⓉ. They're bad for you, your clients, your salon, and your pocketbook. If you're going to spend money on ventilation equipment, get something that will help you, not injure you or make you ill.

IONIZERS AND ELECTROSTATIC AIR CLEANERS

Ionizers are devices that create **negative ions.** These ions put a staticlike charge on dust, soot, pollen, animal dander, and other small solid particles. Once they are charged, these dusts clump together into microscopic clusters. Large clusters are much heavier, so they fall from the air. Unfortunately, ionizers work only on particles in the air. They have absolutely no effect on vapors ⒻⓉ. What good are these devices in salons? By themselves, they don't do very much. Knocking dust particles from the air doesn't remove them from the salon. Just walking around or sweeping can stir them up again. Also, ionizers provide no breathing zone protection and have absolutely no effect on vapors. Ionizers are not useful in salons, even if they are combined with a HEPA filter. HEPA filters combined with activated charcoal are much better. Sometimes ionizers are combined with the ozone generators. These should never be used in the salon for the reasons described above.

Electrostatic air filters have improved efficiency over most filters, but they are not superior to HEPA filter technology. Electrostatic air filters are mostly used with furnaces and air-conditioning to improve air quality for general ventilation systems. Other types of electrostatic air cleaners are sold, but these are both inefficient and may generate ozone as well. These devices are best avoided.

ENZYMES, MAGNETS, AND MORE

There are many devices sold that make unbelievable claims. Generally, they are exactly that . . . unbelievable. These include everything from medical-grade ozone to ultrasound air cleaners, units that supposedly "clean through solid walls," "magnetize air," or use electromagnetic energy to purify breathing air, and even systems that are touted as using enzymes to break down air contaminants. There are a lot of them! They all have two things in common: they are usually sold by marketers who exaggerate the risks hoping to scare people into buying their products, and there is no scientific evidence to back up their performance claims for improving salon air quality.

Some of these devices are simply fraudulent. Some make wildly exaggerated claims that walk a tightrope between truth and fiction. Why bother with any of them? Nothing will work better than the ventilation systems described earlier in this chapter. Save your money and purchase systems that have a long track record. Invest in a ventilation system that uses proven technologies and go with the best you can afford. As with most things, higher quality and efficiency command a higher price. But your investment will reward you with cleaner air and peace of mind.

BEFORE YOU GO

Let the overexposure principle guide you throughout your career. Professional nail products should be used without fear or apprehension, but salon safety takes effort and attention. Why be afraid when you can be safe? It's not hard if you know what to do. Look for techniques and products that lower your exposure. This is the key to working safely. With this knowledge you will join the ranks of the modern, chemically aware nail technician.

FAST TRACK (FT)

(FT) HEPA filters are high-efficiency particle filters.

(FT) HEPA filters work best on dust but have no effect on vapors.

(FT) Activated charcoal is combined with HEPA pre-filters in room air cleaners.

(FT) Activated charcoal is like a chemical sponge, mopping vapors from the air.

(FT) All filters must be changed regularly for proper performance and safety.

(FT) Overused, saturated activated charcoal filters may be a fire hazard.

(FT) Microfilters are highly effective for some applications.

(FT) Room air cleaning units pull contaminated air from the surrounding area and return clean air to the room.

(FT) Roof exhaust ducts must be 10 feet higher than air intake vents within 50 feet.

(FT) Ideally, keep salon humidity between 30 percent and 55 percent.

(FT) Controlling humidity controls the growth of bacteria, mold, and mildew.

(FT) A local HVAC company can help you determine what's best for your salon.

(FT) The best solution to salon vapor control is local exhaust to the outdoors.

(FT) HEPA vacuums are designed with leakproof seals and collection bags.

(FT) Never use any air cleaner that generates ozone.

(FT) Ionizers provide no breathing zone protection and have no effect on vapors.

Review Questions

1. What is the most effective way to prevent inhalation overexposure to dusts in the salon air?

2. What is a microfilter?

3. What does HVAC stand for?

4. What is the most important job of a good ventilation system?

5. What are the risks of using ozone generators?

6. Are HEPA filters useful for controlling vapors? Why?

7. What is the difference between general exhaust and local exhaust?

8. What can happen if activated charcoal filters are overused and become saturated with flammable vapors?

9. Roof exhaust ducts must be _____ feet higher than air intake vents within _____ feet.

10. _____ is like a chemical sponge.

11. _____ _____ can be used to track the flow of salon air.

12. What effect do ionizers and HEPA filters have on vapors in the air?

13. A level of _____–_____ percent humidity is the best range for indoor air.

14. Name the condition caused by improperly cleaned or maintained humidifiers.

15. What is the importance of an EPA registration number on devices such as ozone-generating air cleaners?

Chapter 16

16

Nails Around the World

Objective

In this chapter you will learn about the practices of nail technicians and salons in many different and widely flung parts of the world. You'll also see how different the world can be. But you'll also see that no matter where they are found, nail technicians share many of the same challenges, experiences, questions, needs, dreams, and hopes.

NAILS: JAPANESE STYLE

Education Team
Takara-Belmont
Tokyo, Japan

Nail technicians are called "nailists" in Japan. Nails are getting more popular than ever, and nailists are adored by fashion-conscious consumers. Hip young fashionistas crave art nails with multiple glitters, while older clients prefer conservative shades and round or square shapes. Nail service is typically provided at nail-only salons, usually inside department stores or shopping malls. You can also have your nails done at hair salons or skin care centers that have expanded their business to offer nail services. Japanese culture is well known for its precision, and nails are no exception. You can expect first-rate service and hospitality at almost every salon.

Traditionally, Japanese are not used to body contact, such as hugs or handshakes, so nail service is not as common as hairdressing. It is totally unlike in the United States, where bank tellers can wear long red nails. Japanese culture is much more conservative. Such nails would be viewed as a social taboo in certain workplaces or on certain occasions.

Japanese do not hesitate to pay for expensive designer clothes or bags, but many people still consider nail services as luxuries and something special for certain events such as weddings. Male clients and nail technicians are rare. Natural nail care is the most popular service, generally priced between $30 and $50 (US), including polish. Nail enhancements usually cost more than $100 for a full set. Celebrity nail techs can get more than $300 a set with detailed, sculptured art nails. These high-profile nailists are often featured in beauty and fashion magazines, and consumers are eager to have what they see on the covers. Nail-only magazines with high-level artistry are also available at Japanese bookstores, and they are exported to many Asian countries where Japanese nail arts are worshiped.

Japanese nail technicians love to compete, and many of them have won international competitions. Nail competitions are held about ten times a year in Japan, and both novices and professionals compete for their perfection. Sculptured and fantasy nail competitions are the most respected, but natural nail care competitions are also well recognized. UV gel competitions are getting popular too, as the UV gel nail is the fastest-growing service. Many brands have been launched in the market to appease nailists and customers who do not like the odor and complexity of conventional liquid and powder technology.

There is no state or government license in Japan for nail technicians, as there is for cosmetologists. Nail technician associations and nail schools issue their own diploma or certificate when students finish 200–300 hours of training, but many students choose to learn more by attending advanced classes and participating in the ongoing education that is constantly offered at the nail supply stores or by manufacturers at trade shows. The number of nailists is rapidly increasing in Japan, and they are working hard to meet the very high expectations of savvy Japanese customers.

NAILS: NORWEGIAN STYLE

Hanne Gruer
Octane
Oslo, Norway

Since 2002 my salon has been situated in the central area of Oslo, the capital of Norway. The salon is right next to one of the bigger shopping streets. It is a quite small salon, but there is room for three nail tables and a pedicure chair. My clients are mainly full-time working women in their thirties, but I also have a few teenagers and several elderly clients. About 85 percent of these clients prefer a permanent French manicure with a square nail shape. I do not have any clients with extremely long nails (fortunately). I spend a lot of time and effort educating my clients about design lines and the consequences of wearing nails that are too long for them. When it comes to nail shape, I think clients pick what they are used to and not necessarily because of a fashion preference. My newer clients are more open to trying different shapes and colors. I have been a nail technician for quite a few years now. I find the education has become increasingly interesting and challenging. I take as many classes as possible but still make sure that my clients get the service and help they need.

NAILS: KAZAKHSTAN STYLE

Olga Miroshnichenko
NickOl Beauty and Health Center
Almaty, Kazakhstan

The Republic of Kazakhstan is a secular, democratic, and unitary state situated in the central part of Europe. In land size, Kazakhstan is the ninth largest country in the world and features mountains, hills, and plains. Our population is almost 15 million, of whom 53 percent are Kazakhs and 30 percent are Russians. The official language is called Kazakh, but people also speak Russian. There are eighty-five cities, and Astana is our capital. But the largest city is Almaty, the former capital of Kazakhstan, with 1.1 million people. Temperatures in our country vary widely, from −45°F (−43°C) in the winter to 113°F (45°C) in the summer.

For the last ten years I have owned a beauty and health center called NickOl, and it is located in the center of Almaty. NickOl has a beauty salon, training center, and professional products equipment center (which is a priority in our business). We started our nail service in 1997 and have tried many materials and studied various technologies. So far, acrylic systems are the most popular, although UV gel nails have recently arrived on the Kazakhstani market. Taking into account the local mentality, a woman is considered here as the "keeper of the family fireplace" and usually does the work around the house by herself. That is why her nails must be strong and able to bear much stress. But some are opposed to having nail services. Some religious believers avoid any artificial decorations and only want their nails to look natural.

Approximately 1 percent of the people of our country wear artificial nails, and the approximately 2,000 nail technicians who work in Kazakhstan service them. The most courageous of these nail technicians will participate in the Kazakh Professional Contest for Manicuring, Nail Enhancement, and Nail Art. For the last four years our center has sponsored this contest, which is held during our annual spring show, the KazInterBeauty exhibition. This exhibition is very popular among beauty industry professionals. During the exhibition there are many different contests and shows, as well as demonstrations of new technologies and new products by all the biggest companies in the professional nail industry.

Educational courses for nail enhancement are held six times per year in our training center:

- Basic level: nine days of classes that teach the fundamentals of acrylic salon nails, French, backfill, and spa

- Advanced level: six-day classes that teach techniques such as colored acrylics, UV gels, competitions nails, and design

The groups usually consist of 10–12 students. Our training center is well equipped: equipment, showcases, advertising materials, video equipment (projector, computer, video camera), and so on. Upon completion of the educational course, only 60–70 percent of students continue to work on their specialization, although demand for technicians is continuously rising. More and more salons are being opened. Hand and foot care is becoming more popular as the service spectrum is being enhanced, but there are not enough qualified specialists.

In the last three to four years, acrylic white-and-pink French on forms has become the predominant choice. When UV gel nails are applied, it is usually over artificial tips. Designs with colored acrylics or gels are in demand before holidays and at contests and trainings. They are attractive, but they are not as popular as traditional looks. Classical French has many advantages here: it suits everybody everywhere and is more natural-looking.

The patrons of nail salons are well-to-do people that work in banks, embassies, legal institutions, oil/gas companies, trade representations, and so on. The cost of a nail enhancement service is $15–$70 (US). The duration of the service can vary from 150 to 180 minutes. The cost of a backfill is $8–$35, and the service can last between 120 and 150 minutes. Spa manicures cost $15–$40 for a 40- to 60-minute service, while spa pedicure services are $20–$50 for 60 to 80 minutes. The cost of our training courses is $10–$30 per day. In this country, a nail technician needs to have between 50 and 60 patrons to be fully employed.

As nail technicians and educators, we are proud of the inventions in the nail enhancement industry and looking forward to seeing new achievements! To be a nail technician in our country means not only to make beautiful nails but also to solve our clients' nail problems.

NAILS: UK STYLE

Samantha Sweet

Designer Nails

Leeds, United Kingdom

I am lucky and incredibly proud to have been a part of the UK nail industry for twelve years, thanks primarily to my mum, Gigi Rouse, one of England's first and most famous nail educators. Nails have been the fastest-growing segment of the beauty industry for eight years, and many have jumped onto the nail bandwagon in the United Kingdom for countless differing reasons!

Our company has won numerous accolades over the years, and we are particularly proud of the education that we provide. From the very beginning we wanted to do it right and we have never compromised our beliefs. The United Kingdom does not (as yet) have strict laws regarding the nail industry, but the public is now far more aware. Magazines in the United Kingdom are very aware of the professional nail industry and professional nail products and are giving them their top awards.

Unfortunately, anyone can become a nail technician in the United Kingdom. It doesn't matter if they are trained or not. This is not our philosophy. We teach that professional products should not be sold to nonprofessionals. They have no business using professional products without proper training. Unfortunately, some UK-based companies will sell their products regardless of training. This not only produces poor and unskilled technicians, it also damages the reputation of the professionally trained and skilled nail technicians. A customer will tell at least ten people about a bad experience, so it is our goal to make sure that bad experiences don't happen. In the United Kingdom, most women believed that the only way to wear enhancements was long and square, like they saw on TV or while on holiday in the United States. UK technicians usually persuade their clients to embrace what suits them, and most clients willingly allow themselves to be pushed in the right direction. The United Kingdom is also a celebrity-obsessed nation and celebrity trends have an enormous effect on the British public. If Victoria Beckham or Kylie Minogue is sporting nails, they want nails—simple as that!

The stiletto (long and pointy) and almond-shaped nails have become far more popular over the last two years. Of course, short, neat ovalesque shapes are also popular. I surveyed numerous nail technicians across the United Kingdom and Ireland for their opinions on the most popular length, shape, and color in their areas. Here is what I found. The permanent French manicure look is still winning, hands down. Also, color on toes has become very popular as well. Finally, airbrushing, freehand nail art, and colored acrylics are becoming increasingly popular, but not for everyday wear. Even top-flight career women are not being bashful about their nails—if they want them long, they'll have them long!

Britain is renowned not for its sunshine but instead for its miserable weather. I think this is why we British and Irish women spend so much money on ourselves in the beauty department. It's not uncommon for a salon to have the same loyal clients for ten years. On the other hand, we are lucky that our weather is not too hot or too cold, so nearly all types of artificial nail systems work well. I hope I have spread a little light on the UK nail industry in general. I'd like to thank the Nail Geeks (www.nailgeek.com) across the United Kingdom and Ireland, who gave me wonderful feedback via the site on nail style preferences in their particular areas. Cheers!

NAILS: RUSSIAN STYLE

Galina Zelenova

Ole House

Moscow, Russia

What is it like to be a nail technician in Russia? Five or six years ago, this occupation was considered one of the least desirable and lowest-paid jobs. Now it is all different. Today, nail technicians' salary compares almost on a level with those of people who have bachelor's degrees.

Because of the changes in our society, products and technologies from countries outside of Russia are now allowed for sale. In order to make these new products popular with consumers, we had to first open educational centers and teach nail technicians about these new technologies. We offer different levels of education at different prices, depending on the class. At the end of training, technicians get their diploma. This diploma is very important for getting a job as a technician in a salon. In Russia, nail technicians are not required to get a license. But the salon must be licensed. For the salon to keep their licenses, they must maintain a consistently high level of qualified nail technicians on staff. These nail technicians are allowed to work with their own products and materials. But they may also use products provided by the salon. All items used by nail technicians must be officially certified, and the controlling organizations ensure this by frequently checking salons.

Usually, nail technicians are paid by commission, which may vary from 25 to 60 percent. The average nail technician in Moscow makes between $800 and $1,000 (US) per month. Nail technicians who win nail competitions can charge a much higher rate for their services and have higher incomes. The price for a nail service varies from $70 to $170 in Moscow, but in other regions of Russia the price can vary from $30 to $70. It's very common for Russian salons to offer a wide range of services, such as hair, skin, cosmetics, manicures, and pedicures. There are only a very few salons that specialize in nail services only, probably less than 10. Despite this, the nail salons are becoming more popular. The most popular nail service in Russia is the classic manicure (the one where you get your cuticles cut). This type of service is the oldest of its type and has been around for a very long time in Russia. Not many clients have switched to European-type manicures, but some salons combine the classic manicure with elements of spa. We also have "hot" manicures, which are used for treating nails, and this service is even performed on children. Men are not very frequent guests in manicure salons, but this is changing, and some are beginning to enjoy spa treatments. Russian women like nail enhancements, especially if they have nail problems such as short nail beds, bitten nails, and so on. Colored powders and nail art rapidly became popular and now compete with the ever-popular French manicure nail enhancements.

Nail competitions are a big influence on the popularity of nail enhancements in Russia. Almost every beauty show will have a nail competition. Many cities have semifinal competitions with the finals held in Moscow. Both Russia and our training center, Ole House, could not be more proud of its master nail technicians. Our technicians have even won first place two years in a row in the Düsseldorf, Germany, nail competition—one of the most prestigious nail competitions in the world. What is it like to be a nail technician in Russia? It means to have an interesting and well-paid job, the love and respect of your clients, and an opportunity for professional growth.

NAILS: NAMIBIAN STYLE

Adri Roelofse
Professional Nails
Namibia

The Republic of Namibia is a country situated along the south Atlantic coast of Africa. Namibia is the 31st largest country in the world but very sparsely populated. Namibia is divided into 13 regions, but there are only 1.8 million people and less than 30 percent live in urban areas.

Nail enhancements are not big yet but are growing very fast. The French look is most popular, especially with the younger generation. Older woman prefer a shorter natural look or colored gel. UV gels and light-cured acrylic and silk wraps are the most often performed professional services. Acrylics are getting more and more popular. When I came to Namibia I was the only one doing acrylic nails, and I was welcomed by some very misinformed clients. The general knowledge here was that acrylics are bad for your nails and cause fungus. I started doing UV gels just to get clients. Then I offered them acrylics as an alternative. All my clients are using acrylic now and they are very satisfied. I have a waiting list of people wanting acrylic nails. Toenails and nail art are also very popular. Clients prefer nail art on only two fingers or only on the big toes. Usually they prefer little diamonds or gold and silver stripes or decals.

Nail education is not adequate in Namibia. Aspirant nail technicians must go to South Africa for proper training, and that is very expensive. So most only get training on the few product lines available. These are given by the nail product distributors, who are very misinformed about other products and opportunities. We don't have a nail board in Namibia. At this stage, you don't even need a license to do nails. That sets up a playground for untrained nail technicians who get product from trained nail techs. Then they start doing nails without any knowledge of nail diseases and sanitation. That's one reason why acrylics are not as popular with these nail technicians—it is a much more difficult system to master.

I work from home and have a very relaxed atmosphere in my salon, where I serve coffee, tea, and cool drinks. I also clean my clients' rings for them before they leave . . . yes, for free. Spa manicures and pedicures are also very popular. I started doing waterless manicures and my clients are very impressed.

I am very committed to this industry and would do my utmost to better the nail profession in this country, with the help of a lot other nail techs who feel the same as I do.

NAILS: LOS ANGELES STYLE

Justine Hartel

Paint Shop

Los Angeles, California

Living in Los Angeles has given me many exciting career opportunities. I started with Paint Shop, a nail spa in Beverly Hills for several years and had my first celebrity client, the lovely Dixie Carter. I realized then that I had a skill that's very valuable to beautiful people! Looking good is imperative in LA. So all the beauty business here is cutting-edge and quite competitive. Nail fashionistas want natural, sheer pink manicures or pink-and-white enhancements. And of course, bright, perfect toes are a must to show off those $500 sandals! Everywhere you go you'll see polished, decorated hands and feet—on women of all ages and guys, too! A high-end salon manicure might typically cost $30 (US), spa pedicure $70, full set $65, fill $40.

But the real business is in celebrity outcalls—a visit to the home or hotel suite of someone too famous to go out in public for their grooming. Beauty professionals here spend years finessing hotels and salons, hoping to get the call when Madonna needs a pedicure. House calls start at $150 and go waaaaay up. Then there are films, TV shows, photo shoots, performances . . . and they all need their nails to look good! I've been backstage at the Staples Center for Grammys, the Kodak Theatre for Women Rock, and Chateau Marmont for the Oscars, and I was a guest on Lifetime TV's *Head 2 Toe*. In my work I've met Alicia Keys, Angela Bassett, Dolly Parton, Jennifer Love Hewitt, and the Osbournes. The key to getting these cool gigs is, first, being great at what you do and, second, being in the right place at the right time. Stars want stylists who are highly skilled, available, clean, dependable, fast, and capable of blending in with any surroundings. People are amazed when I tell them about my nail adventures in La-La Land! There aren't enough awesome stylists to go around, so to all you aspiring celebrity nail technicians I say: get good and then get out here! Hollywood is waiting!

NAILS: MIDDLE EASTERN STYLE

Sonette van Rensburg
Nstyle Nail Lounge
Dubai, United Arab Emirates

Dubai is a land of startling contrasts. The beautiful Arabian Gulf coast with its turquoise waters, many uninhabited islands, and coral reefs is surrounded by land that is mostly stark desert and large salt flats called the Sabkha. Here you will find spectacular sand dunes broken by an occasional oasis. Dubai is situated on the northeastern part of the Arabian Peninsula, bordered by Saudi Arabia and Oman. It has a subtropical, arid climate with temperatures ranging between 50°F (10°C) and 118°F (48°C). The population of Dubai is about 1.1 million people, and there are 2.4 men to every woman. The culture is firmly rooted in the Islamic traditions, and Dubai's heritage and culture are tied to its religion. But it's more than just a religion, it's a way of life that governs the minutiae of everyday events, even what to wear and what to eat and drink. Women have to be very conservative with their dress. They often wear long black robes known as *abayas* and scarves to cover their hair and face whenever in public.

When I started my nail career 18 years ago, I realized quickly that this was something I was absolutely born to do. Then, artificial nail enhancements weren't really popular, probably because the nails looked like doorstoppers and were one color with no real design, form, or shape. But after working for almost two years at a nail bar in South Africa, I was convinced I knew quite a lot and should open my own salon. I was mistaken and learned that my education had only just begun. Like others just starting out, I experienced bacterial infections and many other problems. Instead of quitting, I took a beauty therapy course to learn more about health, client care, and the proper procedures for working in a salon environment. My training and qualification as an aesthetician taught me how to take better care of my salon and my clients. I then followed up with a course in nail technology and gained more valuable training. In fact, because of this, I ended up taking first place in South Africa's first major nail competition. I was happy, my clients were ecstatic, and my business was flourishing. I continued my education by becoming an educator for the leading nail manufacturer. I didn't think it was possible to learn so much about nails. But what I have learned has made me a better nail technician and educator. By now, my hunger and passion for this industry had been awakened and there was no turning back. I opened up a nail technology school and salon so I could continue educating and doing clients' nails. That's one thing about this industry—when a client gets used to high-quality work, they will not settle for anyone else. They trust you and literally leave their hands in your hands.

Then everything changed! My husband accepted a position in Dubai, so we moved. I had no idea what lay ahead or what to expect! Fortunately, I found a beauty salon in Dubai where I could set up my own nail business. When I first arrived, the artificial nail market was predominately UV gels. But that has changed and now liquid/powder enhancements dominate. Of course, salons mostly performed natural nail manicures, and to my amazement, women were coming and asking me to cut their cuticles. Even after lengthy explanations telling them why I shouldn't and wouldn't cut the living skin, they still insisted, saying I did not know how to do a manicure! Eventually I was able to educate them with the facts, and I have developed quite a professional reputation as a result. Another hurdle was that Muslim women would not wear nail enhancements. They believe that artificial nails were not proper or allowable, since the natural nail breathes and should not be covered by anything when they pray, as they need to wash their hands, feet, and the other parts of their bodies. They believe it is important for the water to touch their nails. Teaching my clients that the natural nails don't breathe was not as difficult as I thought it would be, and because I took the time to educate them, more Muslim women are now wearing nail enhancements. Some only wear enhancements for a special occasion and immediately soak them off afterward. Others wear them constantly and are happy now that they know the water touches the cuticle area and the small margin of exposed nail plate next to the soft living tissue.

On average clients pay about $18 (US) for a manicure, $25 for a pedicure, and $84 for a full set of artificial nails. The nail industry in Dubai is booming. Some salons and nail lounges are unlike any others I have ever seen: beautifully fitted out, trendy, and very state-of-the-art. Most women here don't work but spend a lot of time outdoors, shopping and socializing. Visiting the local nail lounge is more than just a treat; it has become a social event. Because Dubai is often visited by the rich and famous, I have had the opportunity to enhance the nails of prominent people such as the actress Brenda Vaccaro and the well-known belly dancer Yasmine. I have also worked on international models appearing on the catwalks during Dubai's highly respected Fashion Week. My work up there along with the spectacular designs of Dior, Lacroix, Givenchy, and Ungaro! This was probably one of the most exciting projects I have worked on and it really put a feather in my cap.

Working in Dubai, I have learned so much about different cultures, but I've also learned that women around the world have one thing in common: they all want to have beautiful, well-groomed nails. What I like most about this profession is when a lady walks into your salon devastated with the state of her nails and then two hours later walks out smiling. That gives me such an amazing feeling of self-satisfaction and achievement. I have learned through the years as a nail technician and educator that you must keep an open mind and be always willing to learn more. Learn from your experiences and mistakes, be professional at all times, and work with passion and a love for what you do. You are never too old or too wise to learn, and there is always something new to discover. That's what has kept me so motivated through all the years. The best advice I can give to any nail technician is to remember that education is the key to success!

Today, I spend most of my time continuing to educate others in nail technology, but I still have a small handful of clients that will not let me go as their nail technician. I never dreamed when I first started out that 18 years later I would still be in the nail industry. But I love it, it is in my blood, and I am passionate about what I do.

NAILS: TAIWANESE STYLE

Evelyn Wang
Creative Signature
Taipei, Taiwan

Taiwan is an island of 23 million people, all living within its 25 districts. In our country, the mainstream client wants natural nail care and spa pedicure and spa manicure services, and younger consumers love inexpensive nail art products. There are about 100 salons in Taiwan that offer nail services. Only 30 percent are purely nail salons; the remaining 70 percent are jointly operated within hair, facial, and body salons. About 70 percent of all salons are located around the Taipei metropolitan area, where nearly 5 million people live. I believe about 25 new salons open each year because of the market demand. But 10 to 15 older salons go out of business every year, due to lack of professionalism. The average salary for being a nail tech is from U.S. $750 to $3,500 monthly depending upon skills and whether the nail professional co-owns the salon or not.

Nail enhancements are not yet popular in the Taiwanese market. For a full set of nail enhancements, most salons charge $30 to $150 (US). Unfortunately, the average nail technician's knowledge, information, and technical skills are still too low. Most of the nail technicians are unable to distinguish between good and bad nail enhancement products. Since there is no formal nail education provided by the vocational school system, the only source of nail education is from the nail products' importers or distributors. Thus, the quality of the nail education is not adequate in Taiwan.

In our salon, we offer nail enhancement, spa pedicure, and spa manicure services. In order to create the proper atmosphere for spa services, we separate the nail enhancement area from pedicure and manicure service spaces to prevent the odors that detract from the quality of the spa service. In the spa room, we have flowers, play soft music, and serve handmade cookies, tea, and fresh fruits. There is a VIP room that is big enough for five guests to enjoy the spa services simultaneously; thus the group guests can come to our salon and enjoy talking and laughing together in the VIP room, then go home with their beautiful hands and feet. Our salon is in a high-income residential building located in a high-tech industry business park—thus we are aiming at the high-income customers. Forever French, a usable-length, natural-looking nail, is much more popular than decorated nails. We also make a personal set of tools available for those customers who don't want to share implements with others.

We will keep improving ourselves in our skills and services; hopefully we can expand our market to other locations in the near future. Looking on the bright side, this market is still in the growing stages, thus there is healthy competition going on in areas such as education, service, product quality, and so on. Hence I hope the lack of education described above won't last for much longer.

Chapter 17

Special Topics

DOS AND DON'TS FOR SAFE ELECTRIC FILE USE

Nancy King, Director
Association of Electric File Manufacturers (AEFM)

- Always contact the AEFM for an electric file training course (www.aefm.org).
- Always clean and disinfect bits after each use.
- Never use arbor bands more than one time, even on the same person.
- Always follow manufacturers' instructions for all nail products.
- Always use professional nail machines designed for use in nail salons.
- Always follow the rules and regulations of your state.
- Never use an electric file on a client before taking a safety course.
- Never use bits without cleaning and disinfecting.
- Never use a metal or carbide bit on the natural nail.
- Never apply downward pressure on the nail while filing.
- Craft or hobby tools are not designed for professional salon use.

HOSPITALS, NURSES, AND NAILS: MY OPINION

Doug Schoon, M.S.

In late 2003 some hospitals began prohibiting their employees from wearing artificial nails. Why has this occurred? Here's a brief synopsis of the issue.

Normal, everyday bacteria can collect under the free edge of the nail plate. It's completely normal and can't be avoided. That's life! Bacteria are everywhere. Most are completely safe, but some can cause disease or illness in humans. Bacteria that can cause illness or disease are called pathogens. What can we do about pathogens? The best way to remove these bacteria is by properly scrubbing under the free edge of the natural nail. This isn't surprising and should make complete sense to anyone. Obviously, longer natural nails can harbor more bacteria, since the plate is longer (just like a bigger house can hold more people). The same situation applies to artificial nails, and that is how this issue began.

Scientific studies performed over the past ten years show that on the average, nurses do not properly wash their hands between patients (when they wash at all) and they are in too much of a hurry. Nurses spend only about four to six seconds washing their hands and rarely properly scrub underneath the extended edges of their nails. Experts agree that nurses should wash their hands and scrub their nails for no less than 30 seconds between patients. The same experts also agree that if this was done, there would be a dramatic drop in the number of infections transmitted by nurses from patient to patient, solving one of the most important problems in hospitals today.

This long-standing problem came to national attention when three nurses in a neonatal intensive care unit improperly washed their hands and then used a shared container of hand cream that had been sitting by the sink (strictly against the hospital's policies). This hand cream was contaminated with a common type of bacteria that later caused the death of three infants who had been previously admitted for other serious illness. One of the three nurses had short natural nails, one had long natural nails, and one had long artificial nails. Of course, the grossly sensationalized news headlines suggested that "artificial nails kill babies," which is silly and not what happened at all.

Since then, several other studies confirmed that longer nail plates require more cleaning and scrubbing time to ensure patient safety. Cracked and chipped nail polish was also cited as a factor contributing to increased amounts of bacteria on fingernails. What did the hospitals do with this information? Insist that nurses start washing their hands properly? You would think so, but that's not what happened! Instead, several large hospital chains began telling all employees that they could no longer wear artificial nails. Nail polish is still allowed, but only if it is not cracked or chipped. Of course, this completely ignores the problem, and nurses still do not properly wash their hands!

These hospitals claimed the artificial nail ban was justified, based on recommendations from the Centers for Disease Control (CDC). However, this is not correct. The CDC only recommended that nurses involved in critical care areas (high-risk situations such as surgery wards and intensive care units) should not wear artificial nails or cracked nail polish. Instead, these hospitals overreacted and insisted that all hospital workers must remove their artificial nails, even receptionists and secretaries. They ignore the fact that a doctor's tie can carry as much or more bacteria than artificial nails. Visitors expose patients to even more infection risks than either of these. Personally, I strongly disagree with this "bury your head in the sand" approach. Luckily, organizations such as the Nail Manufacturers Council (NMC) are working closely with both the CDC and the Association for Professionals in Infection Control (APIC) to resolve this misunderstanding. It is hoped that eventually hospitals will redirect their infection control efforts in a more positive way. And hopefully they will finally and successfully address the hand-washing problems that are rampant in health care institutions.

COME GEEK WITH ME

Samuel Sweet, The Nail Geek

www.thenailgeek.com

Let's face it—I'm a geek. A couple of years ago, Mrs. Geek and I were enjoying a lovely glass of wine while playing the typical "dump your name in the search engine and see what pops up" game. We started with my wife's name, and lo and behold, there was actually a samanthasweet.com Web site! That's right, her World Wide Web identity was already taken! Desperate, I plugged in samuelsweet.com, and Lady Luck was on my side. While my wife's name was taken, mine was waiting for someone to lay a claim. So I did what every man with a glass of wine and high-speed Internet access would do—I bought the name. So I had the name. What the heck do I do with it? The site began life as a place to put the articles I've written, as well as the step-by-step guides I've published in various industry magazines around the world. The site was an instant success, and within a few months I found a massive amount of my time was being spent answering technical questions (many of which were of the same nature). I needed a better way of communicating!

On January 9, 2003, I opened the infamous forums on my Web site to allow open public discussion on all things nail-related. Well, it turned into a bit of a phenomenon! In the first 18 months, there were over 41,000 posts and the site had over 2,500 registered users, racking up 200–300 new posts each day (heck, by the time you read this it may well be double that number). Everything was evolving very quickly, so I changed the site's name to better reflect the community that participated in the shared discussions. Within 18 months, thenailgeek.com became the largest worldwide community of professional nail technicians and the largest repository of nail discussions anywhere. What started as a site for posting tutorials and articles has taken on a life of its own. Some of the industry's most prominent educators and competition winners began to regularly contribute, teach, and give advice on the site.

From discussion forums, the site expanded to include photo galleries of some fantastic nail enhancements, as well as astonishing nail art. But that's not all! There are quizzes to test your knowledge, private messaging services, integrated chat rooms, and of course lots of tutorials, articles, and industry Web site links. If you're looking for nail-related information, a quick search of this site will produce countless results.

Why did I start thenailgeek.com? It's my way of staying in touch and being a part of a worldwide community of professional nail technicians while providing a benefit to all that participate. I guess it feels kind of cool to have started something that so many nail technicians firmly believe is their lifeline for the industry. I know it has been my lifeline, too. Hope to see you there sometime!

GET HOOKED!

Debbie Doerrlamm, Webmaster

www.beautytech.com

Roll back time to 1994. I was just moving up from part-time nail technician to full-time. Like most, I had questions. The problem was, who to ask? The logical answer was the instructor who had given me a class three years previously, but she had become ill and was no longer available. The next option is to get help from the local nail supply house. We know how that goes: "The nail stuff? I think it's over there in the corner." Grasping for straws, through my computer I reached out to the online community America Online. What started out as a quest for information grew to be the largest and longest-established portal Web site for beauty professionals, www.beautytech.com. Within that first year, Doug Schoon wandered into the folds of our newly founded group and contributed as well as asked questions until his fingers grew numb. Doug has been a wealth of knowledge over the years and never misses an opportunity to share it all with the masses.

Online forums are a great continuing education resource, and they are as close as your mouse. In 2005, BeautyTech continues to give the professional a place to hang out, complain, brag, and ask the obvious and not-so-obvious questions to a wide array of their peers—seasoned technicians, educators, and students, as well as manufacturers. Help arrives in your in-box almost immediately from all different age brackets, geographical locations, and levels of expertise. Along with the opportunity for networking, you can find class and show calendars, articles galore, a mentoring program, sample student quizzes, and over 1,300 links to professional beauty Web sites.

Said Alice Wallace, a 10-year nail veteran and 8-year BeautyTech networker, "The networking here gives us the courage to try new things or gather new information. We can get feedback or make sure we're not the only ones that are 'getting it' or not getting it. My participation on BeautyTech.com has taught me that I wish to be seen as a professional by my peers, my clients. It's also been great for my own well-being. BeautyTech.com gives you an education like no other. Best of all it's free and you never have to be afraid to ask a question."

It is not only nail technicians who benefit from this networking forum. Salon owners can get a better perspective and better understand that their clients are better serviced by educated nail technicians; trade magazines gain insight and article ideas; manufacturers receive firsthand and first-rate feedback instantly. Of course, friendships blossom between nail techs the world over. Also, they usually increase their income and have fewer problems because of this newfound knowledge. Over 50 percent of the participants in the BeautyTech forums say they have had "immeasurable increase" in their income since they started networking online. So visit www.beautytech.com when you have a night off and no full book the next day—you will be hooked!

Answers to Review Questions

CHAPTER 1

1. What is the definition of *proximal, lateral,* and *distal?*
   Answer: Proximal means "nearest attached end," distal means "farthest attached end," and lateral means "to the side."

2. Which finger has the narrowest matrix?
   Answer: The narrowest matrix makes the narrowest nail plate. Therefore, the little finger must have the narrowest matrix.

3. If a person was born with _____ nails, their matrix must be shorter than normal.
   Answer: Thin.

4. List 10 parts of the nail unit.
   Answer: Matrix, proximal nail fold, lateral nail fold, nail plate, nail bed, hyponychium, eponychium, cuticle, solehorn, onychodermal band, free edge, lunula.

5. _____ carry blood and nutrients from the heart to the nail unit, while _____ carry blood and waste products away from the nail unit.
   Answer: Arteries, veins.

6. Name the guardians of the nail.
   Answer: Eponychium, hyponychium, the two lateral folds. The onychodermal band is also important to the hyponychium seal.

7. Why is the onychodermal band important, and what does it protect?
   Answer: The onychodermal band protects and seals the nail bed from the outside world. It helps prevent infections under the nail plate. It reinforces the hyponychium seal.

8. What chemical substance is the nail plate composed of, and where else on the body is it found?
   Answer: Keratin, found in skin and hair.

9. How are sensations such as pain relayed to the brain?
   Answer: Nerve endings sense pain, pressure, and so on and nerve fibers carry them to the brain for processing.

10. If the nail plate is firmly attached to the nail bed, how can it move when it grows?
    Answer: The nail bed consists of two types of tissue, bed epithelium and dermis. The epithelium is firmly attached to the nail plate, but it is free to glide over the dermis via the ridges and grooves.

11. Which two nail anatomy terms are commonly misused and sometimes used interchangeably even though they are completely different?
    Answer: *Nail bed* and *nail plate*. The nail bed lies underneath and supports the hard keratin nail plate.

12. Where does the cuticle come from?
    Answer: The underside of the eponychium.

13. The fingernail plate is approximately _____ cell layers thick.
    Answer: 100.

14. The nerve endings in the nail bed can detect _____ and _____ very well but cannot detect _____ very well.
    Answer: Pressure, pain, heat.

15. Name the tissue that adheres to the bottom of the nail plate.
    Answer: Bed epithelium.

CHAPTER 2

1. Toenails grow _____ as fast as fingernails.
   Answer: Half.

2. The natural nail plate contains less than ____ percent calcium.
   Answer: 0.1 percent.

3. _____ is a surface's resistance to being scratched or dented.
   Answer: Hardness.

4. Which abrasive material is nearly as hard as diamond?
   Answer: Black silicon carbide.

5. Diffusion is the process that describes how liquids _____.
   Answer: Are absorbed or move through a solid.

6. _____ _____ are the strongest type of chemical linkage.
   Answer: Covalent bonds.

7. _____ _____ are a special type of covalent bond created between two molecules of cysteine found on separate protein chains.
   Answer: Sulfur cross-links.

8. Water diffuses through the nail plate about _____ times faster than through skin.
   Answer: 1,000 times.

9. The nail plate contains about __ percent oil and ___ percent water.
   Answer: 5 percent, 18 percent.

10. Oils have a _____ effect and can noticeably increase flexibility of the plate.
    Answer: Plasticizing.

11. Why do nails tend to peel at the top of the free edge, rather than underneath?
    Answer: The cells on the top side of the plate are approximately two months older than those on the underside.

12. It is much better for nails to be _____, rather than hard.
    Answer: Tough.

13. Besides oils, water, and keratin, name five other substances that are found inside the nail plate.
    Answer: Iron, aluminum, copper, silver, gold, titanium, phosphorus, zinc, sodium, calcium.

14. The hollow junctions between nail cells that rivet them together are called

    _____.

    Answer: Desmosomes.

15. Nail enhancement or polish removers can _____ the skin.
    Answer: Dry.

CHAPTER 3

1. The triceps is an example of an _____ muscle, since it allows the arm to be straightened or extended.
   Answer: Extensor.

2. The biceps is an example of a _____ muscle, one needed to flex or bend a joint.
   Answer: Flexor.

3. When two muscles work as a matched team to extend and contract, they are called an _____ pair.
   Answer: Antagonistic.

4. Define tendonitis.
   Answer: It is an inflammation of the soft tissue that surrounds the tendon.

5. Name the three main layers of tissue on the hand.
   Answer: Epidermis, dermis, subcutaneous fat.

6. In what part of the epidermis are new skin cells created?
   Answer: The basal layer.

7. Which layer is called the "true skin"?
   Answer: The dermis.

8. Which type of muscle do we have in our hands?
   Answer: Skeletal muscle.

9. Fat-filled cells are also called _____ cells.
   Answer: Adipose cells.

10. The carpal tunnel is created by a wide _____ that nearly encircles the wrist.
    Answer: Ligament.

11. Carpal tunnel syndrome is always preceded by which disorder?
    Answer: Tendonitis.

12. What is the best therapy for tendonitis?
    Answer: Ice therapy.

13. Muscles usually become torn by _____.
    Answer: Fatigue or overwork.

14. Name seven symptoms of cumulative trauma disorders.
    Answer: Pain, numbness, aching, stiffness, tingling, weakness, swelling.

15. How often is it recommended to stop and stretch to prevent cumulative trauma disorders?
    Answer: Every 30 minutes.

CHAPTER 4

1. Under most circumstances, nail techs should use __- to __-grit abrasives.
   Answer: 180- to 240-grit.

2. If the delicate tissue between the bed and plate is friction-burned by an abrasive, what nail condition could result?
   Answer: Onycholysis, which can increase the risk of infection.

3. Other than injury or illness, name four main causes of nail discoloration.
   Answer: Dyes, damage, drugs, age.

4. Toughness is the nail plate's ability to _____ cracks and breaks.
   Answer: Resist.

5. What nail products can cause pseudoleukonychia and why?
   Answer: Frequent use of substances such as nail polish remover can cause excessive dryness of the nail plate.

6. _____ is a condition that causes the nail plate to grow with an abnormally white appearance.
   Answer: True leukonychia.

7. What common natural dye can stain your nail plates brown?
   Answer: Henna.

8. How can damage to the nail bed cause brown spots under the nail plate?
   Answer: Damage causes a small amount of blood to ooze out and form a red spot under the plate.

9. Can oils moisturize the nail plate?
   Answer: No, oils can't moisturize the nail plate, because only water can be moisturizing. Oils can seal the surface so that moisture builds up underneath, thereby indirectly causing moisturization to occur.

10. How can excessive washing of your hands dry out nail plates?
    Answer: Cleaners, washes, soaps, shampoos, or detergents all work with water to strip essential oils from the nail plate, which can lead to dryness.

11. *Onycho-* is Latin for _____.
    Answer: Nail.

12. The calcium content of the nail is _____.
    Answer: Less than 0.1 percent.

13. *Leuk-* comes from the Latin word for _____.
    Answer: White.

14. Carbon monoxide poisoning causes nail beds to turn _____.
    Answer: Cherry red.

15. Where is bed epithelium found and what does it do?
    Answer: The rails attached to the underside of the nail plate are made of a specialized tissue called bed epithelium. They allow the nail plate to slide across the bed.

CHAPTER 5

1. What government department prohibits the sale of nonprescription products designed to treat fungus on the nail plate?
   Answer: The Food and Drug Administration (FDA).

2. Fungus eats _____ and bacteria eat _____ on the nail plate.
   Answer: Keratin, oil.

3. Interdigital fungal infections are found where on the feet?
   Answer: Between the toes.

4. What percentage of people with psoriasis have moderate to serious nail problems at some point during their lives?
   Answer: Approximately 90 percent.

5. If your client had been seriously ill three months ago, what symptoms would you expect to see in the nail?
   Answer: Beau's lines.

6. What nail condition could be caused by exposure to solvents or is inherited and can be seen in both mother and daughter?
   Answer: Spoon nails.

7. What nail products can cause pseudoleukonychia and why?
   Answer: Frequent use of nail polish remover can cause excessive dryness of the nail plate.

8. _____ is a condition that causes the nail plate to grow with an abnormally white appearance.
   Answer: True leukonychia.

9. What is the world's most common type of fungal foot infection?
   Answer: The interdigital form of athlete's foot (tinea pedis).

10. What effect do hot oil soaks have on parrot beak nails?
    Answer: None. Water soaks will cause them to straighten, but not oil soaks.

11. What type of foot infection covers the entire bottom of the foot and has a scaly, dry appearance?
    Answer: The moccasin form of athlete's foot (tinea pedis).

12. Warts are an example of pathogens that are _____. In other words, they take advantage of damaged, broken, or abraded skin to start infections.
    Answer: Opportunistic.

13. Which causes more fingernail infections, bacteria or fungus?
    Answer: Bacteria.

14. *Dorsal* means _____.
    Answer: Top side.

15. What is lichen planus?
    Answer: It is a reoccurring skin inflammation that forms tiny, itchy lesions on the wrist and arms.

CHAPTER 6

1. What is a chemical?
   Answer: Everything you can see or touch, except light and electricity (energy), is a chemical. All matter is chemical.

2. What is the difference between matter and energy?
   Answer: Matter occupies space and is made of chemicals; energy is not made of chemicals and doesn't take up any space.

3. What is a molecule?
   Answer: A molecule is a chemical substance in its simplest form.

4. What is the difference between vapors and fumes? Give an example of each.
   Answer: Vapors are formed when liquids evaporate into the air, such as water and solvents. Fumes are solid particles mixed with smoke, such as chimney smoke and welding fumes.

5. What is the cause of all odors in the salon air?
   Answer: All salon odors are caused by vapors in the air. Not fumes!

6. Give three reasons that explain why some vapors smell stronger than others.
   Answer: (1) There are a lot of the vapor's molecules in the air; that is, the substance is very volatile. (2) Because the nerves in the nose are very sensitive to the vapor molecule, even in extremely low amounts. (3) The person may have a smell aversion and think the odor is very strong.

7. Define and give an example of a chemical change.
   Answer: A chemical change occurs when a chemical changes into something different, such as sugar or paper burning.

8. Define and give an example of a physical change.
   Answer: Physical change only changes the outward appearance of the chemical, such as freezing water or dissolving sugar or salt in water.

9. What are catalysts? Why do you think they might be important to nail technicians?
   Answer: A catalyst is a chemical that changes the rate of a chemical reaction. They make a nail technician's work easier and faster. For example, the chemical reactions used to make artificial nail enhancements might take months to happen without a catalyst. A catalyst reduces the time to seconds or minutes.

10. Define solvents and solutes.
    Answer: A solvent is anything that dissolves another substance. The substance being dissolved is called a solute.

11. Why is it wasteful to use a saturated solvent?
    Answer: Solvents only dissolve a certain amount of solute before they become saturated. Then the solvent can no longer dissolve any additional solute. Using a saturated solvent wastes time and needlessly exposes the client's skin to solvents. It's like a sponge that's dripping with water.

12. What is an element and how many types of elements occur in nature? Why are they important?
    Answer: There are 88 naturally occurring elements. They are the building blocks of all molecules. Five of them are considered to be the building blocks of life.

13. What does *ppm* stand for? What is it used for?
    Answer: Parts per million. It is used to describe the amount of vapor molecules per million molecules of air. Note: Although the text didn't delve into this, ppm can also be used as a measure of contaminants in water.

14. What is a corrosive?
    Answer: A chemical that can quickly damage the skin upon contact. They usually have an extremely acid or extremely basic pH.

15. What type of products have no pH?
    Answer: Products that contain no water have no pH. A product must contain water in order to have a pH. pH is a measure of how much acid or base there is in a water-containing mixture.

CHAPTER 7

1. What causes adhesion?
   Answer: Adhesion develops when the molecules on one surface are attracted to the molecules on another surface.

2. If two surfaces are not compatible, they will _____ each other.
   Answer: Repel.

3. _____ are special ingredients that make liquids more compatible with solid surfaces.
   Answer: Wetting agents.

4. _____ are special ingredients that make solid surfaces more compatible with liquids.
   Answer: Primers.

5. What is the area between two adhered surfaces called?
   Answer: The adhesive bond.

6. Define delamination. How is it prevented?
   Answer: When two adhered surfaces peel away from each other it is called delamination. Properly cleaning the surface and correct product application techniques will help prevent delamination.

7. An _____ is a chemical that causes two surfaces to stick together.
   Answer: Adhesive.

8. List three types of artificial nail primer. Which are not corrosive?
   Answer: Acid-based, non-acid, and acid-free. Non-acid and acid-free are not corrosive.

9. Hydrogen bonds form _____ bonds while covalent bonds form _____ bonds.
   Answer: Temporary, permanent.

10. Is it necessary to rough up the nail plate to make high-quality, professional nail products adhere well to the nail plate? Explain why or why not.
    Answer: Scrubbing, properly dehydrating the nail plate, and avoiding skin contact will help ensure good adhesion. These steps, along with proper application technique, will prevent lifting. Roughing up the plate causes dangerous and excessive thinning of the natural nail. This must be avoided at all costs.

11. What causes the heat generated during heavy filing of the natural nail?
    Answer: Friction.

12. Why do nail dehydrators improve adhesion?
    Answer: Even if you thoroughly dry the nails, the surface of the plate will be covered with an invisible, ultra-thin layer of moisture that can block adhesion.

13. Explain how moisture in the nail affects nail polish adhesion.
    Answer: Moisture can build up underneath the coating, creating a "back pressure" that pushes the coating off the nail. Also, moisture-saturated nail plates can change shape when they dry and stretch the film until it breaks.

14. How long will the nail remain dry after nail dehydrators have been used?
    Answer: Up to 30 minutes.

15. Give two examples of an aggressive filing technique.
    Answer: Filing the natural nail with an abrasive under 180 grit, using an electric file on the natural nail, using a heavy downward pressure while filing.

CHAPTER 8

1. What are coatings? Name the two main types.
   Answer: Coatings cover the nail plate with a hard film and include nail polish, topcoats, base coats, treatments, artificial enhancements, and tip adhesives. The two types are (1) coatings that cure or polymerize and (2) coatings that harden upon evaporation.

2. Every type of product used to create nail enhancements does so by a chemical reaction called _____.
   Answer: Polymerization.

3. Polymers created by using two different monomers are called _____.
   Answer: Copolymers.

4. What are monomers and polymers? Define each and explain the differences.
   Answer: Many monomers hook together to make a long polymer chain. Each individual molecule is called a monomer. *Mono-* means "one," *poly-* means "many," and *-mer* means "unit." So polymers are made from many monomers.

5. What is the difference between a simple polymer and a cross-linked polymer?
   Answer: The head of one monomer reacts with the tail of another to create a long chain of monomers called a simple polymer. When many simple chains are hooked together with cross-linking monomers, a netlike structure is created. These polymers are cross-linked (like rungs on a ladder or a cargo net).

6. After the monomers react and a hard polymer is created, have all the chemical reactions finished? Explain your answer.
   Answer: The surface may be hard enough to file, but it will be days before the chains reach their ultimate lengths. So the chemical reaction (polymerization) isn't finished for quite some time. Note that the same is true for UV gels.

7. What are the main two sources of energy for initiator molecules?
   Answer: Light and heat. They are the only types of energy that are useful for making nail enhancements.

8. Why do polymers shrink when they are created?
   Answer: Monomers don't touch each other until they polymerize. After they polymerize they embrace each other tightly. When billions of monomers suddenly come closer together the effect is very noticeable. This is what we call shrinkage.

9. What is an exotherm? How can you tell when it is happening?
   Answer: The term means "heat releasing." This occurs when two monomers join and a small amount of heat is released. This is called an exotherm or exothermic reaction. You can't feel the heat released from two monomers, but the heat released from billions of monomers in the nail enhancement can be quite noticeable.

10. Do nail polishes and topcoats polymerize on the nail? Explain.
    Answer: No, they form coatings strictly by evaporation of solvents.

11. At what salon temperatures do artificial nail products work best?
    Answer: 68–77°F (20–25°C).

12. How can you tell if a product truly cures with UV light?
    Answer: The product will cross-link and will not be easily removed with solvent or removers.

13. Name three products that can cause high amounts of exotherm.
    Answer: Wraps, UV gels, and fast-set monomer systems.

14. How should nail enhancement product brushes be stored?
    Answer: Lay them flat and cover them to protect them from dust and other contaminants.

15. What is the largest container that should be used to refill your monomer dish?
    Answer: 4 ounces.

CHAPTER 9

1. What is the chemical family name for all nail enhancement coatings and tip adhesives?
   Answer: The acrylics.

2. What is a UV absorber and how does it work?
   Answer: UV absorbers are ingredients that prevent discoloration caused by sunlight (a major cause of yellowing). They do this by absorbing damaging UV light and changing it into less damaging blue light or heat.

3. In microns, how large are most polymer powder particles?
   Answer: Most polymer powder particles are around 50–80 microns. But they can be as large as 125 microns or as small as 10 microns (1/10th of a hair's thickness).

4. What effects do excessive amounts of monomer liquid have on nail enhancement durability?
   Answer: Excessive monomer reduces durability and leads to more breakage. The highest level of enhancement toughness is obtained when using the correct ratio of monomer to polymer. Too much monomer can also make the artificial nail more susceptible to discoloration.

5. Why are inhibitors used in nail enhancement products?
   Answer: Inhibitors are ingredients that prevent premature polymerizations. They extend shelf life and help prevent the monomer from gelling in the container.

6. Too _____ a consistency, using brushes that are too _____, or using the _____ polymer powder with the monomer liquid are some of the leading causes of allergic skin reactions to nail enhancement products.
   Answer: Wet, large or oversized, wrong or incorrect or mismatched.

7. When performing the bead test described in this chapter to test a bead mix ratio, describe what a medium bead should look like.
   Answer: The bead should melt out fairly slowly over 10 seconds and then should hold its domed shape. The overall height of the bead should drop a little, about one-quarter of the bead's original height. Also, there should be no ring of excess liquid monomer around the base of the bead. Its appearance could be described as "frosted glass."

8. Why shouldn't products based on methyl methacrylate monomer be used in the salon?
   Answer: MMA causes allergic reactions and can cause serious damage to nail plates if they are accidentally hit, jammed, or incorrectly applied. Problems also develop when the products are improperly removed. The FDA and many other governmental bodies, as well as nail associations, say you shouldn't use it.

9. What should you do if you suspect that someone is selling methyl methacrylate liquid monomer?
   Answer: Call the local state board immediately!

10. A medium-consistency mix ratio contains ___ parts liquid to _____ part powder.
    Answer: 1½, 1.

11. A _____ _____ is an ingredient that reduces brushstrokes and improves workability.
    Answer: Flow modifier.

12. How is MMA physically and chemically different from PMMA?
    Answer: MMA is a liquid monomer. PMMA is a solid polymer made from MMA monomers.

13. Bubbles in the artificial nail product that appeared after the product hardened are probably caused by _____ _____.
    Answer: Excessive shrinkage.

14. The curvature of the natural nail plate focuses the _____ _____ of shrinkage toward the apex.
    Answer: Stress forces.

15. The _____ the mix ratio, the _____ the shrinkage.
    Answer: Wetter, greater.

CHAPTER 10

1. Gel products are based on which family of monomers and oligomers?
   Answer: Monomers/oligomers are based on both the methacrylates and the acrylates—both from the acrylic family.

2. An _____ is a short chain of monomers that is not long enough to be a polymer.
   Answer: Oligomer.

3. List the five factors that determine the degree or percentage of cure in UV gel systems.
   Answer: Thickness of UV gel layer, color and opacity, UV bulb age and condition, position of hand and fingers under lamp, time the product spends curing under the lamp.

4. Which types of UV gels are the most difficult to properly cure?
   Answer: White and colored UV gels.

5. As a rule, every time you double the distance between you and a light source, the intensity drops by what percentage?
   Answer: 75 percent.

6. _____ absorb UV light and convert it into the energy needed for polymerization.
   Answer: Photoinitiators.

7. Which are more likely to cause skin allergies, UV gels, wrap resins, or tip adhesives?
   Answer: UV gels are most likely.

8. Which are less likely to cause skin allergies, UV gels, wrap resins, or tip adhesives?
   Answer: Wrap resins and nail adhesives are less likely.

9. Which type of nail enhancement product is best or safest for the natural nail?
   Answer: No type of nail enhancement product is better or safer for the nail plate than another.

10. What is the chemical name of the wrap resin monomer?
    Answer: Wrap resin monomers are called cyanoacrylates.

11. The initiator for wrap resins is _____.
    Answer: Water (moisture).

12. Which type of artificial nail enhancement product shrinks more: wrap resins or UV gels?
    Answer: Wrap resins.

13. Which is more susceptible to staining, wraps or UV gel nail enhancements?
    Answer: Wraps.

14. What should be done if skin becomes bonded together with wrap resins or nail adhesives?
    Answer: Never attempt to pry the skin apart. Use acetone to dissolve the bond and allow the skin to separate.

15. Name three important pieces of safety equipment required for working with wrap resins.
    Answer: Safety glasses, mist masks, and proper ventilation.

CHAPTER 11

1. What do the overexposure principle and Paracelsus's philosophy have in common?

   Answer: Both say that everything can be dangerous if you overexpose your-self to that substance and that reducing your exposure to safe levels will pro-tect you.

2. List at least five important pieces of information found on an MSDS.

   Answer: Potentially hazardous ingredients found in each product, proper storage, fire prevention and safe handling techniques, ways to prevent haz-ardous chemicals from entering your body, the short- and long-term health effects of overexposure, early warning signs of product overexposure, emer-gency first-aid advice, emergency phone numbers, safe handling techniques.

3. Name the routes of entry.

   Answer: (1) Inhalation of vapors, mists, and dusts, (2) absorption through the skin or broken tissue, (3) accidental or unintentional ingestion.

4. What is the least expensive and easiest way to help keep the vapors out of the salon's air?

   Answer: Keep caps on containers and empty trash often.

5. Why are dust masks ineffective against vapors?

   Answer: Vapors are hundreds of times smaller than dust particles.

6. Name five potential symptoms of chemical overexposure.

   Answer: Overexposure can cause headaches, nausea, angry or frustrated feelings, nosebleeds, coughs, dizziness, tingling fingers and toes, dry or scratchy nose and throat, puffy or red and irritated skin, itching, and many other symptoms.

7. To work safely with chemicals you must lower your _____ to _____ levels.

   Answer: Exposure, safe.

8. What percentage of chemicals in the world are never toxic under any cir-cumstances?

   Answer: 0 percent; all substances can be toxic.

9. Are natural substances safer? Explain.

   Answer: No, natural simply means from nature. Nature is a dangerous place filled with potentially harmful substances.

10. What should you do before flying on an airplane with a large amount of flam-mable products?

    Answer: Check airline regulations.

11. Paracelsus said, "All substances are _____; there is none which is not a _____. Only the right dose differentiates a _____ and a remedy."

    Answer: Poison.

12. _____ solvents are quickly evaporating.
    Answer: Volatile.

13. Give three examples of things that are not organic.
    Answer: Rocks, sand, metals, water, air.

14. Products that are sensitive to UV light should be stored in a _____ location.
    Answer: Dark or out of sunlight.

15. Can clients wear nail enhancements during pregnancy?
    Answer: Yes, they can safely wear artificial nails or polish.

CHAPTER 12

1. What is the most common occupational disease in America?
   Answer: Skin disease.

2. Which is more dangerous to the skin, irritants or corrosives? Why?
   Answer: Not all irritants are corrosive. Corrosives can cause permanent and irreversible damage. Skin irritations (from non-corrosives) will usually disappear when overexposure to the irritant discontinues.

3. Will an ingredient allergy ever go away?
   Answer: Allergies are for life. Once a person is allergic to a substance, he or she is always allergic to that substance.

4. Name two common salon irritants.
   Answer: Water and methacrylic acid primer.

5. Allergic contact dermatitis accounts for _____ percent of cosmetic-related skin problems.
   Answer: 80 percent.

6. What is the best type of disposable glove for nail salons?
   Answer: Nitrile.

7. Why can overly large brushes create skin overexposure?
   Answer: The belly of large brushes contains excessive amounts of monomer liquid and they create overly wet beads. The excess liquid monomer can run into the nail folds and cause skin overexposure. Also, it is nearly impossible to control the mix ratio with these brushes.

8. The substance that causes the allergy is called a _____ or _____.
   Answer: Sensitizer or allergen.

9. What is the best way to avoid allergic reactions and irritations?
   Answer: Avoid prolonged and repeated contact or overexposing the skin to products that are not designed for skin contact.

10. What causes the inhibition layer on top of cured UV gels?
    Answer: Oxygen in the air prevents the gel from hardening on the surface.

11. What two natural ingredients cause most latex glove allergies?
    Answer: Cornstarch powder and proteins found in the rubber used to make latex.

12. How much formaldehyde is found in professional nail enamels containing tosylamide/formaldehyde resin? Can this make clients become sensitive to formaldehyde?
    Answer: Approximately 0.002 percent formaldehyde. There is not enough to cause overexposure under normal circumstances. Clients who are sensitive to nail polish probably first became allergic to formaldehyde-containing nail hardeners.

13. What are the risks of using formaldehyde nail hardeners excessively or improperly?
    Answer: Excessive use of formaldehyde nail hardeners can make nails appear dry and become brittle. It also increases the risk of overexposure and skin allergy.

14. What are the only valid tests for skin allergies?
    Answer: Patch testing, scratch, prick, and RAST.

15. What Internet site will give you the latest information on medical scams?
    Answer: Quackwatch.com.

CHAPTER 13

1. Besides pathogens, name something else that's considered a contaminant in salons.
   Answer: Any visible debris, hair, dust, oil, food, etc.

2. Up to what percentage of contaminants are washed from a surface by proper sanitation alone?
   Answer: 99 percent.

3. How long should you wash your hands if they become heavily contaminated?
   Answer: 60 seconds using a brush.

4. Give two reasons why it's so important to rinse your hands thoroughly and use lukewarm water.
   Answer: Hot water and soap residue can irritate skin.

5. Why are pedicure clients with freshly shaved legs more susceptible to skin infection?
   Answer: Tiny razor nicks provide an opportunity for pathogens to invade the skin and begin to grow.

6. _____, _____, and _____ are three highly effective disinfectants that do not require EPA registration numbers.
   Answer: Bleach, isopropyl alcohol, ethyl alcohol.

7. Quats are both good disinfectants as well as good _____.
   Answer: Cleaning agents.

8. If you cut a client's skin with an abrasive file, what two things should you do?
   Answer: Seal the abrasive in a plastic bag and dispose of it.

9. Why are monomer liquids and nail polish considered to be self-disinfecting?
   Answer: Because pathogens cannot live or grow inside of these products.

10. Name two disinfectants that are not safe for use in the professional salon.
    Answer: Formaldehyde (formalin) and glutaraldehyde.

11. Give an example of a brush used in a salon service that must be disinfected.
    Answer: A nail oil brush.

12. Give two examples of a brush used in salon services that do not require disinfection.
    Answer: Brushes used to apply acrylics, UV gels, primers, nail dehydrators, and polishes.

13. Does an FDA registration ensure that a product will work as promised by the manufacturer? Explain your answer.
    Answer: No, the FDA does not certify cosmetics, cosmetic devices, or implements.

14. If an alcohol hand sanitizer is used, are your hands clean? Explain your answer.
    Answer: No, hands must be washed to remove contaminants. Alcohol does not remove contaminants. It kills pathogens.

15. Is HIV, hepatitis, or tuberculosis transmitted by salon services?
    Answer: No, not a chance!

CHAPTER 14

1. _____ is a condition where your nose can no longer smell certain strong odors.
   Answer: Olfactory fatigue.

2. Your _____ is an invisible sphere about twice the size of a basketball.
   Answer: Breathing zone.

3. Never use a _____ without a lid.
   Answer: Dappen dish.

4. How are fumes different from vapors?
   Answer: Vapors are made from the evaporation of liquids. Fumes are created by burning substances.

5. If you no longer smell strong odors in the salon, you may be suffering from _____.
   Answer: Olfactory fatigue.

6. Should you try to purify the air in the salon?
   Answer: No, it would be practically impossible. Instead, lower air contaminants to safe levels.

7. Why can't we smell certain types of vapors?
   Answer: Their molecules are too large.

8. What two important factors help the brain determine the odor of a vapor molecule?
   Answer: The molecule's shape and size.

9. Why should you wipe your brush on a disposable pad instead of your table towel?
   Answer: Wiping your brush on a table towel puts monomer vapors into the air. If you use a pad, you can throw the pad into a closed waste container and minimize vapors.

10. Why is it important to empty the salon's waste cans throughout the day?
    Answer: Vapors will escape from the waste can into the salon air. These vapors can increase the amount of contaminants in your breathing zone. Also, some salon chemicals are flammable. Trash cans left in the salon overnight are a potential fire risk.

11. If the air smells funny in the salon, why not just use aromatherapy oil or perfume?
    Answer: You can't improve the air quality by putting nice-smelling vapors into the air to cover up the bad-smelling ones.

12. Why not use a wide-mouth dappen dish to hold your monomer liquid?
    Answer: Compared to a dish with a ½-inch opening, a 2-inch opening creates 16 times more vapor and a 3-inch opening creates 36 times more vapor.

13. Is it all right to fill your dappen dish from a 16-ounce bottle of monomer liquid?
    Answer: No, you should only fill dappen dishes from a small container of monomer liquid (4 ounces) to prevent excessive evaporation of the product.

14. Name three disadvantages of leaving caps off of your products for too long.
    Answer: More vapors escape into the air, the product will have a shorter shelf life, and the product might not work correctly.

15. Which is it more important to remove from the salon air, vapors or odors?
    Answer: Vapors. If you remove vapors, you'll remove odors. But if you remove all odors you could still have large amounts of vapors in the air.

CHAPTER 15

1. What is the most effective way to prevent inhalation overexposure to dusts in the salon air?
   Answer: Wear a dust mask.

2. What is a microfilter?
   Answer: Microfilters are highly effective air filters that do not meet the highest HEPA standards. Even so, for some applications such as disposable dust masks, they are the filters of choice.

3. What does HVAC stand for?
   Answer: Heating, ventilation, and air-conditioning.

4. What is the most important job of a good ventilation system?
   Answer: It must keep breathing zones clean.

5. What are the risks of using ozone generators?
   Answer: Even at low concentrations, ozone causes eye, throat, and lung irritation and/or allergy and asthma-like symptoms.

6. Are HEPA filters useful for controlling vapors? Why?
   Answer: No, the biggest vapor molecule is hundreds of times smaller than tiniest dust particles. Vapors whiz right through a HEPA filter.

7. What is the difference between general exhaust and local exhaust?
   Answer: General exhaust brings fresh air into a room and pulls out stale air. Local exhaust captures vapors, mists, and dust at the source and expels them from your breathing zone.

8. What can happen if activated charcoal filters are overused and become saturated with flammable vapors?
   Answer: It may create a fire hazard.

9. Roof exhaust ducts must be __ feet higher than air intake vents within __ feet.
   Answer: 10 feet, 50 feet.

10. _____ is like a chemical sponge.
    Answer: Activated charcoal.

11. _____ _____ can be used to track the flow of salon air.
    Answer: Smoke powder.

12. What effect do ionizers and HEPA filters have on vapors in the air?
    Answer: Absolutely no effect.

13. A level of __–__ percent humidity is the best range for indoor air.
    Answer: 30–55 percent.

14. Name the condition caused by improperly cleaned or maintained humidifiers.
    Answer: Humidifier fever or humidifier lung.

15. What is the importance of an EPA registration number on devices such as ozone-generating air cleaners?
    Answer: This number helps the EPA identify the specific facility where the product was made. It is not an EPA endorsement, nor does it suggest in any way that the EPA has found this product to be either safe or effective.

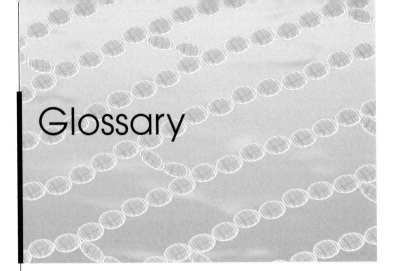

Glossary

Absorption: The movement (migration) of a liquid or gas into a solid substance.

Acid-based: Term referring to primers that contain methacrylic acid.

Acid-free: Primers that contain absolutely no acid components at all.

Acids: Substances with a pH between 0 and 7.

Acrylates: A category of substances belonging to the acrylic family (*see* Acrylics).

Acrylics: A special family of monomers and/or oligomers used to create artificial nail products, including wraps, UV gels, and liquid/powder systems.

Activated charcoal (activated carbon): A substance that can act as a chemical sponge to absorb many types of vapors and impurities from water or air.

Acute effects: Refers to the short-term effects or early warning signs of over-exposure.

Adhesion: A force of nature that causes two surfaces to stick together.

Adhesive: A substance that causes two surfaces to stick together.

Adhesive bond: The small area between two adhered surfaces.

Adipose cells: Fat-filled cells found in the subcutaneous fat layer of skin tissue.

Air balance: The flow of air into or out of the salon.

Air blowers: Designed to move air through ventilation ducts.

Alkaline: *See* Bases

Allergen (sensitizer): A substance causing an allergy, such as pollen.

Allergic contact dermatitis: A condition of heightened immune sensitivity to a particular ingredient.

Aluminum oxide: An abrasive used on nail files.

Amino acids: The building blocks of nature, used to create proteins.

Antagonistic pair: Term used to describe muscles that work together, such as the triceps and biceps.

Antiseptic: Solution designed to prevent infection when skin is cut or damaged.

Apex: The highest point on the nail plate.

Arteries: Blood vessels that carry blood from the heart to many parts of the body, including the fingernail.

Association of Electric File Manufacturers (AEFM): Organization that can help nail technicians find basic electric file training courses, as well as advanced courses for those who wish to further develop their skills.

Athlete's foot (tinea pedis): The most common type of skin infection on the feet.

Autoclaves: Devices used by hospitals to sterilize through the use of highly pressurized steam and powerful disinfectants.

Bacteria: One-celled living organisms that are the biggest cause of fingernail infections.

Bactericidal: Demonstrating the ability to kill bacteria.

Basal layer: The bottom layer of the epidermis, where new skin cells are created.

Bases: Substances with a pH between 7 and 14.

Beau's lines: Depressions or valleys stretching across the width of the nail plate, occurring when nail plate growth is temporarily slowed or halted.

Bed epithelium: A sticky tissue that adheres tightly to the bottom of the nail plate.

Benzoyl peroxide: An initiator used to energize monomers and cause polymerization to occur.

Blood vessels: Small tubes that nourish tissue cells by carrying the food and oxygen needed for growth and reproduction and that remove waste products.

Bones: Give the hand and fingers their structure and supporting framework.

Breathing zone: An invisible sphere about twice the size of a basketball that sits in front of your face. Every breath you take comes from this area.

Brittleness: A condition that causes nail plates to break, crack, or fracture.

Capillaries: Tiny branches in the blood vessels that carry blood to the matrix and nail bed.

Carpal tunnel syndrome: Most common type of cumulative trauma disorder, characterized by pressure on the tendons and nerves in the carpal tunnel.

Catalyst: A substance that changes the rate at which a chemical reaction will occur, making it go faster or slower.

Chemical change: The alteration of matter through chemical reaction.

Chemically organic: Substances with a chemical structure comprised chiefly of the element carbon. According to this definition, all living things are "organic." Governmental regulations for agricultural practices and consumer foods sometimes create more restricted definitions that do not apply to this term.

Chemical reaction: When two or more molecules interact to create a new and different molecule.

Chemicals: Everything you can see or touch, except light and electricity.

Chemophobia: The irrational fear of chemicals.

Chronic effects: Long-term effects of overexposure or misuse, usually occurring after six months or more of overexposure.

Chronic inflammatory pain cycle: Recurrent pain from a cumulative trauma disorder.

Chronic paronychia: A long-lasting bacterial infection causing redness and swelling of the nail fold area.

Class S vacuum cleaners: Term used in Europe to describe vacuum cleaners with HEPA-quality filters.

Clubbing: A condition occurring when blood vessels in the nail bed become enlarged, resulting in a nail plate with an extreme degree of curvature.

Coating: A generic term for any product that covers the nail plate with a hard film. Examples include nail polish, topcoats, base coats, treatments, artificial enhancements, and tip adhesives.

Consistency: The amount of polymer powder mixed with the monomer liquid, also known as the mix ratio.

Contact dermatitis: Inflammation of the skin caused by touching certain substances to the skin.

Copolymers: Polymers made from two different types of monomers.

Corrosives: Severe irritants that can cause rapid, visible, and sometimes irreversible skin damage.

Cosmetic Ingredient Review (CIR): A highly prestigious independent expert panel that renders opinions on the safety of cosmetic ingredients.

Covalent bonds: Special chemical bonds created between two molecules. They are the strongest type of chemical bond.

Cross-link: A link between two polymer chains. In artificial nails, their function is to create strong, netlike polymer structures out of weaker, stringlike polymers.

Cross-linker: A monomer that can join different polymer chains together.

Crystalline: Having a structure that is very orderly and arranged.

Cumulative trauma disorders (CTDs): The fastest-growing type of occupation-related injury involving inflammation of tissues. Each can cause painful and crippling illness that may be permanent if not treated properly.

Cure: A chemical reaction that converts artificial nail products into hardened artificial nail enhancements.

Cuticle: Thin layer of colorless dead tissue between the eponychium and the nail plate, forming a seal to keep pathogens from infecting the matrix area.

Cyanoacrylates: A branch of the acrylic family (*see* Acrylics). The monomers from this branch are primarily used as wraps, no-light gels, and tip adhesives.

Cysteine: A type of amino acid that forms cross-links. Cysteine forms the sulfur cross-links in hair that make it curly.

Decontamination: A process that removes harmful pathogens and visible debris from implements or other surfaces.

Dehumidifier: A device that dries the air by pulling moisture from the air and depositing it in a holding tank or reservoir for disposal.

Delamination: A process that involves the separation of two or more layers, such as the separation of the natural nail plate into thin sheets or layers.

Dermatitis: A condition with symptoms such as dry, itchy, or inflamed skin.

Dermis: The lower layer of skin, located between the epidermis (above) and the subcutaneous fat layer (below).

Desmosomes: Ringlike junctions that act like tiny rivets between two nail cells.

Diffusion: A process that describes how molecules move through different substances, such as liquids being absorbed through a solid substance, vapors moving through air, or colored dye spreading out in water.

Disinfectant container: A term used to describe any container used to disinfect salon implements.

Disinfection: A process that, when properly performed, kills all living pathogens on a surface after it has been properly sanitized.

Distal nail plate: The part of the nail plate that grows beyond the free edge of the fingertip.

Dorsal pterygium: An abnormal growth of skin on the top surface of the nail plate.

Durability: A property of tough materials that occurs when strength and flexibility are properly balanced and maintained.

Dust/mist masks: Masks specially designed to provide protection from both dusts and mists. These masks are thicker and better-fitting on the face. They will not block vapors and are not a replacement for proper ventilation.

Dyes: Substances that fully dissolve into cosmetic formulations to impart a color.

Electrostatic air filters: Filters used with furnaces and air-conditioning to improve air quality for general ventilation systems.

Elements: The basic building blocks of all matter, such as carbon, oxygen, hydrogen, nitrogen, sulfur, helium, gold, silver, and so on. There are 88 naturally occurring elements.

Energy: Has no substance, is not made of matter, and is the only thing that is not made of chemicals.

EPA registration number: Official registration numbers given by the Environmental Protection Agency to disinfection products that successfully pass a series of tests designed to prove their effectiveness.

Epidermis: The top, translucent layer of skin tissue that covers the body and sits on top of the dermis. It is this upper layer that you shed when the skin is exfoliating. In the case of natural nails, it is the upper layer of the nail bed.

Eponychium: The area of living skin that borders the base of the nail plate and usually covers all of the nail matrix except the lunula.

Ethyl methacrylate (EMA): The most widely used monomer in the nail industry and the ingredient of choice for liquid/powder systems.

Exotherm: The heat produced when monomers and/or oligomers polymerize (form polymers).

Exothermic: A term that means "heat-releasing."

Exothermic reaction: A chemical reaction that produces heat, such as when two monomers or oligomers are joined together.

Extensor: Muscle that allows arms, legs, et cetera to straighten or extend. An example is the triceps.

Fibrils: Tiny fibers created by dozens of coiled keratin strands stacked neatly into tight bundles.

Film former: Ingredients used to create a continuous coating on the nail plate, such as nitrocellulose.

Flexibility: The property that allows a substance to band without suffering damaging cracks or breaks.

Flexor: Muscles that are needed to flex or bend a joint, such as the biceps.

Flow modifier: An ingredient used to change the way a product spreads or moves.

Formaldehyde: A reactive chemical ingredient often used to cross-link nail keratin to improve hardness, but due to its inherent instability this ingredient must be stabilized (*see also* Formalin).

Formalin: A stabilized form of formaldehyde that is used in nail hardener products.

Free edge: The part of the nail plate that extends beyond the fingertip.

Free radical: Highly energetic molecules that can trigger many types of chemical reactions.

Fumes: Tiny, solid particles suspended in gases. Examples include car exhaust, smoke from chimneys, and welding fumes.

Fungi: Plural form of fungus.

Fungicidal: Demonstrating the ability to kill fungi.

Fungus: Parasitic organisms that cause infection. Fungi belong to their own kingdom of organisms, which includes yeast, molds, smuts, and mushrooms, and reproduce by forming spores. Not all forms or types of fungus can cause infections in humans.

Gelling: Partial, premature polymerization of monomer liquids, UV gels, wraps, or adhesives while they are still in their original container. Inhibitors are often put in these products to prevent this from occurring and thereby extend a product's shelf life.

General ventilation: Ventilation systems designed to exchange old, stale air with new, fresh air while maintaining the room temperature.

Glues: A type of adhesive made from plants or animal parts.

Glutaraldehyde: Disinfectant that is neither safe nor appropriate for salon use. Skin contact with the liquid or inhalation of the vapors can cause serious allergic reactions and breathing difficulties.

Guardian seal: A fold of skin pushing up against the nail plate and creating a tight seal that prevents bacteria and chemicals from getting underneath.

Hardness: Resistance of a substance to being scratched or dented.

Heating, ventilating, and air-conditioning (HVAC): Experts who can give advice on how to improve air quality and better control the salon environment.

HEPA filters: High-efficiency particle filters that remove the tiniest floating dusts and pollens from the air.

HEPA-rated vacuum cleaners: Specially designed to have leakproof seals and collection bags to provide a dramatic improvement over conventional vacuum cleaners, which can leak large amounts of dusts back into the room.

Hepatitis: A disease that does not pose any significant risk of transmission by salon implements or services. Hepatitis A is transmitted in foods, whereas other forms (B, C, D, etc.) are bloodborne.

Histamines: Substances that cause the blood vessels around the injured tissue to enlarge.

HIV: The virus that causes acquired immune deficiency syndrome (AIDS).

Hives: Smooth, slightly elevated area on the skin. Also sometimes referred to as *wheals* or *welts*.

Humidifier: Designed to evaporate moisture into dry air and increase the humidity.

Humidifier fever (humidifier lung): Caused by improperly cleaned and maintained humidifiers. Typical symptoms are flulike, with fever, chills, loss of appetite, headache, and cough.

Humidity: The amount of moisture in the air.

Hyponychium: The seal of living tissue between the nail plate in the nail bed. One of the guardian seals.

Immune response: The reaction of the immune system to protect the body from foreign substances.

Infrared light: The light energy level just beneath the red on the color spectrum. This type of light cannot be seen by the human eye but is felt on the skin as heat.

Ingestion: A route of entry that allows substances to enter your body by unintentional or accidental swallowing.

Inhalation: A route of entry that allows chemical substances to enter your body by breathing vapors, mists, or dusts.

Inhibition layer: A gooey layer on freshly cured artificial nails that is caused when oxygen prevents proper surface curing.

Inhibitors: Ingredients that prevent monomers and/or oligomers from prematurely hardening (gelling) while still in the original container.

Initiator: A molecule that absorbs extra energy and uses it to cause chemical reactions to occur.

Interdigital infections: Fungal infections that occur between the toes.

Interface: Where two surfaces meet and touch.

Inverse pterygium: An abnormal growth of skin under the free edge of the nail plate.

Involuntary muscles: Muscles not under voluntary control, including cardiac and smooth muscles.

Irritant contact dermatitis: A skin condition caused by exposure to substances that are damaging to the skin.

Keratin: A super-tough protein made in the nail matrix. It is a main component in the natural nail's structure.

Keratin cells: The building blocks that create the layers of the nail plate.

Keratin strand: Long-chain protein usually containing 300 to 500 amino acids linked together.

Lateral fissures: Small cracks in the nail plate caused when the free edge is sharply impacted.

Lateral nail folds: The two skin folds that form tight seals along the sidewalls of the nail plate.

Leukonychia: Any condition that causes abnormal whitening of the nail plate.

Leukonychia spots: Large groups of immature nail cells trapped inside the nail, usually because of a previous injury to the nail matrix.

Lichen planus: A recurring skin inflammation that forms small, itchy lesions on the wrists, arms, and elsewhere.

Ligaments: Specialized tissues that link bone to bone.

Load: Forces exerted on artificial or natural nails that may cause damage if they become excessive.

Local exhaust: Systems that capture and control vapors, dusts, and mists right at the source, so that they never escape into the salon air.

Lunula: A bluish-white, opaque area that is visible through the nail plate. This area is the front part of the nail matrix.

Material Safety Data Sheets (MSDS): Documents that provide valuable safety and storage information to product users. Each MSDS contains information on safe handling, first aid, emergency response, early warning signs of overexposure and ventilation, and other topics.

Matrix: A small area of living tissue directly below the eponychium where nail cells are created.

Matter: Anything that takes up space or occupies an area; all solids, liquids, or gases.

Melting range: The range over which a solid substance will melt into a liquid. A narrow range is 1–2°, a broad range is 3–10°, and a very broad range is 11–50°.

Methacrylates: A category of substances belonging to the acrylic family (*see* Acrylics).

Methacrylic acid: An acidic and corrosive substance used in most types of acid-based nail primers.

Methyl methacrylate (MMA): A monomer that is prohibited by many state and government regulations since it creates too much damage to the natural nail when used in high concentrations as an artificial nail enhancement.

Methyl methacrylate polymer (PMMA): A solid polymer substance that has very different chemical and physical properties than MMA monomer. This substance is not harmful to the natural nail, nor is it the same substance that is prohibited by many state and government regulations.

Microfilters: Highly efficient air filters that make excellent pre-filters for air conditioners and heating systems.

Microns: A unit of measure for very small items; a thick human hair is about 100 microns in diameter.

Microorganisms: Microscopic living creatures such as bacteria, fungi, and viruses.

Mildew: Term that is sometimes incorrectly used to describe infections of the nail plate, but mildew is not likely to cause nail plate infections.

Mists: Tiny liquid droplets that are temporarily suspended in the air.

Mix ratio: The amount of polymer powder mixed with the monomer liquid; also known as *consistency*.

Moccasin: The most common form of athlete's foot. Covers the entire bottom of the foot. Usually the skin is scaly with a dry appearance.

Mold: Term that is sometimes incorrectly used to describe infections of the nail plate, but mold is not likely to cause nail plate infections.

Monomers: Molecules that can join together to create polymer chains.

Mucoid cysts: A large, mucus-filled lump that is usually found under the eponychium.

N95-certified: A certification given to masks that have been tested and shown to have vastly superior abilities (when compared to standard masks) to filter dusts from the air.

Nail bed: An area of pinkish tissue that supports the entire nail plate.

Nail plate: The hard keratin structure growing over the tip of the finger or toe.

Nail unit: Each of your finger- or toenails can be divided into several major sections. Each of these separate parts cooperates with the others to form the nail unit.

Natural: Occurs in nature. Does not mean a product is safe, wholesome, or better.

Natural nail: Also known as the nail plate.

Negative air balance: A situation in which the air pressure inside the salon or room is less than outside, causing the outside air to flow into the salon.

Negative ions: Ions create a staticlike charge on dust, soot, pollen, animal dander, and other small, solid particles, causing them to clump together in clusters.

Nerve endings: Nerves that end near the skin's surface; they are highly sensitive and able to create sensations such as pain, pressure, and warmth.

Nerve fibers: Nerves that carry sensations from the sensitive nerve endings all the way to the brain for processing.

Nerves: Provide the sensations of touch, pain, and warmth, and stimulate movement in the muscles in the fingers and hands.

Nitrocellulose: A naturally occurring simple polymer that produces very hard shiny surfaces in nail polish and treatments.

Non-acid: Primers that actually do contain an acid, but not methacrylic acid; they are based on other, less corrosive or non-corrosive acids.

Noncrystalline: Having a structure that is less orderly and more random.

Odorless: Term used when vapors have odors that are difficult to smell.

Odors: Sensations that result when specialized cells in the nose (olfactory glands) are stimulated by particular chemicals in gaseous form.

Olfactory fatigue: A condition that occurs when the olfactory glands are overwhelmed by certain smells and quit detecting them.

Olfactory glands: A concentrated area of olfactory nerves that is located in the nose.

Olfactory nerve: Smelling cells in the nose use this nerve to send messages directly to the brain.

Oligomers: Short chains of monomers that are usually very thick and/or stringy and often have a gel-like appearance.

Onychodermal band: A narrow band of bunched-up tissue located behind the hyponychium. This band proves the ability of the hyponychium to prevent pathogens from infecting the nail bed.

Onycholysis: A condition in which the nail plate and bed become detached and separate to form a small space under the nail plate.

Opportunistic pathogens: Disease-causing microorganisms that invade and grow in damaged, broken, irritated, or abraded tissue.

Optical brightener: Ingredient used to make colors look brighter.

Organic: Carbon-containing substances. All living things are organic.

Outdoor venting system: These systems vent the air outdoors instead of back into the salon.

Overexposure principle: Principle stating that every chemical has a safe and unsafe level of exposure and that you won't be harmed unless you repeatedly exceed the safe levels.

Ozone: A potentially dangerous substance (to inhale) that chemically reacts with certain vapor molecules and converts them into new and different substances, usually with a lower or different odor.

Paronychia: Bacterial infection causing redness, swelling, and tenderness of the eponychium and/or lateral sidewalls.

Parrot beak nails: Nails with extreme curvatures that go in the opposite direction of spoon nails.

Parts per million (ppm): A measurement that is often used to show the level of contamination found in air or water.

Patch testing: The most medically reliable method for identifying skin allergens. A tiny amount of the suspected allergen is diluted, applied to a small spot on the skin, and covered with a bandage. After a fixed period of time (24–48 hours), the exposed site is examined to determine if a skin reaction has occurred.

Pathogen: Any microorganism that causes disease or illness in humans.

Permeability: The ease by which a liquid or gas moves through a porous substance.

Phalanges: The fingertip bones, which determine the overall length, shape, curvature, and spread of the nail unit.

Phenolics: A type of chemical substance used to disinfect salon implements.

Photoinitiators: Ingredients that absorb light (usually UV) and convert it into the energy needed to drive the polymerization process.

pH scale: A scale (0-14) used to measure the amount of acid or base in water mixtures.

Physical change: An alteration in the physical appearance of a substance.

Pigments: Insoluble, finely ground substances that are used in cosmetics to impart a color.

Plasticizers: Additives that can improve the flexibility of solid substances, including both artificial and natural nails.

Polish thinners: Solvents used to combat the premature thickening of nail polish and treatments.

Polymerization: A chain reaction between monomers and/or oligomers that produces a hardened artificial nail or adhesives. Also referred to as *cure* or *curing*.

Polymers: Very long chains of individual molecules that have been chemically linked together.

Polypeptides: Many amino acid molecules linked together into polymer chains.

Porosity: The measure of how many voids or spaces there are in a solid substance. The more voids, the greater the porosity.

Positive air balance: The air pressure inside the salon or room is greater than the pressure outside, causing air to flow out of the salon.

Primers: Substances used to modify the surface of the natural nail to improve adhesion.

Proteins: Naturally occurring polymers formed from amino acids.

Proximal nail fold: The part of the eponychium where the skin meets the emerging nail plate.

Pseudoleukonychia: Condition caused by stripping oils or moisturizer from the nail plate, causing surface layers to develop a dried-out, white, or flaky appearance.

Psoriasis: A chronic skin condition characterized by inflamed, red, raised areas that develop silvery scales. This disease also causes pitting, splitting, and discoloration of the nail plate.

Pterygium: Any abnormal, winglike structure of skin.

Quaternary ammonium compounds (quats): A commonly used type of salon disinfectant that is relatively safe and very effective.

Resin: Any solid or semisolid polymer (natural or synthetic) that melts over a broad temperature range.

Room air cleaning units: Units designed to remove air contaminants from a room.

Routes of entry: A passageway for chemical substances to gain entry into the body. There are three such routes: inhalation, absorption, and ingestion.

Salmon patches: Dark yellow to red patches appearing on the nail plate that are usually caused by psoriasis.

Sanitation: A procedure that leads to proper and thorough cleaning of an object or surface.

Saturated: A solvent that is unable to dissolve any more solute.

Scanning electron microscope (SEM): Highly advanced scientific tool used to greatly magnify images.

Self-disinfecting: Products that prevent the growth of bacteria, viruses, or fungi.

Sensitization: The process of developing an allergy to a particular substance.

Sensitizer (allergen): A substance causing an allergy, such as pollen.

Serrations: Ragged appearance of the free edge of the natural nail plate.

Sick building syndrome: Occurs in offices and buildings across the country as a result of chemicals escaping from building materials or office supplies. Symptoms range from sore eyes, fatigue, dermatitis, headaches, and nausea to coughing or frequent lung and throat irritations.

Silicon carbide: A crystalline mineral used on nail abrasives because it is inexpensive and nearly as hard as diamond.

Simple polymer: Non-cross-linked polymers that form into single chains.

Smell aversion: A fairly common occurrence where a person develops a strong dislike of a particular smell, even though the vapor may be perfectly safe to breathe.

Smoke powders: Extremely fine white powders used for testing ventilation.

Solehorn: A thin layer of cloudy, yellowish tissue that can be seen closely by examining the underside of the free edge.

Solute: A substance that is dissolved by a solvent.

Solvent: A substance, usually a liquid, in which other substances are dissolved. The most common solvent is water.

Splinter hemorrhages: Red areas or spots of blood under the nail plate, usually caused by some trauma or damage to the nail bed.

Spoon nails: An abnormally large upward curvature of the nail plate.

Spores: A highly resistant form of bacteria or fungi that are coated with a waxy, protective layer, making them difficult to kill with disinfectants. Once they become reactivated, spores develop into their mature form and may cause infections or create new spores.

Sterilization: Use of very high temperatures and pressurized steam to kill pathogens.

Strength: The ability to resist breaking under a heavy load.

Structural protein: A protein that creates a hardened or solid structure, such as the keratin found in hair and fingernail plates.

Subcutaneous fat: A layer of fatty tissue located under the dermis and containing large blood vessels and nerves.

Sulfur cross-links: Specialized linkages between two strands of protein. In hair and nails the amino acid cysteine is responsible for these linkages.

Surfactants: The cleansing agents used in shampoos, hand and body washes, and other products. Also used in low amounts as wetting agents to improve adhesion.

Suspension agents: Finely ground clays or polymers that are added to products to prevent solid particles from settling.

TAF resin: A special copolymer used to improve adhesion and toughen nail polish and treatments.

Tendonitis: A painful condition caused by microscopic tears in overfatigued muscles. Symptoms include inflammation and swelling, especially around joints.

Tendons: Thick, inflexible bands of fibrous tissue that link muscles to bones.

Thixotropic: A property that allows certain full-bodied liquids, such as nail polish, to become thinner when shaken, mixed, or stirred.

Toughness: A property of materials that depends on a balance of strength and flexibility.

Transverse fissures: Small cracks in the stress area of a nail plate that is severely bent.

True leukonychia: A fairly rare condition in which the nail plate may turn completely white and opaque or may have an opaque white band running the entire length of the nail.

Tuberculosis: Bacterial infection of the lungs that is only transmitted by coughing and inhaling the bacteria.

Ultraviolet (UV) light : The energy level of the light that is directly above violet in the color spectrum. This type of light cannot be seen by the human eye.

Universal sanitation: Concept stating that salons should always be clean, sanitary, and presentable.

UV light absorbers: Special ingredients that absorb UV light and convert it into harmless blue light and heat (infrared energy), thereby preventing discoloration or damage to the nail coating.

Vapor: A form of matter created when liquids evaporate into the air.

Vaporization: The process by which a liquid changes into a vapor.

Veins: Vessels that collect blood from the capillaries and return it to the heart.

Ventilation ducts: Tubing or enclosed channels that move fresh air in and out of the salon.

Virucidal: Demonstrating the ability to kill viruses.

Virus: Extremely simple and extremely small type of parasite that infects plants, animals, and bacteria and often cause disease. They are unable to reproduce unless they invade a host cell to use it as an incubator to create copies of themselves. Because of this, viruses are not considered living organisms.

Visible spectrum: The colors of the rainbow that make up sunlight.

Voids: Large, irregularly shaped bubbles that can appear almost anywhere in solid substances, including artificial nails.

Volatile: Quickly evaporating.

Voluntary control: The ability to move muscles at will.

Wattage: The amount of electrical power that an electrical device (such as a lightbulb) will consume.

Wear resistance: The ability of a material to resist abrasion or rubbing.

Wetting: An effect causing liquids to spread out and cover more of a surface.

Wetting agents: Substances designed to make liquids more compatible with a surface and less likely to be repelled.

Index